The Springer Series on Demographic Methods and Population Analysis

Volume 46

AF806269

Series Editor
Kenneth C. Land, Duke University

In recent decades, there has been a rapid development of demographic models and methods and an explosive growth in the range of applications of population analysis. This series seeks to provide a publication outlet both for high-quality textual and expository books on modern techniques of demographic analysis and for works that present exemplary applications of such techniques to various aspects of population analysis.

Topics appropriate for the series include:

- General demographic methods
- Techniques of standardization
- Life table models and methods
- Multistate and multiregional life tables, analyses and projections
- Demographic aspects of biostatistics and epidemiology
- Stable population theory and its extensions
- Methods of indirect estimation
- Stochastic population models
- Event history analysis, duration analysis, and hazard regression models
- Demographic projection methods and population forecasts
- Techniques of applied demographic analysis, regional and local population estimates and projections
- Methods of estimation and projection for business and health care applications
- Methods and estimates for unique populations such as schools and students

Volumes in the series are of interest to researchers, professionals, and students in demography, sociology, economics, statistics, geography and regional science, public health and health care management, epidemiology, biostatistics, actuarial science, business, and related fields.

More information about this series at http://www.springer.com/series/6449

Christos H. Skiadas • Charilaos Skiadas
Editors

Demography and Health Issues

Population Aging, Mortality and Data Analysis

Springer

Editors
Christos H. Skiadas
ManLab, Technical University of Crete
Chania, Crete, Greece

Charilaos Skiadas
Department of Mathematics/Computer Science
Hanover College
Hanover, IN, USA

ISSN 1389-6784 ISSN 2215-1990 (electronic)
The Springer Series on Demographic Methods and Population Analysis
ISBN 978-3-030-09376-1 ISBN 978-3-319-76002-5 (eBook)
https://doi.org/10.1007/978-3-319-76002-5

© Springer International Publishing AG, part of Springer Nature 2018
Softcover re-print of the Hardcover 1st edition 2018
This work is subject to copyright. All rights are reserved by the Publisher, whether the whole or part of the material is concerned, specifically the rights of translation, reprinting, reuse of illustrations, recitation, broadcasting, reproduction on microfilms or in any other physical way, and transmission or information storage and retrieval, electronic adaptation, computer software, or by similar or dissimilar methodology now known or hereafter developed.
The use of general descriptive names, registered names, trademarks, service marks, etc. in this publication does not imply, even in the absence of a specific statement, that such names are exempt from the relevant protective laws and regulations and therefore free for general use.
The publisher, the authors and the editors are safe to assume that the advice and information in this book are believed to be true and accurate at the date of publication. Neither the publisher nor the authors or the editors give a warranty, express or implied, with respect to the material contained herein or for any errors or omissions that may have been made. The publisher remains neutral with regard to jurisdictional claims in published maps and institutional affiliations.

Printed on acid-free paper

This Springer imprint is published by the registered company Springer International Publishing AG part of Springer Nature.
The registered company address is: Gewerbestrasse 11, 6330 Cham, Switzerland

Preface

This book deals with demography and health issues with special attention on population aging, mortality, and data analysis. Emphasis is done on the introduction and use of quantitative methods and advanced data analysis methods in various aspects of demography and health.

The quantitative methods, with the aid of informatics and computing, received special attention in the last decades of the twentieth century and have further developed and applied in the first part of the twenty-first century. These methods already have done considerable changes in various scientific fields and of course in estimating vital aspects of demography and health.

Mortality, population aging, and data analysis are further developed while the tools used are friendly to end user. Accordingly, a large number of people are "ready" to understand and apply the new tools, thanks to the fastgrowing literature both theoretical and applied along with many "computer packages" and visual support.

The interdisciplinary works are considered as an important task of the new era along with the development of fields like Data Science and Big Data Analysis important to handle large data sets familiar in international studies in demography and health sciences. In a view the twenty-first century is already characterized by an optimistic way of data analysis approaches. We have a large number of people educated and trained to collect and store data sets and vast and expanded networks to disseminate information. Demography and health have most benefited and more developments are in progress.

Accordingly we have edited this book by selecting and providing the material in order to support the quantitative data handling along with qualitative study and analysis. This book covers very important topics on demography and health issues organized in six chapters.

Chapter one focusses on Demography and Related Applications in Health Status and the Lifespan Limit, including three papers on modeling and estimation of the health state and the healthy life expectancy of a population and a paper on exploring the limits to human life span, a challenging subject renewed last years after several publications in Nature.

Chapter two on Mortality Modeling and Applications includes four contributions including the establishment and development of a mortality database for developing countries, an application in Brazil, and two methodological papers for forecasting mortality and evaluation of the health trends with application in Greece.

Chapter three on Statistical Models and Methods in Biostatistics and Epidemiology includes a contribution on the cumulative rate of kidney cancer statistics in Australia, a paper on the reliability of mortality shifts in the working population in Russia, and a three-way data analysis applied to specific mortality trends. All papers focus on important statistical methodologies and related applications.

As far as new methods and tools are introduced in demography and health issues, the four papers included in Chapter four on Stochastic and Neuro-Fuzzy Methods provide interesting information on handling and applying advanced methodologies. Space-time variables, stochastic distance estimation, Monte Carlo methods in health research, and attitude measurement by a neuro-fuzzy approach are analyzed and applied.

Chapter five on Data Analysis in Demography includes six papers covering important topics on data handling and related statistics. Data decomposition, statistical analysis of health risks, an inference system for mortality data, a study on the Jackson exponentiality test, intervention analysis, and special statistics are the main topics studied.

Health Sciences, Demography, Risk, and Insurance is the topic presented in Chapter six in the seven papers included. Risk factors and risk estimates, job insecurity measurement, health estimates of some countries of the rapid developing world, social capital, income inequality and the health of the elderly, retirement scheme from the Italian mortality experience, and application of a Probit model for analyzing the death clustering of the Tribes of Central and Eastern India are presented and further analyzed.

We thank all the contributors and especially the authors of this book and of course the Springer team for help and support.

Chania, Crete, Greece
Hanover, IN, USA
December 2017

Christos H. Skiadas
Charilaos Skiadas

Contents

Part I
Demography and Related Applications: Health Status and the Lifespan Limit

Chapter 1
The Health Status of a Population Estimated: The History of Health State Curves

Christos H. Skiadas and Charilaos Skiadas

1.1 The Main Parts of the Stochastic Theory Needed

The Health State of an individual is a stochastic process by means that is highly unpredictable in the time course while fluctuates from higher to lower values. However, we have detailed and accurate data sets for deaths over time, that is we know the distribution of people reaching the end (the death distribution of a population) when the health state of an individual is reaching the zero level.

In a modeling approach the problem can be set as a first exit or hitting time modeling of a stochastic process crossing a barrier. Technically the stochastic theory was developed during last two centuries with the observation of the so-called Brownian motion and proved experimentally by Jean Perrin while the mathematical modeling of this classical stochastic process was due to several scientists including Thorvald N. Thiele, James Clerk Maxwell, Stefan Boltzmann, Albert Einstein, Marian Smoluchowski, Paul Lévy, Louis Bachelier. Mathematically the simple stochastic process of the Brownian motion is presented as a Wiener stochastic process in honor of Norbert Wiener. In nowadays the Wiener process is included in the majority of computing devices and programs thus giving the opportunity to generate stochastic paths and simulate processes as the health state of an individual.

So far after almost 150 years of quantitative works on stochastic theory the problem remains unsolved in the microscopic level. It is not possible to know exactly

C. H. Skiadas (✉)
ManLab, Technical University of Crete, Chania, Crete, Greece
e-mail: Skiadas@cmsim.net

C. Skiadas
Department of Mathematics/Computer Science, Hanover College, Hanover, IN, USA
e-mail: Skiadas@hanover.edu

© Springer International Publishing AG, part of Springer Nature 2018
C. H. Skiadas, C. Skiadas (eds.), *Demography and Health Issues*,
The Springer Series on Demographic Methods and Population Analysis 46,
https://doi.org/10.1007/978-3-319-76002-5_1

the development of the health state of an individual in the course of time as it is not possible to know the place and speed of a particle in a gas.

Fortunately that we have learned is that we can find "mean properties" of "large ensamples". We can estimate the pressure of a gas in a box, the temperature, the "mean speed" of the molecules and so-on. Accordingly we can find the "health state" or the "operational state" or the "viability" of a population as the "mean health state" of the total number of individuals. That we know is the effect on the population when the health state of an individual is zero that is the death distribution per age. *The task is to find the "mean health state" per age when we know the death distribution.*

Finding the Mean Health State as a summation of the stochastic processes of individuals could follow the lessons learned from the developments in Kinetic Theory in Physics. However, several new findings are needed. Especially as in the case of the human health, the data provided from the death distribution are produced from the health stochastic paths of the individuals when for the first time hit the zero health state barrier set at zero level or the X axis of a diagram.

That we search is first to find a distribution for the health state and then to estimate the final distribution when the health state paths hit for the first time the zero barrier. Then we can generate stochastic paths by stochastic simulations and verify the validity of our estimates. Both the direct and inverse problems are important tools to establish the Health State Theory.

1.2 The Health State Defined, Modeled and Estimated

That all people know by experience is that the health state is decreasing with age. By questioning we can have a scale for the health state ranging from 0 to 10 or as a percentage from 0 to 100. However, technically is simpler to accept the health state ranging from 0 to 1, with 1 been the "mean health state" of a population in the first years of the childhood and 0 at the age of the mean zero health of the population. This is the point where the number of deaths to the right is analogues to the number of deaths to the left of a graph.

An interesting comparison of the linear health state curve for the Mediterranean Flies studied by Weitz and Fraser and the curved with a negative slope for the human populations is also done along with stochastic simulations.

Torrance in the middle of 70s proposed a Health Status Index model suggesting the level of functioning of the health state of an individual at 1 for the perfect health state and lower values after injuries or diseases recovering after treatment to the perfect level in the first period of the life span. Then the level of functioning or health state is dropping down until the zero health level at the age of death (see Fig. 1.1).

Accordingly the health state of a population will be the average of a large ensemble of individuals, usually the total population of a country or a territory. Clearly this approach overcomes several shortcomings the main being the lack of a health state or health status unit of measurement. He accepts unity as the measure of the perfect health state for every individual. Clearly assuming unity as the maximum health state of an individual is not correct. Instead the "mean health state" should be

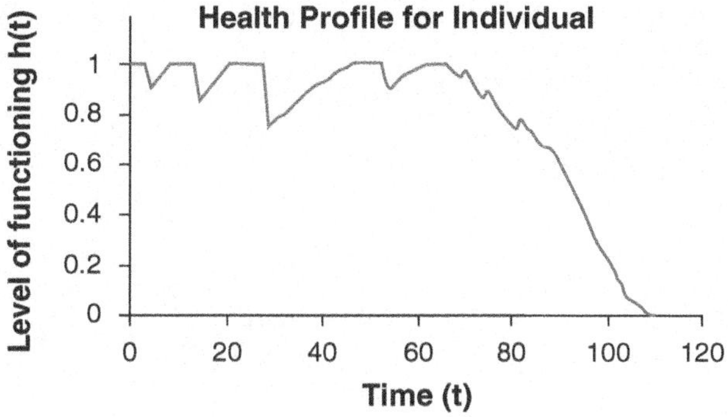

Fig. 1.1 Based on: G. W. Torrance. "Health Status Index Models: A Unified Mathematical View", Management Sci., 22(9), 1976: 990–1001

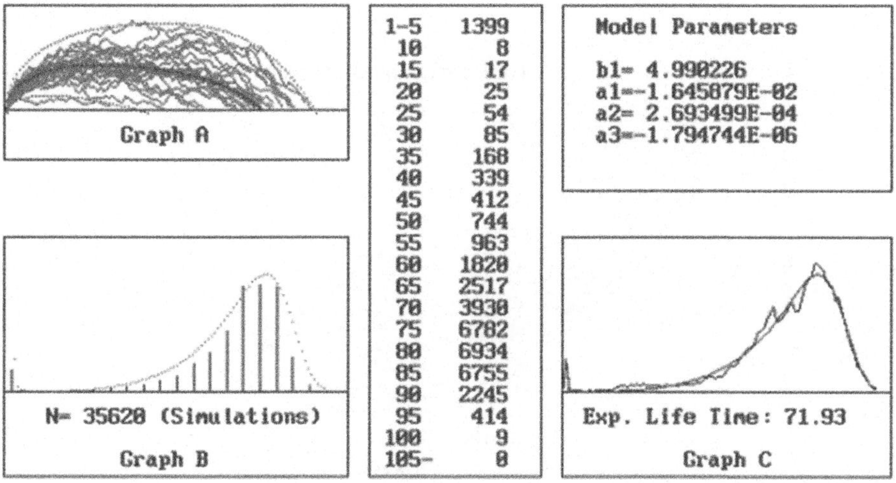

Fig. 1.2 Based on: Janssen, Jacques and Skiadas, Christos, H. Dynamic modelling of life-table data, Applied Stochastic Models and Data Analysis, 11, 1, 35–49 (1995)

expected to be at a unity level at maximum health state. The individual health state levels are expected to be at higher at lower values as it was the case of our modeling approach in 1995.

Fortunately, whereas the health state paths for the individuals is not possible to be estimated, the mean health state for the population can be found if we know the distribution of deaths that is the distribution that it is formed by counting the number of deaths at every age (usually estimated in yearly time periods). Then the first exit time theory of a stochastic process (expressing our health) crossing a barrier (here is the X axis representing the zero health level) provides the mean health state curve that is the health state of the population as a relatively smooth curve starting from a low level at birth reaching a maximum level and then gradually declining until zero (see Fig. 1.2). This was solved in 1995 by Janssen and Skiadas. In the same publication the inverse problem was approached that is to find the death probability density by generating a large number of stochastic paths by stochastic simulations.

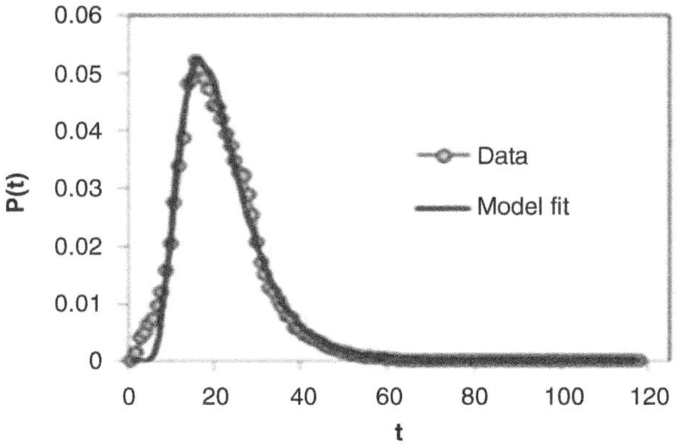

Fig. 1.3a Based on: Weitz, J.S. and Fraser, H.B. Explaining mortality rate plateaus, Proc. Natl. Acad. Sci. USA, 98(26), 15,383 (2001)

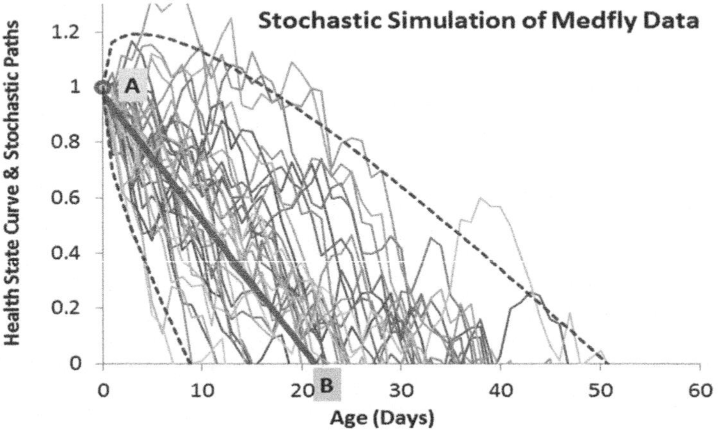

Fig. 1.3b Our Simulations from the book "Skiadas, C.H. and Skiadas, C. Exploring the Health State of a Population by Dynamic Modeling Methods, Springer, 2017"

The general theory was developed in order to apply in the case of human mortality data.

Few years later (2001) Weitz and Fraser applied the simpler first exit time model to the death data provided by Carey in a publication in Science. The health state curve for this case is a line starting from the level one and declining until the zero level (see Fig. 1.3a). We have done stochastic simulations (see Fig. 1.3b) to reproduce the data whereas we have estimated the parameters by fitting the model to data.

The stochastic simulations for USA 2010 (females) are provided based on a model published in 2010. In this model the simple linear case of the Weitz and Fraser is expressed with $c = 1$ whereas higher values for the exponent c account for human mortality modeling (see Fig. 1.4a) to compensate for the repairing mechanisms of the human body. While the linear decline with $c = 1$ is acceptable for medflies higher values for c are accepted for humans thus the mean health state tends to follow a rectangular like form well known in demography as rectagularization.

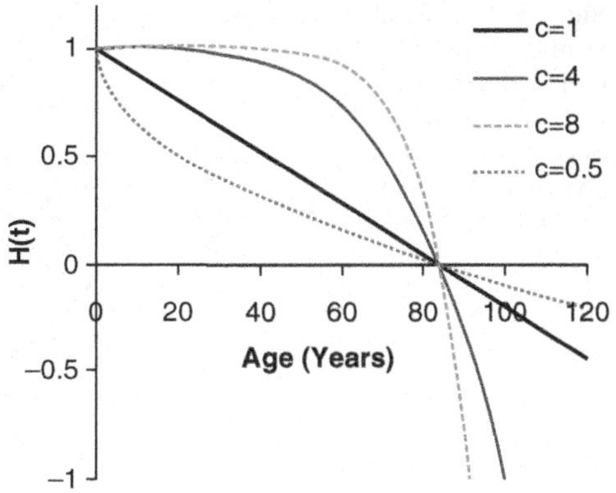

Fig. 1.4a Based on: Skiadas, C. and Skiadas, C.H. Development, Simulation and Application of First Exit Time Densities to Life Table Data, Communications in Statistics 39, 2010: 444–451

Fig. 1.4b Health State Model and Distribution of Deaths as a function of Health State *H*(*x*) at age *x*. From Skiadas and Skiadas 2010, 2014, 2015, 2016, 2017

Health State Function

$$H(x) = 1 - (bx)^c$$

Death Distribution

$$g(x) = \frac{|H_x - xH'_x|}{\sigma\sqrt{2\pi x^3}} e^{-\frac{H_x^2}{2\sigma^2 x}}$$

$$g(x) = \frac{|1+(c-1)(bx)^c|}{\sigma\sqrt{2\pi x^3}} e^{-\frac{\left(1-(bx)^c\right)^2}{2\sigma^2 x}}$$

The very simple equation form (see Fig. 1.4b) for the mean health state versus age x or operational state is: $H(x) = 1-(bx)^c$. The related distribution function for deaths $g(x)$ is included in Fig. 1.4b where σ stands for the standard deviation or the stochastic parameter. This parameter is important to reproduce the stochastic paths (see Figs. 1.3b and 1.5). Note that the derived distribution function is a new one perfectly fitting to the human mortality datasets. Technically, given the death distribution $g(x)$ we fit the model to data by nonlinear regression to estimate the parameters b, c and σ.

The main parts of the theory are illustrated in Fig. 1.5 presenting how starting from the death distribution function (blue curve) we can estimate the Health State parameters.

The figure includes the Health State Function expressed by the heavy magenta curve, hitting the zero line at 85.49 years of age. This age is smaller to the modal age at death that is the age year with the maximum number of deaths. The heavy dark blue curve expresses the death density without the infant mortality cases.

Although the Survival Curve (cyan dashed curve) is known as long as the life tables have introduced, the Health State Curve was calculated after the introduction of the advanced stochastic theory of the first exit time.

The health state curve is illustrated by the heavy magenta line. The corresponding survival curve for the related case is presented by the cyan curve. The blue curve expresses the death distribution. The light curves with various colors are the stochastic paths from the related simulation. The two dashed black curves express the

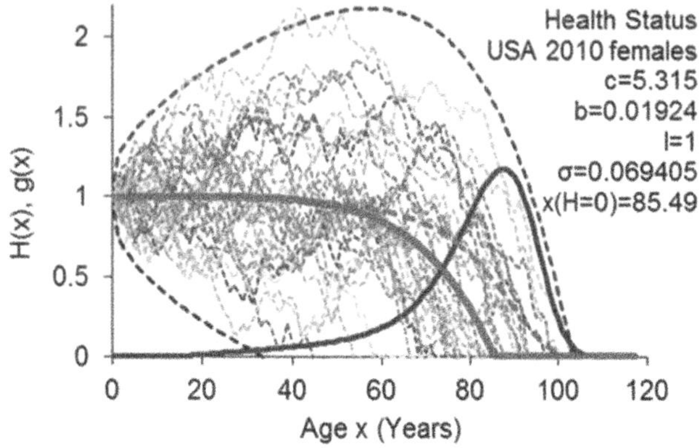

Fig. 1.5 Our Simulations from the book "Skiadas, C.H. and Skiadas, C. Exploring the Health State of a Population by Dynamic Modeling Methods, Springer, 2017"

confidence intervals. Further to the Health State and the Life Expectancy, the age at mean zero health state is also estimated.

Figure 1.6a presents an alternative method to reproduce the death probability density from stochastic paths and Fig. 1.6b provides the death probability density simulated (see Skiadas and Skiadas 2010).

As it was expected the introduction of a new tool as the health state function would lead to new advancement. The health state function estimated is a smooth declining function as is presented for males and females in USA (2010). We have estimated at which age the curvature is at maximum level. This is very important because this point is related with the maximum level of the human deterioration stage. In USA (2010) males this is achieved at 76.45 years of age and at 78.37 years for females (See Fig. 1.7). The next graph illustrates the Health State Curve (red line), the Survival Curve (cyan line) and several survival cases for various values of the standard deviation σ. In the total rectangularization case the survival curve approaches the ABDC blue line (See Fig. 1.7b).

Note that the deterioration function has the form of a non-symmetric distribution function as in the above case for Italy (1950, females) rising slowly at the first ages and exponentially from the middle ages with a maximum at high ages close to 80 years and then declining at very high ages with an asymptotic decay explaining the Greenwood and Irwin (1939) argument for a late-life mortality deceleration or the appearance of mortality plateaus at higher ages (See Fig. 1.8).

Another important point is to find the full form of the human health state (see the figure for USA males the year 2000). The health state starts from a low level at birth grows to the maximum level one at 12 year of age declines to a local minimum at 22 years of age; then a local maximum is reached at age 32 and a continuous decline follows (See Fig. 1.9a). In Fig. 1.9b the two stage estimation is presented. The Health State Simple model H(x) is illustrated by the dashed orange curve whereas the blue curve represents the final form of the estimates (Note that in this case the Health State is estimated for a model with $\sigma = 1$).

The total health state is found by estimating the area under the health state curve (see Fig. 1.10). The result is expressed as years of age that is 68.22 for males and

Fig. 1.6a An alternative method to reproduce the death probability density from stochastic paths

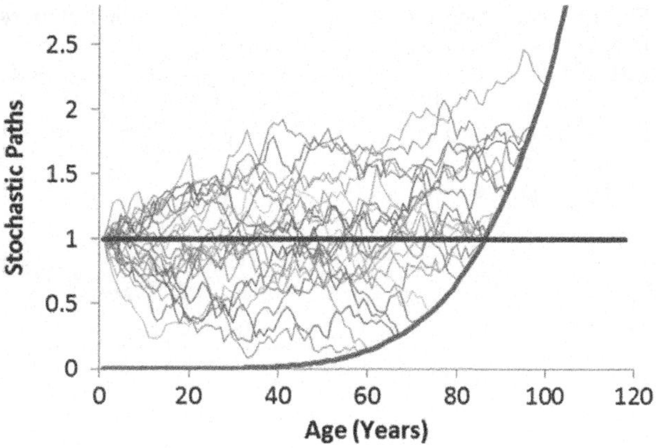

Fig. 1.6b Death probability density simulated (USA 2010, females)

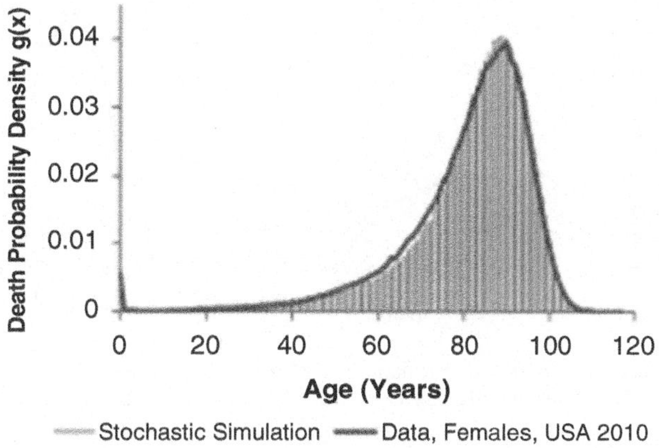

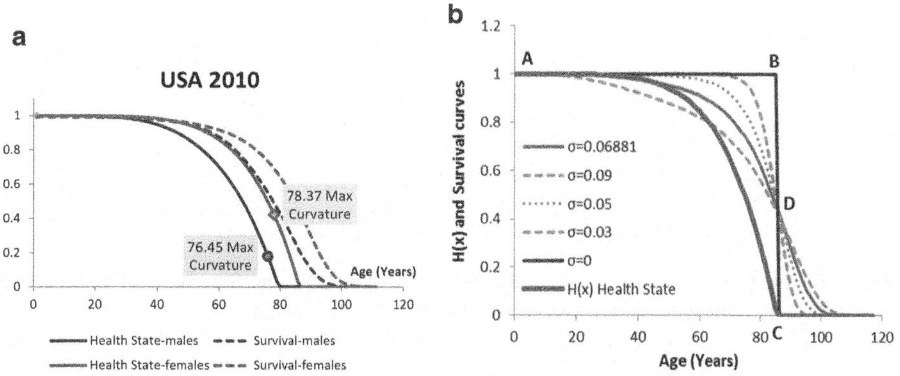

Fig. 1.7 (**a**, **b**) Our estimations from the book "Skiadas, C.H. and Skiadas, C. Exploring the Health State of a Population by Dynamic Modeling Methods, Springer, 2017"

Fig. 1.8 Our estimations from the book "Skiadas, C.H. and Skiadas, C. Exploring the Health State of a Population by Dynamic Modeling Methods, Springer, 2017"

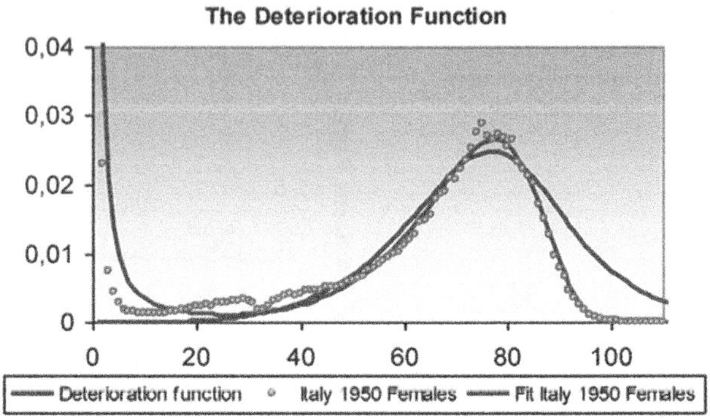

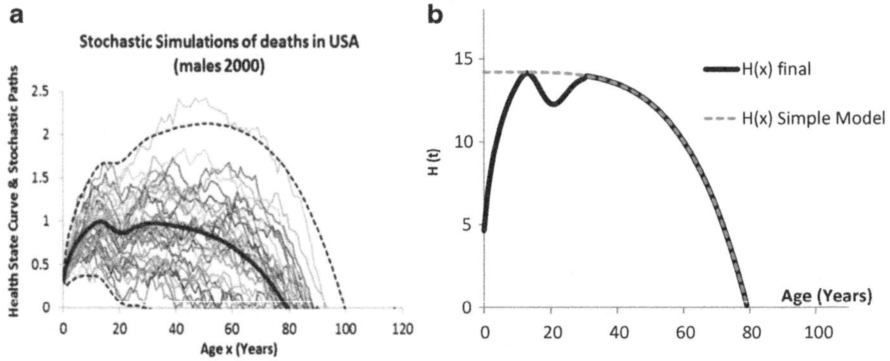

Fig. 1.9 (**a**, **b**) Our estimations from the book "Skiadas, C.H. and Skiadas, C. Exploring the Health State of a Population by Dynamic Modeling Methods, Springer, 2017"

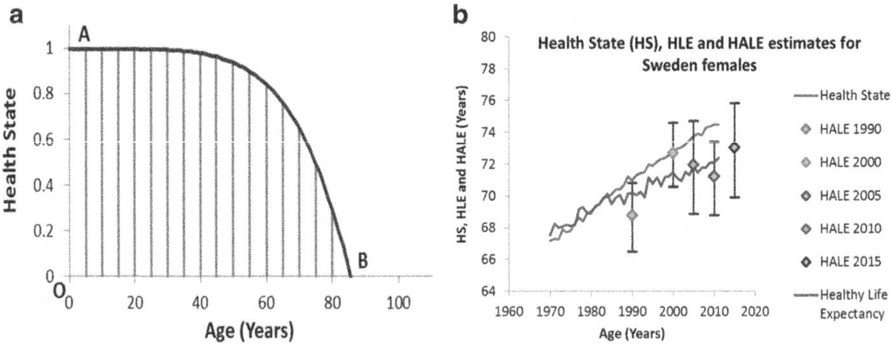

Fig. 1.10 (**a**, **b**) Our estimations from the book "Skiadas, C.H. and Skiadas, C. Exploring the Health State of a Population by Dynamic Modeling Methods, Springer, 2017"

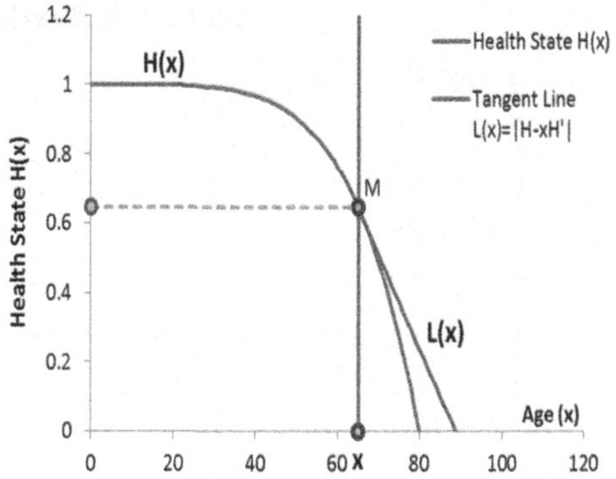

Fig. 1.11a Derivation of the Health State probability density function from the Inverse Gaussian

Fig. 1.11b Health State Model and Distribution of Deaths as a function of Health State $H(x)$ at age x. From Skiadas and Skiadas 2010, 2014, 2015, 2016, 2017

Health State Function

$$H(x) = 1 - (bx)^c$$

Death Distribution

$$g(x) = \frac{|L(x)|}{\sigma\sqrt{2\pi x^3}} e^{-\frac{H_x^2}{2\sigma^2 x}}$$

$$g(x) = \frac{|H_x - xH'_x|}{\sigma\sqrt{2\pi x^3}} e^{-\frac{H_x^2}{2\sigma^2 x}}$$

72.33 for females for USA 2010. The total health state (cyan curve) for females in Sweden (1970–2010) is presented (See Fig. 1.10b) along with our estimates for the healthy life expectancy (red curve) and the HALE estimates of the World Health Organization (rhombus with confidence intervals).

After introducing the Health State Function for the human population a very important point arises of finding a simple method to derive the probability density function based on the simple Inverse Gaussian presented earlier in the application of Weiss and Fraser for Medflies and already known from more than a century. A detailed methodology based on the stochastic theory is already presented in our publications mentioned above and in the references. The very simple transformation comes from the above Fig. 1.11a where by moving the coordinate of the X axis to the point of age x, the probability density function $g(x)$ arises as a first approximation of a simple linearization of the Health State Curve at point M where the curve is replaced by the Tangent Line $L(x) = |H - xH'|$ that is by a linear part of $H(x)$ in the vicinity of the point M. Then the Inverse Gaussian applies for a small interval around the point M thus obtaining the function presented in Fig. 1.11b. This is the extended form we already have derived and applied for the health state of the human population. The related part will be included in a book in progress to appear in The Springer Series on Demographic Methods and Population Analysis.

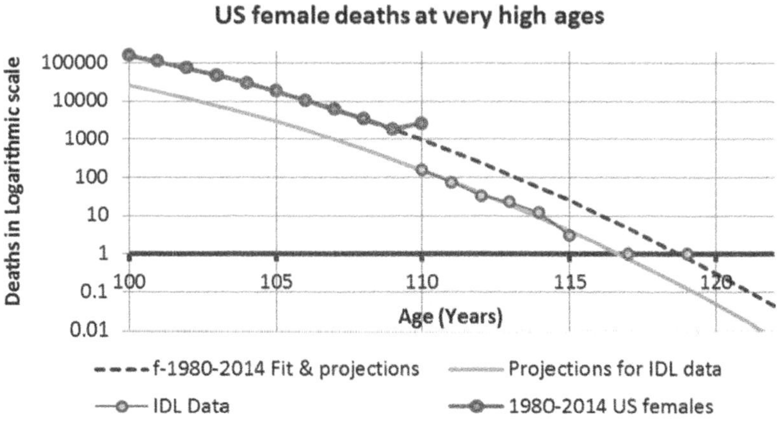

Fig. 1.12 Female supercentenarian deaths, fit and forecasts in USA

1.3 Further Applications and Results

We have developed a method for estimating the Health State or the Viability of a Population in a time period from the distribution of deaths by applying the stochastic theory for the first exit time of a stochastic process. The theory developed is included in our recently published book by Springer along with other interesting applications as the estimation of the healthy life years lost to disability and the maximum human life span. A part of the latter study is illustrated in Fig. 1.12 related to the female supercentenarian deaths, fit and forecasts in USA. The fit and projections for the 1980–2014 female deaths in USA approach the maximum year of female supercentenarian in USA at 119 years of age (IDL is the International Database on Longevity).

References

Greenwood, M., & Irwin, J. O. (1939). The biostatistics of senility. *Human Biology, 11*(1), 1–23.

Janssen, J., & Skiadas, C. H. (1995). Dynamic modelling of life-table data. *Applied Stochastic Models and Data Analysis, 11*(1), 35–49.

Skiadas, C., & Skiadas, C. H. (2010). Development, simulation and application of first exit time densities to life table data. *Communications in Statistics, 39*, 444–451.

Skiadas, C. H., & Skiadas, C. (2014). The first exit time theory applied to life table data: The health state function of a population and other characteristics. *Communications in Statistics-Theory and Methods, 43*, 1985–1600.

Skiadas, C. H., & Skiadas, C. (2015). Exploring the state of a stochastic system via stochastic simulations: An interesting inversion problem and the health state function. *Methodology and Computing in Applied Probability, 17*(4), 973–982.

Skiadas, C. H., & Skiadas, C. (2016). *The health status of a population: Health state and survival curves and HALE estimates*. www.ArXiv.org

Skiadas, C. H., & Skiadas, C. (2017). *Exploring the health state of a population by dynamic modeling methods*. Springer. https://doi.org/10.1007/978-3-319-65142-2 (see at: https://link.springer.com/book/10.1007/978-3-319-65142-2).

Torrance, G. W. (1976). Health status index models: A unified mathematical view. *Management Science, 22*(9), 990–1001.

Weitz, J. S., & Fraser, H. B. (2001). Explaining mortality rate plateaus. *Proceedings of the National Academy of Sciences of the United States of America, 98*(26), 15383–15386.

Chapter 2
Remarks on "Limits to Human Lifespan"

Christos H. Skiadas

2.1 Introduction

Following the debate emerged after the publication in Nature of the paper by Dong et al. 2016 on "Evidence for a limit to human lifespan" many interesting remarks came out for further investigating and exploring the supercentenarians population in the time course (see Brown et al. 2017; De Beer et al. 2017; Hughes and Hekimi 2017; Lenard and Vaupel 2017; Rozing et al. 2017).

A part of the debate was related to the data handling, another on the methodological aspects of the statistical methods and techniques used whereas remarks from cases from several scientific fields could also be considered along with beliefs and personal opinions on the existence or not of a lifespan limit. Perhaps, sooner or later, the studies on expanding the lifespan of simpler species will solve the problem. Until then we have summarized in 12 points the main approaches we can handle with today's knowledge on theoretical and applied tools and methods (more details at Janssen and Skiadas 1995; Skiadas and Skiadas 2010a, b, 2014, 2015, 2017).

1. The first we have noticed is that a clearer and "stronger" data handling is needed.
2. Perhaps we have to "see" the same data from a different viewpoint.
3. High dispersion data sets are not very well presented with a linear trend. Even the nonlinear representation is not good as well.
4. Handling and applying Life Table data sets for over 90 years of age is dubious.
5. Simpler is to use the raw death data instead of the death probability data.
6. Next, a data transformation is important before to start more data handling. This is the lesson learned from Gompertz days (Gompertz 1825). A visual inspection in graphs could be more informative.

C. H. Skiadas (✉)
ManLab, Technical University of Crete, Chania, Crete, Greece
e-mail: Skiadas@cmsim.net

© Springer International Publishing AG, part of Springer Nature 2018
C. H. Skiadas, C. Skiadas (eds.), *Demography and Health Issues*,
The Springer Series on Demographic Methods and Population Analysis 46,
https://doi.org/10.1007/978-3-319-76002-5_2

7. Another important future is to inspect the distribution of deaths and especially the tail at the right hand side (Skiadas and Skiadas 2017).
8. As the number of death cases in the tail sharply declines according to age the case could be studied with one of the methods proposed under the term: "extreme value distributions".
9. By these methods relatively simpler logarithmic expressions replace the formulas for the distribution of deaths and are fitted to the data to the last periods of the life span.
10. These distribution methods include a first and frequently a second logarithm of the logarithm, when the decline in the tail is very sharp. Thus by starting the study by first transforming the data in a logarithmic form the complexity of the logarithmic equation form is reduced.
11. Another point is how to handle exceptional cases as that of Jeanne Calment clearly lying at the very edges of Maximum Reported Age at Death (MRAD).
12. We search in the majority of cases that belonging to the normal trajectories with a high probability. But how about the cases with very small probability as for Jeanne Calment? In France with a total centenarians population of 38.712 in the period 1990–2014 we need a thousand times larger population to have a MRAD at 122 years of age. Or simpler the probability is only 1/1000 for the appearance of one MRAD at this age.

2.2 Data Transformation and Application in United States

The very important point when we handle centenarian and supercentenarian data sets is to bring into light the data from over 100 years of age that is data in the extreme right of the death distribution. These data mainly disappear in the right tail of the death distribution as is presented inside the red circle in the right hand side of Fig. 2.1.

The upper part A of Fig. 2.1 illustrates the distribution of female deaths in USA for the period 1990–1999. The data are provided by the Human Mortality Database (HMD). The main part of particular interest for the centenarian and supercentenarian case is located by a red circle. It includes the data sets from 100 to 110 years of age. However, as the data for 110 years include all the data from 110 years of age and higher, these figures are not used for the applications that follow. Instead the applications and projections done allocate the data form 110 years and higher to appropriate years of age based on the trend followed in the previous years from 100 to 109. The method used needs the transformation in logarithmic scale as presented in the following.

The middle part B of Fig. 2.1 illustrates the same data presented in the A part but in a logarithmic scale chart. The very important point here is that every level presented by the horizontal lines in the B part of the graph characterizes the number of persons dead at this age with the very important level one for the dead at the higher age level. The clear advantage is the presentation of the critical part included

Fig. 2.1 (**a**) Distribution of deaths in USA (female, 1990–1999). (**b**) Deaths in logarithmic scale in USA (female, 1990–1999). (**c**) Logarithm of deaths in USA (female, 1990–1999)

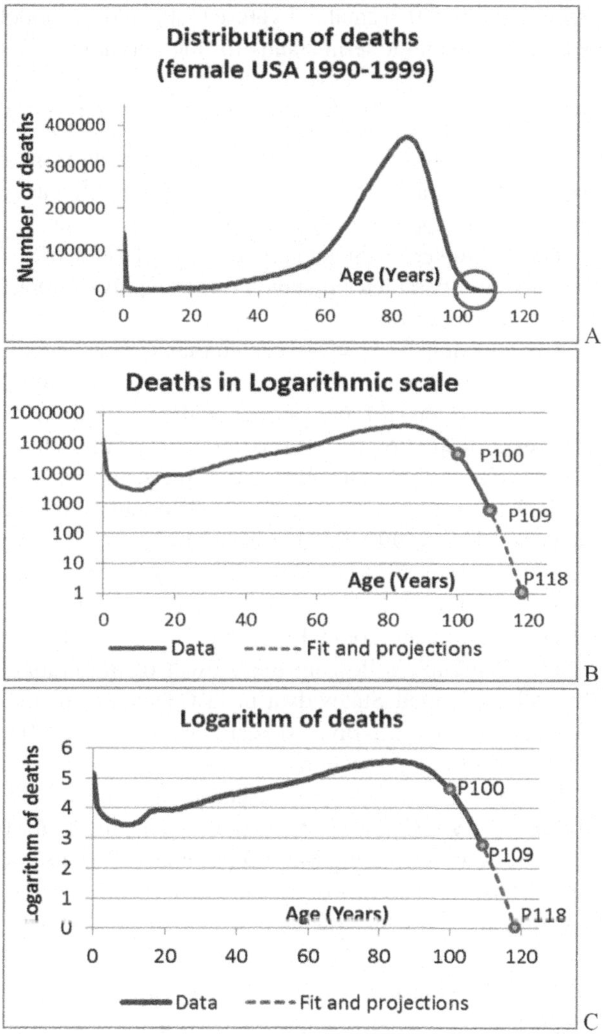

into the circle of the part A of the figure in a convenient form for fitting a model and make projections until level one where the maximum reported age at death (MRAD) is found. For the case studied here this is at year 118 (P118 point in the graph).

The lower part C of Fig. 2.1 presents the logarithms of the death data. This is a simpler illustration with the MRAD of 118 years of age found at zero level on the X axis.

Several models could fit to the total curve expressing the number of deaths. However, for the last part to the right of the death curve a simple quadratic model for the logarithm of the number of deaths could be more appropriate. This is in accordance to the extreme value theory presented by Gumbel and others. The final part of the curve to the right, as it is expressed by the logarithm in Fig. 2.1c, is a smooth graph with a small curvature that could be modeled by a function of the form (where the quadratic term stands for the curvature).

$$\log(g(x)) = a(x - 100)^2 + b(x - 100) + c \tag{2.1}$$

We fit the above model to the 10 data points from 100 to 109 years of age. We estimate the parameters of this model by a nonlinear regression analysis algorithm and make the appropriate projections.

The parameters estimated are: $a = -0.005348$, $b = -0.15905$, $c = 4.651$, where, the quadratic parameter a stands for a negative curvature and the linear parameter b for a negative slope.

The appearance of super centenarians is related to the number of deaths as is illustrated in Table 2.1. The middle column includes the projections for the supercentenarians for the period studied (1990–1999). The MRAD is found at 118 years of age. Note that this number should come from the following relation 0.5 < MRAD<1.5. The 100 years projection is given in the third column of Table 2.1, by assuming that the death population follows the same pattern as for the period 1990–1999. In this case a MRAD equal to 121 years of age is expected in 2100, whereas a MRAD equal to 116 years of age should be found for 1 year death data selection (see the first column of Table 2.1).

These estimates could be correct for a continuing growth of the number of supercentenarians following the growth of the number of centenarians. However, the case of United States data in last decades do not support this argument as is illustrated in Fig. 2.2. Five 10 year periods from 1960 to 2009 are selected from the HMD and fit and projections are done.

It should be noted that by selecting 5 characteristic periods for the death distribution in USA (female), fit to the data from 90 to 109 years of age and doing projections an interesting MRAD point at 117 years is estimated for the 4 cases and one MRAD at 118 years of age, the latter resulting from the 1990–1999 period. The equation applied is analogous to the previous one:

Table 2.1 Supercentenarians estimated

	Average of 10 years	1990–1999	2000–2100
Age	1 year	10 years	100 years
110	34	335	3355
111	18	180	1796
112	9	94	938
113	5	48	478
114	2	24	238
115	1	12	115
116	1	5	55
117		3	25
118		1	11
119			5
120			2
121			1

$$\log(g(x)) = a(x-90)^2 + b(x-90) + c \qquad (2.2)$$

These results for United States females are in favor of the argument for a stagnation of the MRAD development and for the maximum achieved MRAD during 1990–1999 period of time, here found at 118 years of age whereas, a MRAD at 117 years of age for the other periods studied is estimated.

The number of deaths of centenarians is increasing from 1950 and onwards though the growth is slower from 1995 to 2014 as it is expressed in Fig. 2.3. However, this growth could be compensated by the growing negative shift for the logarithm of deaths during time presented in Figs. 2.2 and 2.4. It looks out to be a

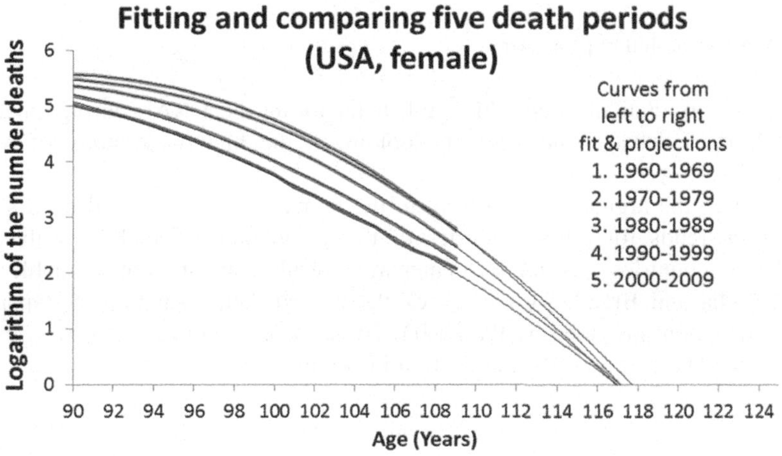

Fig. 2.2 Fitting and comparing five deaths periods in USA (female)

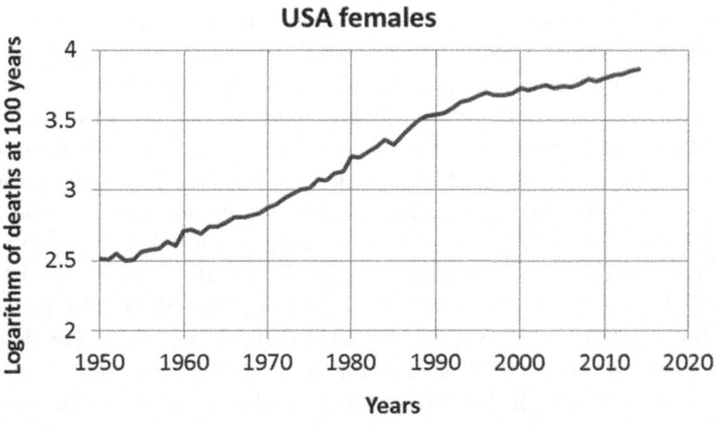

Fig. 2.3 Number of deaths of centenarians from 1950 to 2014 (USA, female)

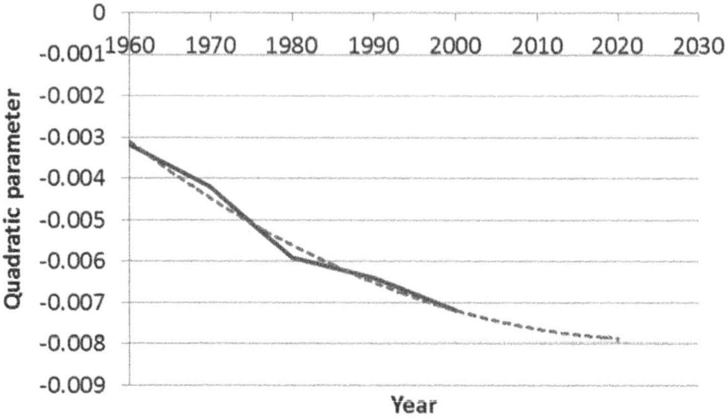

Fig. 2.4 Negative shift of parameter *a*

very hard work to define a possible stable behavior for the MRAD during time. This could lead to debates and conflicts looking at the high uncertainty of related projections.

However, the argument for a limit to the human life span should need similar stagnation trends for other countries of the world and especially for the large population countries. As far as centenarian death data are not available from China, India and Brazil, we can check the related data from France, Japan and United Kingdom provided by the HMD. These three countries and USA were the basis of the Dong et al. 2016 publication in Nature.

2.3 The Case of Japan

The Japan female deaths at 100 year of age steadily increase from 1950 and onwards as is illustrated in Fig. 2.5 (the number of deaths is expressed in logarithmic scale). This is a good result indicating a possible increase of the number of centenarians and supercentenarians (aged 100+ years of age) and thus increasing the probability of finding MRAD at higher ages. However, another indicator is needed to apply coming from the MRAD trend over time. As for the USA case presented in Fig. 2.2, five ten year time periods are selected and the model (2) is fitted to data. The MRAD for each case is found by estimating the year where the projections line crosses the X axis. The estimates for the 5 periods studied are 1970–1979 (MRAD = 109.8), 1980–1989 (MRAD = 111.3), 1990–1999 (MRAD = 112.4), 2000–2009 (MRAD = 115.3) and 2010–2014 (MRAD = 116.3). See also Fig. 2.6 where the period 2010–2014 stands for a 5 year period. The linear model MRAD = 0.1774*YEAR-240.53 is fitted to the 5 MRAD data points (see Fig. 2.7) with a fairly good $R^2 = 0.991$, and projections are done. Accordingly a

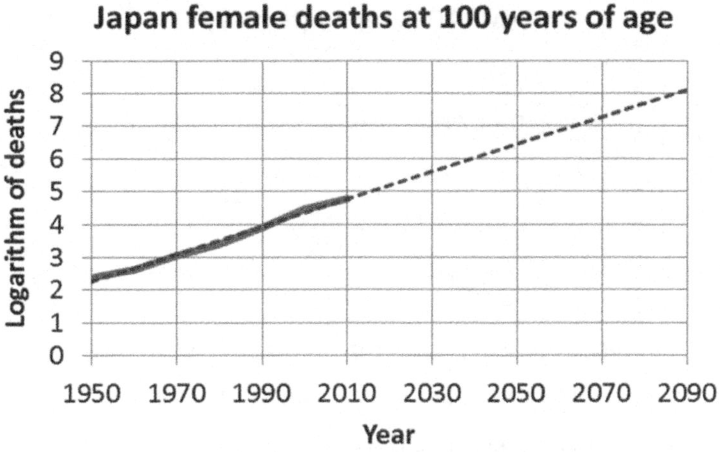

Fig. 2.5 Logarithm of Japan female deaths at 100 years of age

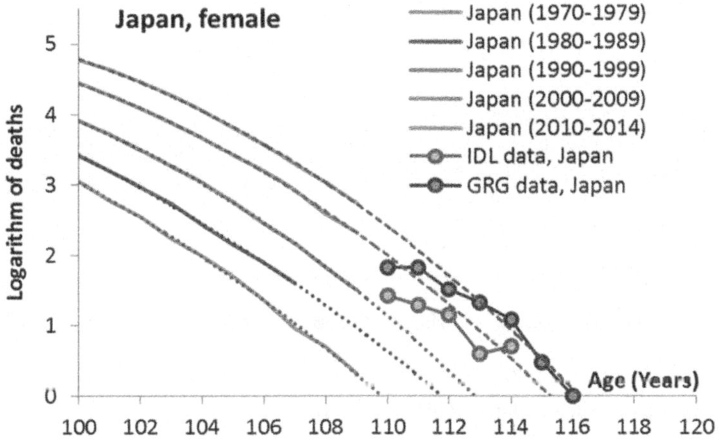

Fig. 2.6 Five year periods for the logarithm of deaths in Japan along with IDL and GRG data

MRAD at 118 years of age is expected by 2020, the 122 years of age should be reached by 2045 and a MRAD at 125 years of age is expected by 2060.

Figure 2.6 illustrates and the female supercentenarians for Japan as are provided by the IDL (1996–2005) and GRG (1998–2014) databases. For both databases (IDL and GRG) the cases collected cover two different time periods, 1996–2005 for the IDL database and a larger for the GRG database. For the latter the time period 1998–2014 was collected for our study. There is a 30 years period, 1966–1996, with only 11 supercentenarian in 205 cases. We have excluded these figures keeping the rest 194 instances from 1998–2014 for the study. This is clear from Fig. 2.8 that the first period 1966–1996 should be excluded. The IDL data points for the 1996–2005

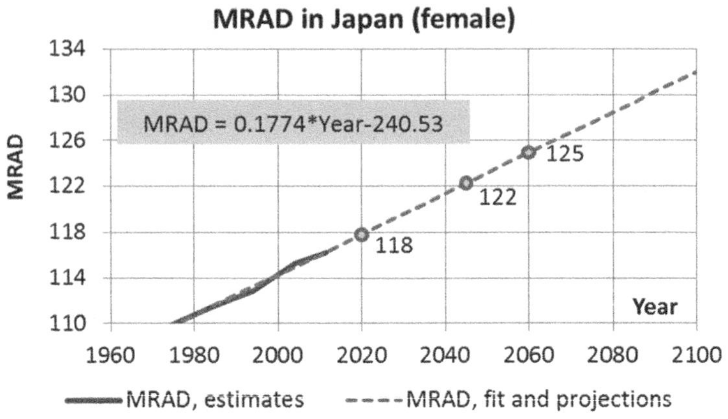

Fig. 2.7 Fit and projections for MRAD in Japan ($R^2 = 0.991$)

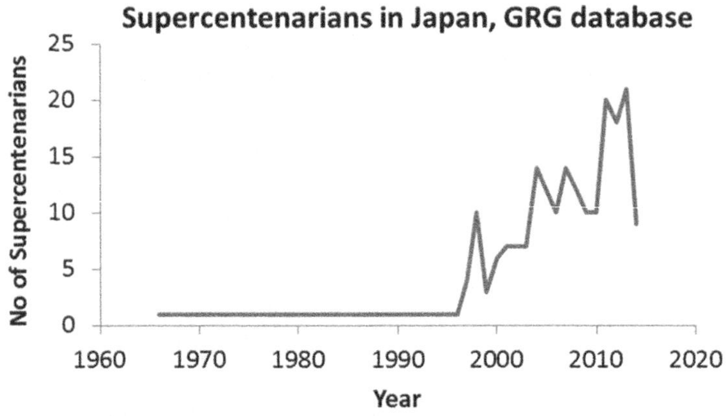

Fig. 2.8 Supercentenarians in Japan (GRG database)

period are located between the trajectories for (1990–1999) and (2000–2009) whereas, the GRG data points are close to the projected lines for the periods (2000–2009) and (2010–2014). Especially for the GRG data providing a MRAD at 116 years of age, the projected line for the period (2010–2014) fits perfectly to the same point for MRAD.

2.4 The Case of France

The France case has similarities with Japan application as the trajectories for the 10 year periods studied tend to keep a parallel like movement to the right hand side of the graph thus suggesting a growing process for the MRAD for the

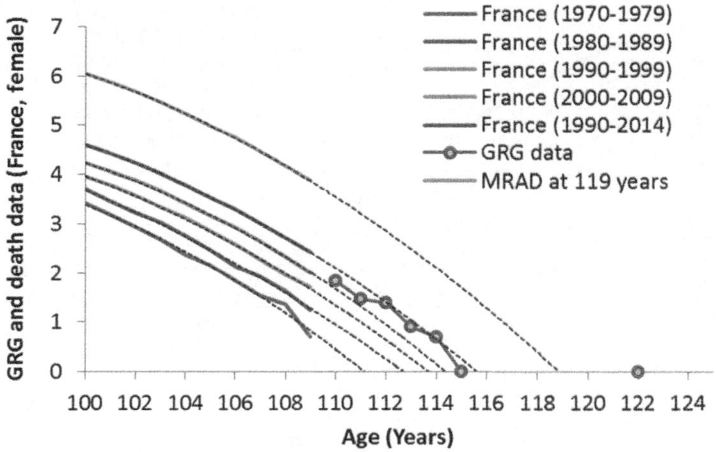

Fig. 2.9 France application for various time periods

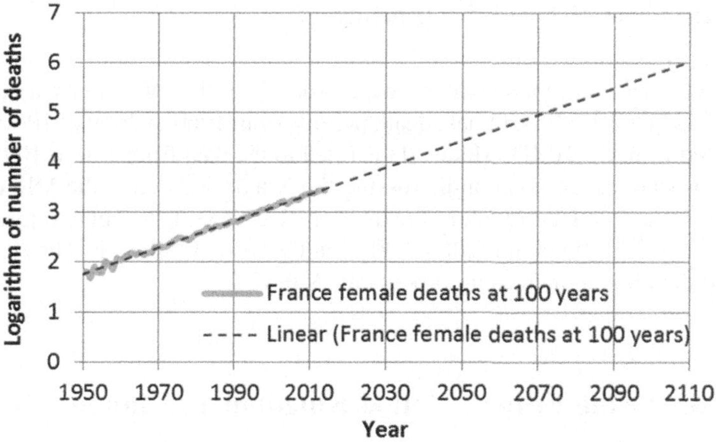

Fig. 2.10 Logarithm of France female deaths at 100 years of age (fit and predictions)

supercentenarians. The GRG data corresponding to the period 1990–2014 are close to the projections of the death data for this period (Fig. 2.9). That is far away from any short of prediction is the single point for the world record MRAD at 122 years. The trend for the deaths at 100 years of age in France steadily increases from 1950 and onwards in an exponential trend thus providing a linear trend for the logarithm of the number of deaths (see Fig. 2.10). The logarithm for the number of deaths in 2110 is 6, corresponding to 1.000.000 persons and to a MRAD at 119 years of age (see the related Fig. 2.9).

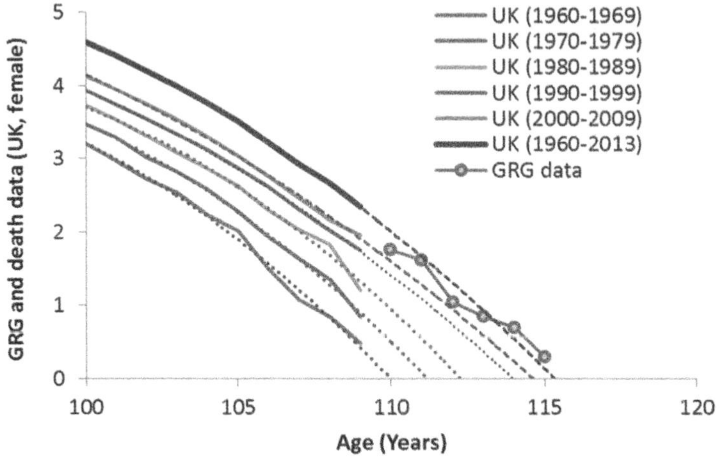

Fig. 2.11 Centenarian and supercentenarian fit and projections for UK (female)

2.5 The Case of United Kingdom

Similar to France and Japan is the growing process for the supercentenarians in UK presented in Fig. 2.11. Five female death periods from 1960 to 2009 of 10 years each are selected from the HMD. Model (1) is fitted to the data from 100 to 109 years of age and projections are done until crossing the X axis and define the MRAD. Very important for estimating the future trends for MRAD are the last two trajectories for the periods (1990–1999) and (2000–2009). In the case of UK both follow a parallel like trend defining an increasing process for MRAD.

2.6 Comparing France, United Kingdom and Japan

That it is demonstrated from these 3 countries (see Fig. 2.12) the number of centenarians is steadily growing while the supercentenarian trend is growing during time as well leading to higher MRAD.

2.7 The IDL Application

Supercentenarian female death data from 15 countries are downloaded from the IDL database as for 20 July 2017. Similar data are included in the Human Mortality Database (HMD) in the death tables for the years 100+ and presented as a single number for the deaths at 100 years of age and over. Though no further analysis is given in these death tables the information for the number of supercentenarians per

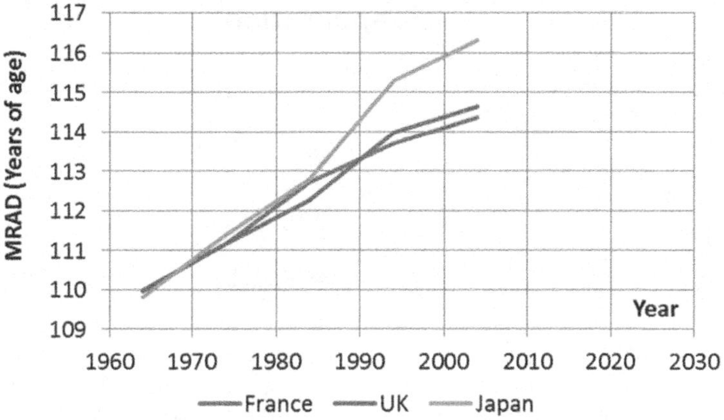

Fig. 2.12 France, UK and Japan comparisons for MRAD estimates

country at specific time periods (the yearly data are available) is vital for the calculations performed here. These death tables include all the age period from zero age to 109. The last 10 data points from 100 to 109 are used to estimate a trajectory for the future paths (projections) that define the supercentenarian trend per year of age from 110 years and onwards.

IDL and HMD-data include completely different number of data points for the supercentenarians as the IDL database covers the confirmed cases. Thus we have found 598 supercentenarians in the IDL database and 3066 in the HMD-data the latter providing more than five times (5.127) higher estimates. However, the HMD-data supercentenarian data are very important because we can arrange these data in the projection curve arising from the fit of a good model of the logarithmic form of Eq. (2.1).

This model fits to the 10 data points from 100 to 109 almost perfectly with a $R2 = 0.99998$. The projection presented in the Fig. 2.13 provides the MRAD at 119 years of age that is exactly the age of the second supercentenarian after Jeanne Calment. The next step is the find a trajectory appropriate for the IDL data in view that these data could follow a parallel like path than that provided from HMD-data for the same time period and for the same 15 countries selected. This is achieved very easily by moving the HMD-data trajectory in a lower position by dividing its element by an appropriate number so that to minimize the sum of squared errors. The new position is illustrated in the figure as HMD-data adapted to IDL. Now the trajectory for IDL provides a MRAD at 117 years of age. The IDL data points are illustrated with red circles and are fairly well adapted to the related trajectory with $R2 = 0.9906$. For both cases the outsider, the point at 122 years of age is far away from any estimate. It could be found with a probability 0.01 for the IDL case and 0.04 for the HMD-data case by means that we can find a MRAD for a population 100 times larger for the IDL case and 25 times larger for the HMD-data case. The trajectory adapted to 122 years of age is presented in Fig. 2.13. The estimation results are given in the next Table 2.2. Note that the MRAD will appear for a number 0.5 or

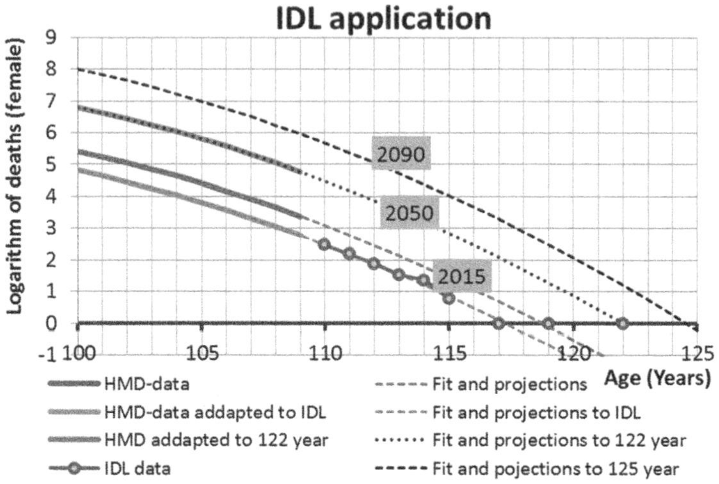

Fig. 2.13 Fit and projections for supercentenarians (IDL and HMD data bases)

Table 2.2 Supercentenarians estimated for IDL, HMD and HMD* databases (HMD* results from HMD-data adapted to a MRAD at 122 years of age)

Age	IDL	HMD	HMD*
110	308	1208	30,195
111	153	601	15,021
112	74	290	7257
113	35	136	3404
114	16	62	1551
115	7	27	686
116	3	12	295
117	**1**	5	123
118	**0.51**	2	50
119	0.20	**1**	20
120	0.08	0.30	7
121	0.03	0.11	3
122	0.01	0.04	**1**
Total	598	2345	58,613

higher by means that the logarithm should be approximately less than −0.3 thus shortening the population needed for at least one MRAD. For the case of 122 years of age the population needed is the half of that estimated to have exactly one in the estimates.

The related death female data for the periods selected are downloaded from the Human Mortality Database (HMD) and summarized as to form one unique database termed here as HMD-data. The periods for collecting the data per country are found from the explanatory details in the IDL database and are presented in parentheses as follows: Australia (1990–2004), Belgium (1990–2002), Canada (1962–2002), Switzerland (1993–2000), Germany (1994–2005), Denmark (1996–2000), Spain

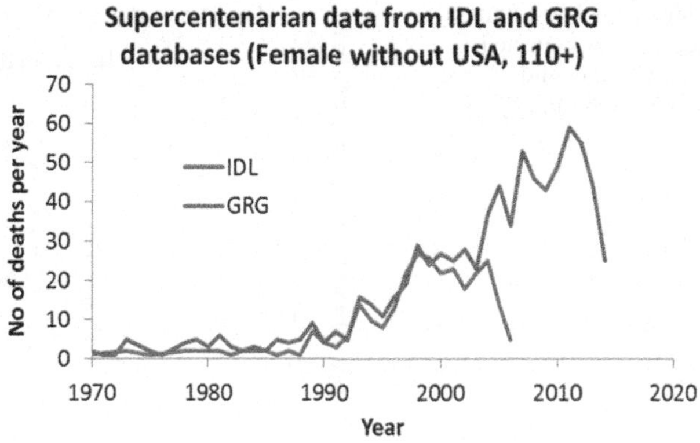

Fig. 2.14 IDL and GRG data series

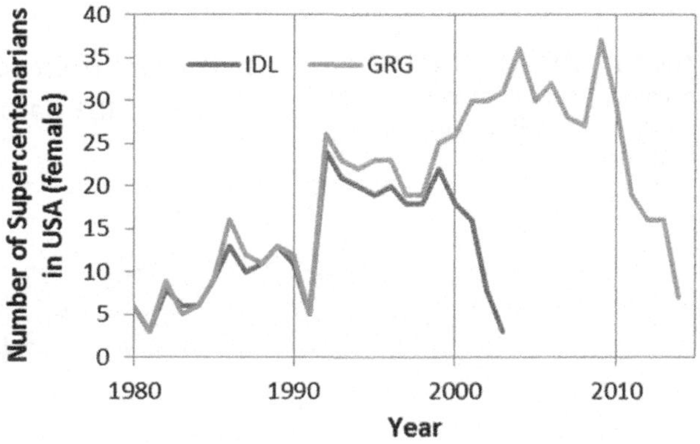

Fig. 2.15 Supercentenarians in USA (female). IDL and GRG data sets

(1989–2007), Finland (1989–2006), France (1987–2003), UK (1968–2006), Italy (1973–2003), Japan (1996–2005), Norway (1989–2004), Sweden (1986–2003) and USA (1980–2003).

Both IDL and GRG databases (see Figs. 2.14 and 2.15) are similar until 2003 and then the GRG database includes data until 2014.

Accordingly we use the IDL dataset for the applications that follow (see Fig. 2.16). The IDL data base provides the super-centenarian data until 2003.

The IDL group of countries without USA includes 13 countries for various periods of time. For the same periods we have downloaded the deaths from the Human Mortality Database and summarized all data to form a unique death distribution presented in Fig. 2.18 in continuous line. We fit the quadratic model to the data from 100 to 109 years of age and then a projection is done. The estimated MRAD is at 116.4 years of age. Similar are the results by applying the GRG data as well (see the dark circles in Fig. 2.17).

The application for USA (female) includes fit to the HMD death data in logarithmic scale, projections and comparisons with the GRG (Fig. 2.18a) and IDL

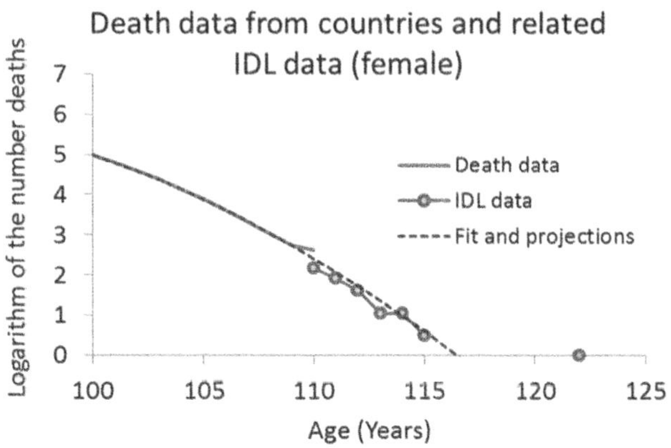

Fig. 2.16 Logarithm of deaths from selected countries, fit and projections, and IDL data

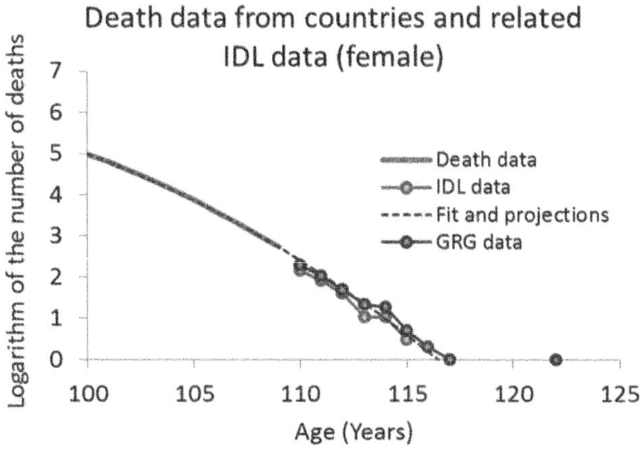

Fig. 2.17 HMD data for countries selected, fit and projections and IDL and GRG figures

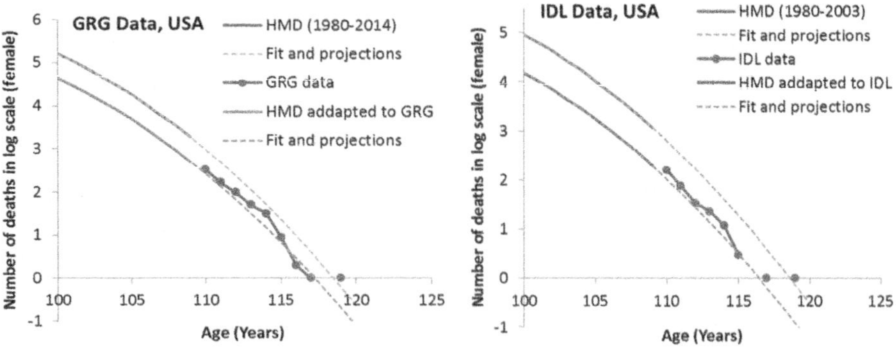

A

R^2=0.955

B

R^2=0.904

Fig. 2.18 HMD data, fit and projections and GRG (**a**) and IDL (**b**) data sets for USA (female)

(Fig. 2.18b) data sets. The adaptation from GRG to HMD data base and IDL to HMD data base and vise-versa provide enough evidence for the use of both data bases in supercentenarian projection studies.

2.8 Summary

So far we have replied to the fundamental question regarding a limit to the human life span by providing methods and tools and make related applications.

While a stagnation appears for USA, the data for France and Japan clearly indicate a continuing growth for the level of supercentenarian trajectories and accordingly for the level of MRAD the latter growing with time.

The expected MRAD is closely related to the number of centenarians. The latter is growing fast in an exponential trend thus ensuring a quite large pull for the expected supercentenarians.

References

Brown, N. J. L., Albers, C. J., & Ritchie, S. J. (2017). Contesting the evidence for limited human lifespan. *Nature, 546*. https://doi.org/10.1038/nature22784.

De Beer, J., Bardoutsos, A., & Janssen, F. (2017). Maximum human lifespan may increase to 125 years. *Nature, 546*. https://doi.org/10.1038/nature22792.

Dong, X., Milholland, B., & Vijg, J. (2016). Evidence for a limit to human lifespan. *Nature, 538*, 257–259. ISSN: 1476-4687. https://doi.org/10.1038/nature19793.

Gompertz, B. (1825). On the nature of the function expressive of the law of human mortality, and on the mode of determining the value of life contingencies. *Philosophical Transactions of the Royal Society of London A, 115*, 513–585.

Hughes, B. G., & Hekimi, S. (2017). Many possible maximum lifespan trajectories. *Nature, 546*. https://doi.org/10.1038/nature22786.

Janssen, J., & Skiadas, C. H. (1995). Dynamic modelling of life-table data. *Applied Stochastic Models and Data Analysis, 11*(1), 35–49.

Lenart, A., & Vaupel, J. W. (2017). Questionable evidence for a limit to human lifespan. *Nature, 546*. https://doi.org/10.1038/nature22790.

Rozing, M. P., Kirkwood, T. B. L., & Westendorp, R. G. J. (2017). Is there evidence for a limit to human lifespan? *Nature, 546*. https://doi.org/10.1038/nature22788.

Skiadas, C. H., & Skiadas, C. (2010a). Comparing the Gompertz type models with a first passage time density model. In C. H. Skiadas (Ed.), *Advances in data analysis* (pp. 203–209). Boston: Springer/Birkhauser.

Skiadas, C., & Skiadas, C. H. (2010b). Development, simulation and application of first exit time densities to life table data. *Communications in Statistics-Theory and Methods, 39*, 444–451.

Skiadas, C. H., & Skiadas, C. (2014). The first exit time theory applied to life table data: The health state function of a population and other characteristics. *Communications in Statistics-Theory and Methods, 43*, 1985–1600.

Skiadas, C. H., & Skiadas, C. (2015). Exploring the state of a stochastic system via stochastic simulations: An interesting inversion problem and the health state function. *Methodology and Computing in Applied Probability, 17*, 973–982.

Skiadas, C. H., & Skiadas, C. (2017). *Exploring the health state of a population by dynamic modeling methods.* https://doi.org/10.1007/978-3-319-65142-2. (see at: https://link.springer.com/book/10.1007/978-3-319-65142-2).

Chapter 3
Exploring the Health Status of a Population: A Simple Health State Model vs the Gompertz Model

Christos H. Skiadas

We present a method to formulate the Health State or Health Status curve of a population from the Gompertz model thus providing a useful tool to demographers, actuaries, policy makers, health people and organizations and sociologists. The model is presented along with a simple first exit time model and another "Best Fit" model. A method of finding the corrected health state or health status is also presented.

3.1 Introduction

The Gompertz 1825 model is a quite reliable tool to express demographic indicators related to the human life table. The corresponding probability density function $g(t)$ of a 3-parameter model is of the form:

$$g(t) = e^{-k+bt-e^{-l+bt}} \tag{3.1}$$

Where b, k, l are parameters and t is the time or age of an individual or population. The very interesting future of this model was that it is easily handled and fited to data sets using logarithms, a technique very important in the days of Gompertz (he had proposed the model in 1825). More important is that this model suggests a linear form for the logarithm of mortality thus providing a very easy handling tool for actuaries. The model provides good estimates for a relatively large part of the life span (in many cases covers a range from 30 to 90 years of age as is illustrated in Fig. 3.1).

C. H. Skiadas (✉)
ManLab, Technical University of Crete, Chania, Crete, Greece
e-mail: skiadas@cmsim.net

© Springer International Publishing AG, part of Springer Nature 2018

C. H. Skiadas, C. Skiadas (eds.), *Demography and Health Issues*,
The Springer Series on Demographic Methods and Population Analysis 46,
https://doi.org/10.1007/978-3-319-76002-5_3

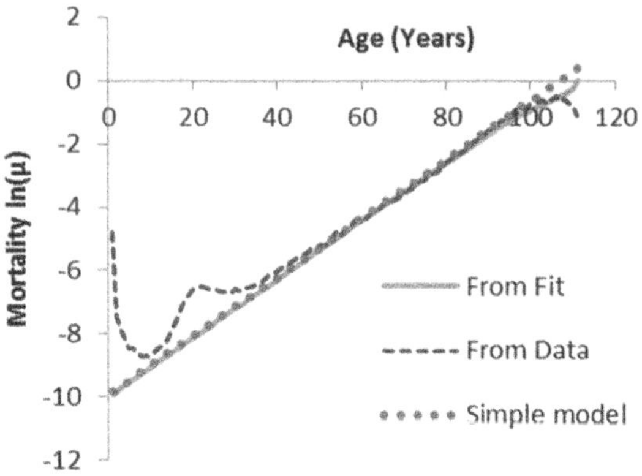

Fig. 3.1 Mortality curves for USA males (2000). Continuous line (Gompertz model fit), dotted line (Simple model), dashed curve (from Data)

3.2 How to Find the Health State Curve of the Gompertz Model

The Health Status index of the population was proposed from the sixties and seventies by Sanders (1964), Sullivan (1966, 1971), Torrance (1976) and others. Sullivan proposed a method for estimating the health status index from information related to disability data collected. Torrance proposed an estimate of the health status of the population based on the summation of the health status of the individuals. Our approach (Janssen and Skiadas 1995 and many studies by Skiadas 2011 and Skiadas and Skiadas 2010a, b, 2013a, b, 2014, 2015 was to find the Health State or Health Status from the outcome that is the distribution of deaths $g(t)$. This approach based on the advanced findings of the first exit or hitting time theory is difficult to handle but it can estimate the health state $H(t)$ of a population from $g(t)$ and vice versa. According to this theory simple or complicated models are proposed and applied to life table data. The simpler model is an extension of the so-called Inverse Gaussian. The probability density function $g(t)$ is given by:

$$g(t) = \frac{|l + (c-1)(bt)^c|}{\sqrt{2\pi t^3}} e^{-\frac{(l-(bt)^c)^2}{2t}} \tag{3.2}$$

Where b, l, c are parameters and $c = 1$ for the Inverse Gaussian. The Health State or Health Status Function $H(t)$ is given by:

$$H(t) = l - (bt)^c \tag{3.3}$$

The model (3.2) is a special form of the more general model proposed by Jennen (1985), Lerche (1986) and Jennen and Lerche (1981) of the following form

$$g(t) = \frac{|H - tH'|}{\sqrt{2\pi\, t^3}} e^{-\frac{(H_t)^2}{2t}} \tag{3.4}$$

Following the above theory and applying models (3.1) and (3.2) and (3.5) to data for USA males and females (1960 and 2000) we find the results presented in the next Tables 3.1, 3.2, 3.3 and 3.4. The first two Tables include the estimated parameter values for the same model (3.2) the "First exit time model-I". This model provides two distinct minima when fitted to data sets related to the first estimates for the parameter *l* to start the non-linear regression analysis. Clearly the global minimum accounts for the case including infant mortality as is illustrated in Fig. 3.1b, whereas the local minimum accounts for a case not including infant mortality (IM). The sum of squared errors (SSE) and the R^2 are almost similar in recent years (USA 2000) and differ considerably in the past when the infant mortality was high (USA 1960).

Table 3.1 Parameter estimates for first exit time model-I

	First exit time model-I					
	b	l	k	c	SSE	R^2
Males						
USA 1960	0.02922	13.914	0.3643	3.475	0.0010286	0.904
USA 2000	0.02198	13.119	0.3725	4.640	0.0001184	0.991
Females						
USA 1960	0.02270	14.055	0.3670	4.523	0.0006195	0.954
USA 2000	0.02017	14.362	0.3768	5.065	0.0000859	0.994

Table 3.2 Parameter estimates for the first exit time model with infant mortality

	First exit time model with infant mortality					
	b	l	k	c	SSE	R^2
Males						
USA 1960	0.01948	0.03220	0.8394	5.259	0.0001456	0.986
USA 2000	0.01686	0.009105	0.8278	6.441	0.0000896	0.993
Females						
USA 1960	0.01674	0.02574	0.8129	6.667	0.0001222	0.991
USA 2000	0.01536	0.00752	0.8233	7.432	0.0000651	0.996

Table 3.3 Parameter estimates for the Gompertz model

	Gompertz					
	b	l	k	c	SSE	R^2
Males						
USA 1960	0.07977	6.035	8.594		0.001001	0.907
USA 2000	0.09282	7.619	10.032		0.000151	0.988
Females						
USA 1960	0.09708	7.937	10.320		0.000635	0.953
USA 2000	0.10344	8.963	11.267		0.000121	0.992

Table 3.4 Parameter estimates for the first exit time model simple

	First exit time model simple					
	b	l	k	c	SSE	R^2
Males						
USA 1960	0.01960		0.8469	5.218	0.0010142	0.910
USA 2000	0.01688		0.8334	6.368	0.0001266	0.990
Females						
USA 1960	0.01672		0.8171	6.622	0.0006314	0.955
USA 2000	0.01536		0.8266	7.382	0.0000975	0.994

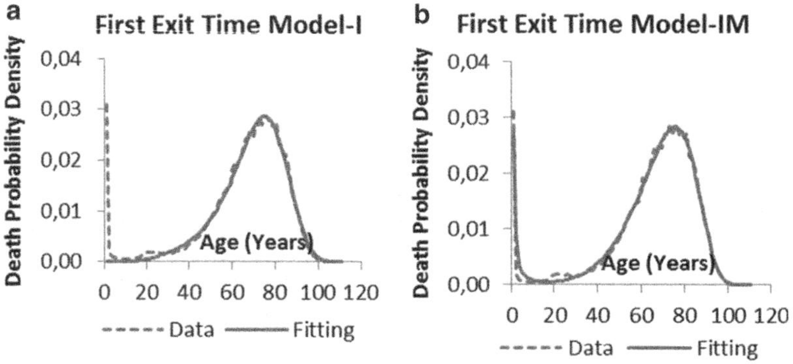

Fig. 3.2 (**a**) Model without infant mortality (USA 1960, males). (**b**) Model with infant mortality (USA 1960, males)

However, the simple case without infant mortality gives similar results with the Gompertz model and is very useful in our study. The IM version of the first exit time model as it is illustrated in Table 3.2 shows relatively small values for the parameter l and, in the limit, it is possible to reduce the model to the simpler 3 parameter form

$$g(t) = \frac{|(c-1)(bt)^c|}{\sqrt{2\pi t^3}} e^{-\frac{(bt)^{2c}}{2t}} \tag{3.5}$$

Of course we cannot model the infant mortality by applying this model. This is the simplest 3-parameter first exit time model (Fig. 3.2a and b)

3.3 A Very Interesting Property of the Gompertz Function

That came to be a very serious reason for the popularity of the Gompertz model was the simple but yet quite accurate modeling of the law of mortality for the ages from 30 to 90 years by the simple exponential function form $m_t = \exp(bt)$ or the simpler logarithmic form $\ln(m_t) = bt$ providing a simple linear equation for the logarithm of the human mortality and consequently a useful tool for actuaries, demographers and policy planners.

From the other point of view the Gompertz model provided a probability density function *g*(*t*) expressing the distribution of deaths over age for a population at a specific period of time. So far we can construct the m_t from *g*(*t*) or vice versa.

The next point is related to our knowledge that the probability density function *g* (*t*) expresses the first exit time density of a stochastic process expressing the health state or health status of a group of individuals or a population during the age development (Skiadas and Skiadas 2013a, b, 2014).

The inverse of (3.4) will provide the unknown Health State or Health Status form. Formula (3.4) cannot be solved directly for the unknown state function *H*(*t*) given *g* (*t*). However, by adding a correction term f_t we can find an approximation of the form (*k* is a constant):

$$g(t) = \frac{k}{\sqrt{2\pi t^3}} e^{\frac{-(f_t + H_t)^2}{2t}} \tag{3.6}$$

Now, inversion of (3.6) yields immediately the following form

$$H_t + f_t = \pm \left(-2t \ln \frac{g(t)\sqrt{2\pi t^3}}{k} \right)^{1/2} \tag{3.7}$$

The estimation of *H*(*t*) from the last formula is presented in Skiadas and Skiadas (2013a, b, 2015).

We can use the right hand part of (3.7) to compare the Health Status estimates from Data, the Gompertz model and the Simple Mortality model proposed. Clearly these estimates overestimate the Health State as it is presented in Fig. 3.3. As the estimates based on the Simple Model provide a fair estimate for the middle stages of the life span, we can use it as a basis of the estimates based on various models. We expect that all the successful models have to provide similar figures in the area of the maximum death rate corresponding to zero health state. In earlier works we have presented a method of estimating the correction function based on stochastic simulations and another based on analytic methods. Here we propose a relatively simple method providing satisfactory results for smooth data sets. In almost all the continuous models the nonlinear regression could provide acceptable smooth data from life table data.

The method starts by estimating *g*(*t*) by nonlinear fitting of the selected model to life table data sets. Then, we estimate the parameter *k* to fulfil the requirements set in the right hand side of (3.7) that is continuity and negative values for the logarithm. As we already have proved (Skiadas and Skiadas 2010a, b, 2013a, b, 2014, 2015, 2017) the only accepted value is given by

$$k = \max\left(g(t)\sqrt{2\pi t^3}\right) \tag{3.8}$$

Then with (3.7) and (3.8) we can estimate the uncorrected $H_{unc} = H(t) + f(t)$. We proceed to find the correction parameter k_{cor} from:

$$k_{cor} = \max\left(\frac{g(t)\sqrt{2\pi t^3}}{|H_{unc} - tH'_{unc}|}\right)$$

The approximation for $H(t)$ is provided by the following formula

$$H_t \cong \pm\left(-2t\ln\frac{g(t)\sqrt{2\pi t^3}}{k_{cor}}\right)^{1/2}$$

The resulting uncorrected health state of the Gompertz model is presented with the dotted curve in Fig. 3.3 where the corresponding corrected health state is illustrated with the dash-dotted curve. The corrected Gompertz curve, the best fit curve and the Simple Model curve for the health state have a common point at $H = 0$ achieved at age $t = 79$ years. The corrected Gompertz model provides a maximum at 30 years of age. The best fit model provides the maximum health state at 34 years. From the same model we estimate a local maximum at the age of 14 years and a local minimum at 20 years of age.

As it is presented in Fig. 3.3 both corrected and uncorrected Gompertz model cases provide an almost quadratic curve form for the health status of the population. The health status starts from low levels at birth and gradually increases until a maximum level in ages from 30 to 40 years and then continuously declines until the end.

However, the above estimations cover partially the full form of the human health state as underestimate the expected maximum health state at early years of age. The correct form is presented in Fig. 3.4A for USA males the year 2000. The health state starts from a low level at birth grows to the maximum level one at 12 year of age declines to a local minimum at 22 years of age; then a local maximum is reached at age 32 and a continuous decline follows. In Fig. 3.4B the two stage estimation is presented. The Health State Simple model H(x) is illustrated by the dashed orange curve whereas the blue curve represents the final form of the estimates (results and figures from Skiadas and Skiadas 2017).

3.4 Conclusions

We provided a method for using the classical Gompertz model to express the health state or health status of a population. The results were compared with findings from other models. It is demonstrated that the Gompertz model expresses the growth and decline of the health status of the population and can be used in simple applications.

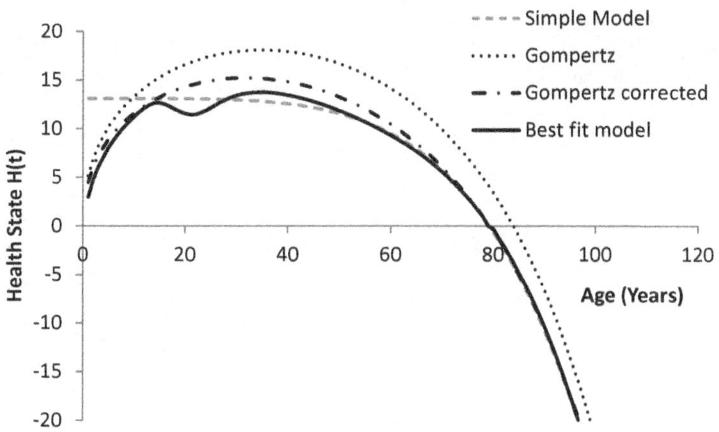

Fig. 3.3 Health State for USA, males (2000) from the Gompertz model, the corrected Gompertz model, the Simple model and the Best Fit model

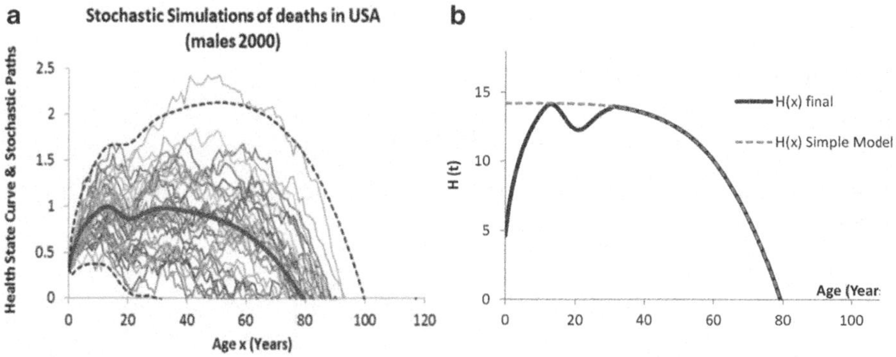

Fig. 3.4 (**a**) and (**b**). Our estimations from the book "Skiadas, C.H. and Skiadas, C. Exploring the Health State of a Population by Dynamic Modeling Methods, Springer, 2017"

More accurate results are produced from the best fit model with the cost of more parameters added in the models.

Appendix

After introducing the Health State Function for the human population a very important point arises of finding a simple method to derive the probability density function based on the simple Inverse Gaussian presented in the application of Weiss and Fraser for Medflies and already known from more than a century. A detailed methodology based on the stochastic theory is already presented in our publications mentioned above and in the references. The very simple transformation comes from

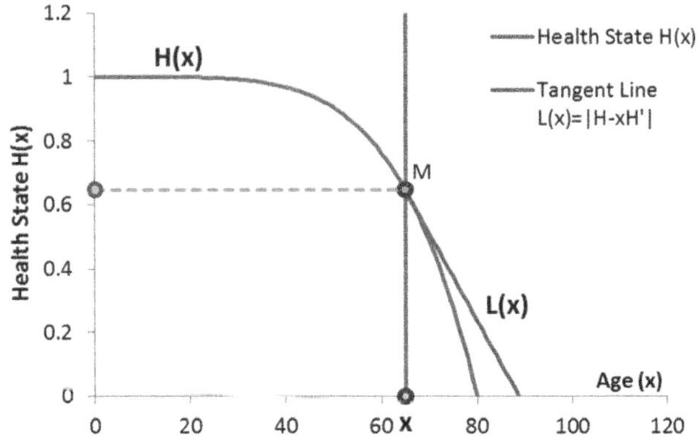

Fig. 3.5 Derivation of the Health State probability density function from the Inverse Gaussian

the next Fig. 3.5 where by moving the coordinate of the X axis to the point of age x, the probability density function $g(x)$ arises as a first approximation of a simple linearization of the Health State Curve at point M

$$H(x) = 1 - (bx)^c,$$

where the curve is replaced by the Tangent Line

$$L(x) = |H - xH'|,$$

that is by a linear part of $H(x)$ in the vicinity of the point M. Then the Inverse Gaussian

$$g(x) = \frac{|\, L(x) \,|}{\sigma\sqrt{2\pi x^3}} e^{-\frac{H_x^2}{2\sigma^2 x}}$$

applies for a small interval around the point M thus obtaining the function

$$g(x) = \frac{|\, H_x - xH'_x \,|}{\sigma\sqrt{2\pi x^3}} e^{-\frac{H_x^2}{2\sigma^2 x}}$$

This is equivalent with (3.4) presented earlier. Note that in (3.4) $\sigma = 1$.

This is the extended form we already have derived and applied for the health state of the human population.

References

Gompertz, B. (1825). On the nature of the function expressing of the law of human mortality. *Philosophical Transactions of the Royal Society, 36*, 513–585.

Janssen, J., & Skiadas, C. H. (1995). Dynamic modelling of life-table data. *Applied Stochastic Models and Data Analysis, 11*(1), 35–49.

Jennen, C. (1985). Second-order approximation for Brownian first exit distributions. *Annals of Probability, 13*, 126–144.

Jennen, C., & Lerche, H. R. (1981). First exit densities of Brownian motion through one-sided moving boundaries. *Zeitschrift Wahrscheinlichkeitstheorie und verwandte Gebiete, 55*, 133–148.

Lerche, H. R. (1986). *Boundary crossing of Brownian motion.* Berlin: Springer.

Sanders, B. S. (1964). Measuring community health levels. *American Journal of Public Health, 54*, 1063–1070.

Skiadas, C. H. (2011, October 1). *A life expectancy study based on the deterioration function and an application to Halley's Breslau data.* arXiv:1110.0130v1 [q-bio.PE].

Skiadas, C. H., & Skiadas, C. (2010a). Comparing the Gompertz type models with a first passage time density model. In C. H. Skiadas (Ed.), *Advances in data analysis* (pp. 203–209). Boston: Springer/Birkhauser.

Skiadas, C. H., & Skiadas, C. (2010b). Development, simulation and application of first exit time densities to life table data. *Communications in Statistics, 39*, 444–451.

Skiadas, C. H., & Skiadas, C. (2013a). *The health state function of a population.* Athens: ISAST.

Skiadas, C. H., & Skiadas, C. (2013b). *Supplement: The health state function of a population.* Athens: ISAST.

Skiadas, C. H., & Skiadas, C. (2014). The first exit time theory applied to life table data: The health state function of a population and other characteristics. *Communications in Statistics-Theory and Methods, 43*(7), 1585–1600.

Skiadas, C. H., & Skiadas, C. (2015). Exploring the state of a stochastic system via stochastic simulations: An interesting inversion problem and the health state function. *Methodology and Computing in Applied Probability, 17*(4), 973–982.

Skiadas, C. H., & Skiadas, C. (2017). *Exploring the health state of a population by dynamic modeling methods*. Springer. http://www.springer.com/us/book/9783319651415

Sullivan, D. F. (1966). *Conceptual problems in developing an index of health* (U.S. Department of HEW, Public Health Service Publication No. 1000, Series 2, No. 17). Washington, DC: U.S. Department of Health, Education and Welfare.

Sullivan, D. F. (1971). (National Center for Health Statistics): A single index of mortality and morbidity. *HSMHA Health Reports, 86*, 347–354.

Torrance, G. W. (1976). Health status index models: A unified mathematical view. *Management Science, 22*(9), 990–1001.

Chapter 4
Estimation of the Healthy Life Expectancy in Italy Through a Simple Model Based on Mortality Rate

Christos H. Skiadas and Maria Felice Arezzo

4.1 Introduction

The debate in Europe is currently paying considerable attention on healthy life expectancy (HALE), focusing on some important subpopulations like those of the elderly and/or those of the females and males. Following the approach of the World Health Organization (WHO), health should be considered as having a dynamic nature, and should be taken into consideration in the context of life, as the ability to fulfill actions or to carry out a certain role in society. This is the so-called functional approach, taken by the WHO in the elaboration of the international frame of reference on the matter.

The most suitable indicator to measure the state of health of a population is health expectancy, which measures the length of life spent in different states of health.

There are several methods to estimate health expectancies. Among them the most commonly used are the Sullivan and the multi-state, respectively based on classical life table and longitudinal data.

The first method was pioneered by Wolfbein on the length of "working life" (Wolfbein 1949) and is described in details in Sullivan (1971); as it is well known, it combines the prevalence of disability obtained through a cross-sectional survey and a period life table.

The second method, named multi-state tables, was pioneered by Rogers (1975) and Willekens for migration and marital status (Willekens 1979; Hoem and Fong

C. H. Skiadas (✉)
ManLab, Technical University of Crete, Chania, Greece
e-mail: Skiadas@cmsim.net

M. F. Arezzo (✉)
Università di Roma "La Sapienza", Rome, Italy
e-mail: mariafelice.arezzo@uniroma1.it

© Springer International Publishing AG, part of Springer Nature 2018
C. H. Skiadas, C. Skiadas (eds.), *Demography and Health Issues*,
The Springer Series on Demographic Methods and Population Analysis 46,
https://doi.org/10.1007/978-3-319-76002-5_4

1976) for the multi-state table of working life and Brouard for the introduction of the period prevalence of labor participation (Brouard 1980; Cambois et al. 1999; Giudici et al. 2013). Multi-state models are based on the analysis of the transitions between states in competition with the probabilities of dying from each state.

The information necessary for this type of analysis derives from longitudinal surveys. The result, in this case, is the so called period (or stable) prevalence and can be interpreted analogously to the stationary population of a period life table, as the proportion of the disabled amongst the survivors of successive fictitious cohorts, subject to the flows of entry on disability, recovery and death observed in the period under examination.

Thus, the period health expectancy is the expected number of years to be spent in the healthy state by this fictitious cohort.

In the classical life table analysis, the survivors of any age are supposed to be at the same risk of dying. When taking heterogeneity into account, the simplest model consists in considering two states (healthy vs unhealthy, enabled vs disabled), but assuming that the population in each state is homogeneous over time, i.e. at each age they are at the same risks of changing their status. This corresponds to the common Markov hypothesis.

Starting from the late 80's a Global Burden of Disease (GBD) study was applied in many countries reflecting the optimistic views of many researchers and policy makers worldwide to quantify the health state of a population or a group of persons. In the time course they succeeded in establishing an international network collecting and providing adequate information to calculate health measures under terms as Loss of Healthy Life Years (LHLY) or Healthy Life Expectancy (HALE).

So far the process followed was towards statistical measures including surveys and data collection using questionnaires and disability and epidemiological data as well (McDowell 2006).

However, a serious scientific part is missing or it is not very much explored that is to find the model underlying the health state measures. Observing the health state measures by country from 1990 until nowadays it is clear that the observed and estimated health parameters follow a rather systematic way. The lessons learned during the last centuries were towards the introduction of models in the analysis of health and mortality. The classical examples are Edmund Halley for Life Tables and Benjamin Gompertz for the law of mortality and may others. Today our ability to use mass storage tools as the computers and the extensive application of surveys and polls to many political, social and economic activities directed the main health state studies. In other words we give much attention to opinions of the people for their health status followed by extensive health data collection. However, it remains a serious question: can we validate the health status results? As it is the standard procedure in science a systematic study as the Global Burden of Disease should be validated by one or more models. Especially as these studies are today the main tool for the health programs of many countries the need of verification is more important.

4.2 Estimation with a Model

We test a simple model proposed by Skiadas (2015) and Skiadas and Skiadas (2017), which we briefly describe in the following, using Italian data and compare the results with those provided by the Italian National Institute of Statistics (ISTAT) and by the GBD.

The model is based on two parameters, b and T, and it is:

$$\mu_x = \left(\frac{x}{T}\right)^b$$

T represents the age at which $\mu_x = 1$ and b is a crucial health state parameter expressing the curvature of μx. As the health state is improved b gets higher values.

Figure 4.1 represents a mortality diagram and illustrates the idea behind the methods proposed.

The main task is to find the area *Ex* under the curve OCABO in the mortality diagram (see Fig. 4.1) which is a measure of the mortality effect. This is done by estimating the following integral:

$$E_x = \int_0^T \left(\frac{x}{T}\right)^b dx = \frac{T}{b+1}\left(\frac{x}{T}\right)^{b.}$$

The resulting value for Ex in the interval [0, T] is given by the simple form:

$$E_{mortality} = \frac{T}{b+1}$$

The total information for the mortality is the area provided under the curve μx and the horizontal axis. The total area *Etotal* of the healthy and mortality part of the life

Fig. 4.1 Mortality diagram

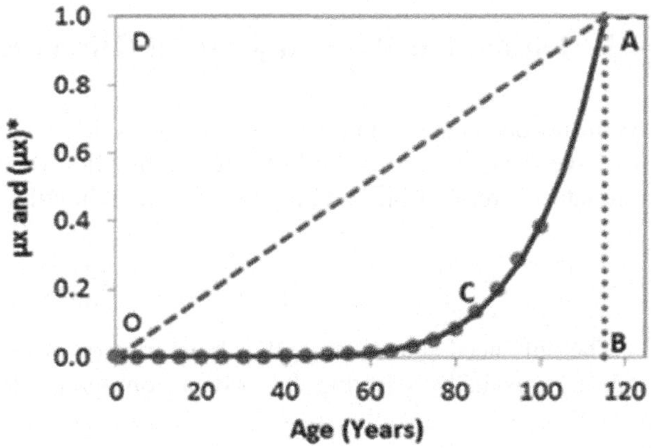

span is nothing else but the area included into the rectangle of length T and height 1 that is *Etotal* = *T*. The health area is given by:

$$E_{health} = T - E_{mortality} = \frac{bT}{b+1}$$

It then follows that:

$$b = \frac{E_{health}}{E_{mortality}}$$

This is the simplest indicator for the loss of health status of a population. Another interesting and closely related estimator is in the form:

$$b + 1 = \frac{E_{total}}{E_{mortality}}$$

This indicator is more appropriate for the severe and moderate disability causes. It provides larger values for the disability measures as the *Etotal* is larger or the *Emortality* area is smaller by means that as we live longer the disability period becomes larger.

This method suggests a simple but yet interesting tool for estimating the loss of healthy life years (LHLY). A correction multiplier λ should be added for specific situations so that the estimator is in the form:

$$LHLY = \frac{E_{total}}{E_{mortality}} = \lambda(b + 1)$$

4.3 Estimation Without a Model (Direct Estimation)

As the needed data sets in the form of mx or qx data are provided from the life tables, we have developed a method of direct estimation of the loss of healthy life year estimators directly from the life table by expanding the life table to the right.

$$b = \frac{E_{total}}{E_{mortality}} = \frac{xm_x}{\sum_0^x m_x}$$

The only need is to estimate the above fraction from the life table data. A similar indicator results by selecting the *qx* data from the life table and using the:

$$b = \frac{E_{total}}{E_{mortality}} = \frac{xq_x}{\sum_0^x q_x}$$

In both cases the results are similar. The estimates from *mx* are slightly larger than from *qx*. In both cases the *b* estimators growth to a maximum at old ages and then decline. The selected *b* indicator for the life years lost from birth is that of the maximum value. A smoothing technique is used to avoid sharp fluctuations in the maximum range area. Both the estimation of the *b* indicator by this direct method and the method by using a model give similar results.

4.4 Applications

Our preliminary results for the Italian data are encouraging as shown in Fig. 4.2a, b. For both cases we have estimated the Healthy Life Expectancy (HLE) by the Direct Method (without a model) and by the Fit Method (with the simple model). Both methods provide close estimates and mainly for the males case. The HALE estimates (Salomon et al. 2012; Murray et al. 2016; WHO 2001, 2002, 2004, 2013, 2014) are also close to ours especially for the latest years.

Three of the nearby countries with Italy are also studied in Fig. 4.3. For all countries, Switzerland, France and Austria, the estimates are close to the related HALE figures.

It should be noted that our methods based on the Life Table data sets are easy to apply even for time periods when health and disease estimates are not collected. Even more the needed second method to straighten the HALE estimates is proposed and applied along with a third one to support the previous (Skiadas 2015, 2016). Another three parallel methods based on Gompertz, Weibull and a Stochastic model (Skiadas and Skiadas 2010, 2014, 2015) provide similar and supporting estimates.

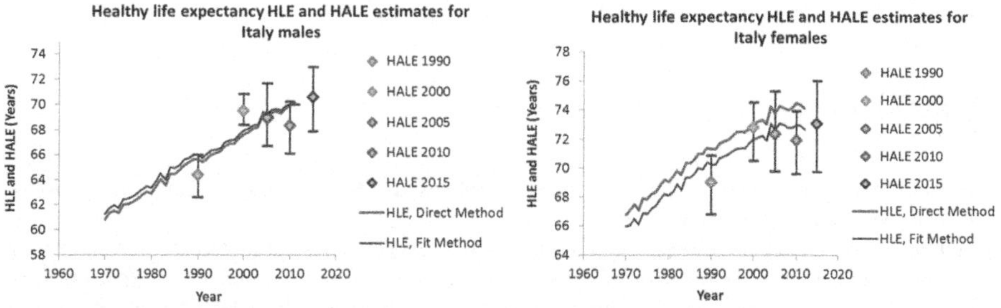

Fig. 4.2 HLE estimates and HALE estimates and confidence intervals for Italian males (left) and females (right)

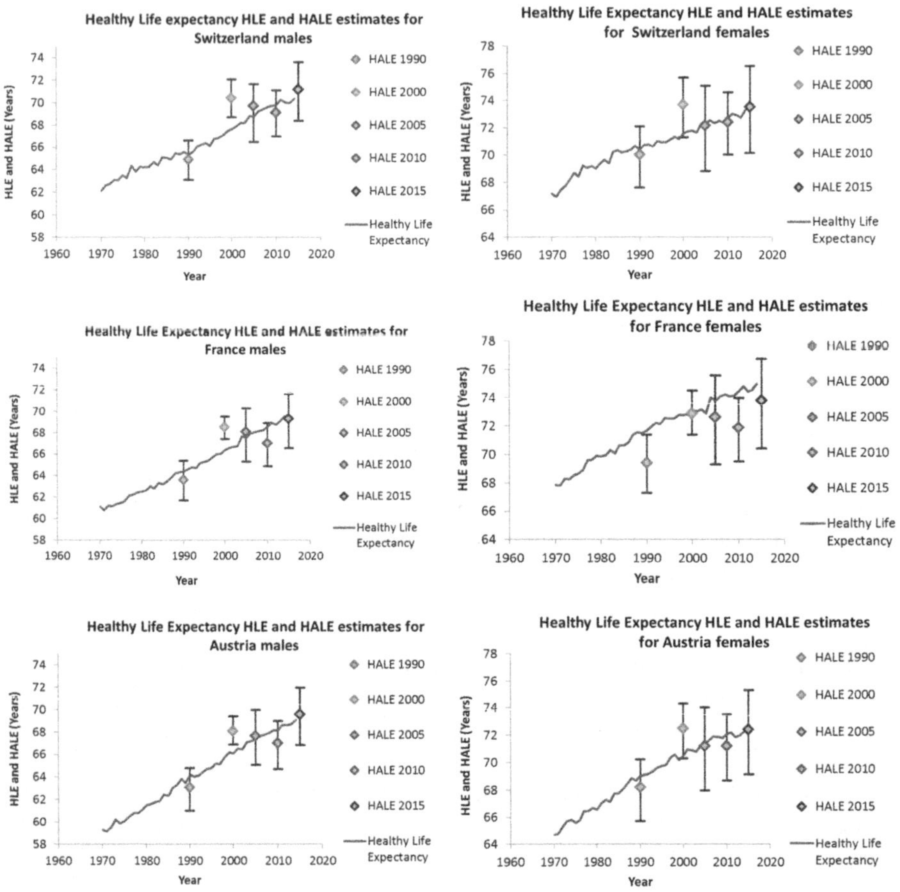

Fig. 4.3 HLE estimates and HALE estimates and confidence intervals for Switzerland, France and Austria males (left) and females (right)

References

Brouard, N. (1980). Espérance de vie active, reprises d'activité féminine: un modèle. *Revue économique, 31*, 1260–1287.

Cambois, E., Robine, J. M., & Brouard, N. (1999). Life expectancies applied to specific statuses. A history of the indicators and methods of calculation. *Population: An English Selection, 11*, 7–34.

Giudici, C., Arezzo, M. F., & Brouard, N. (2013). Estimating health expectancy in presence of missing data: An application using HID survey. *Statistical Methods and Applications, 22*, 517.

Hoem, J., & Fong, M. (1976). *A Markov chain model of working life tables* (Working paper 2 Laboratory of Actuarial Mathematics). Copenhagen: University of Copenhagen.

McDowell, I. (2006). *Measuring health: A guide to rating scales and questionnaires* (3rd ed.). Oxford/New York: Oxford University Press.

Murray, C. J. L., et al. (2016). Global, regional, and national disability-adjusted life-years (DALYs) for 315 diseases and injuries and healthy life expectancy (HALE), 1990–2015: A systematic analysis for the global burden of disease study 2015. *Lancet, 388*, 1603–1658.

Rogers, A. (1975). *Introduction to multi regional mathematical demography*. New York: Wiley.

Salomon, et al. (2012). Healthy life expectancy for 187 countries, 1990–2010: A systematic analysis for the global burden disease study 2010. *Lancet, 380*, 2144–2162.

Skiadas, C. H. (2015, October). *Verifying the global burden of disease study: Quantitative methods proposed.* ArXiv.org. http://arxiv.org/abs/1510.07346

Skiadas, C. H. (2016). *Exploring the HALE estimates of the global burden of disease study by a simple, Gompertz, Weibull and an advanced IM model.* 28th REVES conference, Wien, Austria, 8–10 June 2016.

Skiadas, C., & Skiadas, C. H. (2010). Development, simulation and application of first exit time densities to life table data. *Communications in Statistics – Theory and Methods, 39*(3), 444–451.

Skiadas, C. H., & Skiadas, C. (2014). The first exit time theory applied to life table data: The health state function of a population and other characteristics. *Communications in Statistics-Theory and Methods, 34*, 1585–1600.

Skiadas, C. H., & Skiadas, C. (2015). Exploring the state of a stochastic system via stochastic simulations: An interesting inversion problem and the health state function. *Methodology and Computing in Applied Probability, 17*, 973–982.

Skiadas, C. H., & Skiadas, C. (2017). *Exploring the health state of a population by dynamic modeling methods*. The Springer Series on Demographic Methods and Population Analysis book series (PSDE, Vol. 45), Springer. https://doi.org/10.1007/978-3-319-65142-2., https://link.springer.com/book/10.1007/978-3-319-65142-2

Sullivan, D. (1971). A single index of mortality and morbidity. *HSMHA Health Reports, 86*(4), 347–354.

WHO. (2014). *WHO methods for life expectancy and healthy life expectancy*. Global Health estimates technical paper WHO/HIS/HSI/GHE/2014.5. March, 2014. http://www.who.int/healthinfo/statistics/LT_method.pdf

WHO. Department of Health Statistics and Information system. (2013). *WHO methods and data sources for the global burden of disease estimates 2000–2011*. Global health estimates technical paper WHO/HIS/HSI/GHE/2013.4. November, 2013.http://www.who.int/healthinfo/statistics/GlobalDALYmethods_2000_2011.pdf

WHO. The World 132 Health Report. (2004). *Statistical annex, annex table 4 healthy life expectancy (HALE) in all WHO member states, estimates for 2002*. annex_4_en_2002.pdf

WHO. The World Health Report. (2001). *Statistical annex, annex table 4 healthy life expectancy (HALE) in all member states, estimates for 2000.* annex4_en_HALE_2000.pdf

WHO. The World Health Report. (2002). *Statistical annex, annex table 4 healthy life expectancy (HALE) in all member states, estimates for 2000 and 2001.* whr2002_annex4_2001.pdf

Willekens, F. (1979). *Computer program for increment-decrement (multistate) life table analysis: A user's manual to lifeindec.* Working papers of the international institute for applied systems analysis.

Wolfbein, S. (1949). The length of working life. *Population Studies, 3*, 286–294.

Part II
Mortality Modeling and Applications

Chapter 5
Using Child, Adult, and Old-Age Mortality to Establish a Developing Countries Mortality Database (DCMD)

Nan Li, Hong Mi, and Patrick Gerland

5.1 Introduction

Empirical data used in estimating life tables are collected from three types of source: (1) death registration that counts deaths by sex and age in a certain period, usually a calendar year; (2) census that enumerates the numbers of population by age and sex at a certain time point, and sometimes also death by age and sex during a period before the census time; and (3) sample survey that, in principle, could collect data on both death and population but cover only a small portion of the population in a country. Censuses are conducted in almost all the countries of the world. Besides providing middle-year populations to compute death rates for countries with reliable death registration, some developing countries rely also on census to obtain life tables directly. Since census interviewers must visit every household in a country to enumerate the number of residents at a certain time point, they could also ask just one more question about whether there was a death, or were deaths, in the household in past year; and if yes what is the gender and age of the death, or the genders and ages of the deaths (United Nations Statistics Division (UNSD) 2008). Furthermore, using population data of two successive censuses, some mortality indicators of the period between the two censuses could be estimated, especially for old ages at which the effect of migration is negligible (Li and Gerland 2013). For many countries, census data

The views expressed in this paper are those of the author and do not necessarily reflect those of the United Nations.

N. Li · P. Gerland
Population Division, Department of Economic and Social Affairs, United Nations, New York, NY, USA
e-mail: li32@un.org; gerland@un.org

H. Mi (✉)
School of Public Affairs, Zhejiang University, Hangzhou, Zhejiang, P. R. China

© Springer International Publishing AG, part of Springer Nature 2018

C. H. Skiadas, C. Skiadas (eds.), *Demography and Health Issues*,
The Springer Series on Demographic Methods and Population Analysis 46,
https://doi.org/10.1007/978-3-319-76002-5_5

on population by age and sex can be found from the United Nations Demographic Yearbook (e.g., UNSD 2013a). Occasionally, surveys using large sample size could also provide life tables.

Typical sample surveys often collect information only from a small portion of the population. Subsequently, they cannot produce life tables. This is because death rates at some ages, for example 10–20 years, could be very low, and hence require a large population to be estimated reliably. Nonetheless, sample surveys could provide reliable indicators of mortality for certain age groups when death is not a rare event or when the age group is wide enough. The most commonly sampled mortality indicator is child mortality, which is the probability of dying between birth and age 5, and is often denoted as ${}_5q_0$. The United Nations Children's Fund (UNICEF) as part of the United Nations Inter-agency Group for Child Mortality Estimation (IGME) has been regularly collecting, analyzing, and publishing child mortality for most of the countries back to the 1970s or earlier (see United Nations Children's Fund 2013; http://www.childmortality.org). Based on the same principles used to estimate child mortality using birth histories, surveys such as the Demographic and Health Surveys (DHS, http://www.measuredhs.com/) have been collecting sibling histories since the 1990s to measure adult mortality, allowing to derive the probability of dying between age 15 and 50 or 60 years, namely ${}_{35}q_{15}$ or ${}_{45}q_{15}$, respectively, for an increasing number of developing countries (Timæus 2013). Combining data of surveys and other sources, Wang et al. (2012) at the Institute for Heath Metrics and Evaluation (IHME) estimated adult mortality for 187 countries from 1970 to 2010.

Mortality databases have been established for developed countries (e.g., Human Mortality Database (HMD) 2016) and effectively used for various purposes. For developing countries of which the deaths counted 78% that of the world in 2010–2015 (United Nations Population Division (UNPD) 2015), however, reliable life tables can hardly be found. Indirect estimates of life tables have been provided by the UNPD (2015) and IHME (Wang et al. 2012) for developing countries, using empirical data on child mortality (${}_5q_0$) and adult mortality (${}_{45}q_{15}$). But more than half of all deaths already occurred at age 60 and higher in developing countries in 2010–2015. Thus, estimating old-age mortality (${}_{15}q_{60}$), and using it together with the ${}_5q_0$ and ${}_{45}q_{15}$ estimated by the UNICEF and IHME mentioned above, to establish a mortality database for developing countries is a relevant and urgent task. To fulfil this task, this paper introduces two methods: (1) the Census Method that uses populations enumerated in census to estimate ${}_{15}q_{60}$, and (2) the three-input model life table that utilizes ${}_5q_0$, ${}_{45}q_{15}$, and ${}_{15}q_{60}$ to calculate life tables. Compared to using only child and adult mortality, applying the two methods to the data of HMD after 1950, the errors of fitting old-age mortality are reduced for more than 70% of all the countries. To be more specific to developing countries, the errors are reduced by 17% for Chile, 48% for Japan, and 17% for Taiwan, for two sexes combined, which are the three non-European-origin populations in Human Mortality Database. These results indicate that, in order to establish a mortality database for developing countries, the methodology is adequate and the empirical data are available.

5.2 Methods

The methods include the Census Method and the three-input model life table (three-input MLT).

5.2.1 The Census Method

The Census Method utilizes populations enumerated from census to estimate ${}_{15}q_{60}$, and includes two models. The first is the Census Method with variable-r model (Bennett and Horiuchi 1981; Li and Gerland 2013), which is more suitable when the period between the two successive censuses is not close to 10 years; and the second is the Census Method with survival model, which should work better when the period is close to 10 years.

The Census Method with Variable-r Model

The variable-r model (Bennett and Horiuchi 1981) assumes zero migration and evenly distributed enumeration errors over age. Let $p(x, t)$ be the observed number of population in age group $[x, x+5)$ enumerated from a census conducted at time t, where $x = 60, 65, 70$. The growth rates at age x are computed as

$$r(x) = Log\left[\frac{p(x,t_2)}{p(x,t_1)}\right] / (t_2 - t_1), x = 60, 65, 70, \quad (5.1)$$

where t_1 and t_2 represent the date of the first and second census, respectively. And the accumulated growth rates are

$$\begin{aligned} s(60) &= 2.5r(60), \\ s(65) &= 5r(60) + 2.5r(65), \\ s(70) &= 5[r(60) + r(65)] + 2.5r(70). \end{aligned} \quad (5.2)$$

Further, the middle-point population in age group $[x, x+5)$, $N(x)$, are estimated as

$$N(x) = \sqrt{p(x,t_1)p(x,t_2)}, x = 60, 65, 70. \tag{5.3}$$

Furthermore, the person-years lived in 5-year age group *[x,x + 5)*, L_x, in the underlying stationary population, are obtained as (Bennett and Horiuchi 1981).

$$L_x = N(x)\exp[s(x)], x = 60, 65, 70. \tag{5.4}$$

At old ages such as 60 and over, migrants are negligible comparing to deaths. Thus, the zero-migration assumption is naturally satisfied. In developing countries, however, the errors in enumerating population often occur unevenly across age. A typical example is age heaping. When such errors are severe, the L_x resulted from (5.4), would show implausible patterns of increasing with age, which cannot occur in a stationary population. When such implausible situations occur, adjusting L_x is necessary. Li and Gerland (2013) proposed such an adjustment as is shown in the appendix A, which provides the adjusted $\widehat{L}_x$. After adjusting the age-reporting errors, the number of survivors at age x, l_x, can be estimated using nonlinear optimization and a Gompertz model (Li and Gerland 2013), or it can be estimated locally linearly as below:

$$\begin{aligned} l_{65} &= \frac{\widehat{L}_{60} + \widehat{L}_{65}}{2.5} \frac{\widehat{L}_{65}}{\left(\widehat{L}_{60} + 2\widehat{L}_{65} + \widehat{L}_{70}\right)}, \\ l_{70} &= \frac{\widehat{L}_{65} + \widehat{L}_{70}}{2.5} \frac{\widehat{L}_{65}}{\left(\widehat{L}_{60} + 2\widehat{L}_{65} + \widehat{L}_{70}\right)}, \\ l_{60} &= \frac{\widehat{L}_{60}}{2.5} - l_{65}, \\ l_{75} &= \frac{\widehat{L}_{70}}{2.5} - l_{70}. \end{aligned} \tag{5.5}$$

In (5.5), the $\frac{\widehat{L}_{60} + \widehat{L}_{65}}{2.5}$ and $\frac{\widehat{L}_{65} + \widehat{L}_{70}}{2.5}$ are the first-step estimates of l_{65} and l_{70}, which are linear interpolations between $\widehat{L}_{60}$, $\widehat{L}_{65}$ and $\widehat{L}_{70}$. The $\frac{\widehat{L}_{65}}{\left(\widehat{L}_{60} + 2\widehat{L}_{65} + \widehat{L}_{70}\right)}$ is an adjustment that makes $2.5 \cdot (l_{60} + l_{65}) = \widehat{L}_{65}$. The last two lines in (5.5) are linear formulas of calculating $\widehat{L}_{60}$ and $\widehat{L}_{70}$.

Finally, after estimating l_x, ${}_{15}q_{60}$ is obtained as

$${}_{15}q_{60} = 1 - \frac{l_{75}}{l_{60}} \tag{5.6}$$

The Census Method with Survival Model

When the period between the two successive censuses is close to 10 years, the populations between the period of exactly 10 years can be reliably estimated assuming over-time constant growth rates and using (5.1). Consequently, the 10-year survival ratio of the stationary population is estimated as

$$S = \frac{L_{70}}{L_{60}} = \frac{p(70-74, t_2)}{p(60-64, t_1)}. \tag{5.7}$$

Assuming that the over-age survival ratio is constant, the 1-year and 15-year survival ratios are therefore $S^{\frac{1}{10}}$ and $S^{\frac{15}{10}}$, respectively. Subsequently, the 15-year probability of death between age 60 and 75 can be estimated as

$$q = 1 - S^{\frac{15}{10}}. \tag{5.8}$$

The assumption of constant over-age survival ratio can be adjusted using the United Nations general model life table (UNPD 1982), which leads to a more accurate estimate of old-age mortality as

$$_{15}q_{60} = \begin{cases} q \cdot (1.021 - 0.0002 \cdot q + 0.0002 \cdot q^2), R^2 = 0.999, \textit{female}, \\ q \cdot (1.0153 - 0.0003 \cdot q + 0.0002 \cdot q^2), R^2 = 0.999, \textit{male}. \end{cases} \tag{5.9}$$

5.2.2 *The Three-Input Model Life Table*

The three-input model life table is an augmentation of the flexible two-dimensional model life table (two-input MLT, Wilmoth et al. 2012), which is expressed as

$$\log(m_x) = a_x + b_x \cdot \log({}_5q_0) + c_x \cdot [\log({}_5q_0)]^2 + v_x \cdot k, \tag{5.10}$$

where m_x stands for the five-year age-specific death rates with $x = 0,1,5,10,\ldots$; coefficient vectors a_x, b_x, c_x, and v_x are obtained from fitting mortality data of the Human Mortality Database; and parameter k is flexible, which can be solved to fit an additional ${}_{45}q_{15}$. Obviously, the two-input MLT can be used to produce a life table when ${}_5q_0$ and ${}_{45}q_{15}$ are used as two inputs.

How to utilize the estimated old-age mortality (${}_{15}\widehat{q}_{60}$)? A simple answer (Li 2014) can be found by following the logic of the Logit transformation: $\log[{}_x\widehat{q}_0/(1 - {}_x\widehat{q}_0)] = \alpha + \beta \log[{}_xq_0/(1 - {}_xq_0)]$, in which the standard ${}_xq_0$ is naturally that of the two-input MLT, and level α and pattern β can be chosen to fit some function of observed probability of death ($_x\widehat{q}_0$). When there is only $_{15}\widehat{q}_{60}$, a customary is to set $\beta = 1$ and solve α to fit $_{15}\widehat{q}_{60}$ (see Preston et al. 2001, p. 200). The rationale for using the Logit transformation is that $\log\left[{}_xq_0/\left(1 - {}_xq_0\right)\right]$ would be close to linear at all the ages. It is worth noting that, at old ages, $\log\left(\widehat{m}_x\right)$ would be close to linear according to the Gompertz law. Thus, at old ages, the linear relationship of the Logit transformation can be simplified as:

$$\log\left(\widehat{m}_x\right) = \alpha + \log(m_x). \tag{5.11}$$

Because

$$_{15}\widehat{q}_{60} \approx 1 - \exp\left[-5 \cdot \left(\widehat{m}_{60} + \widehat{m}_{65} + \widehat{m}_{70}\right)\right], \tag{5.12}$$

α is solved by inserting (5.11) to (5.12):

$$\alpha \approx \log\left[\frac{\log\left(1 - {}_{15}\widehat{q}_{60}\right)}{\log\left(1 - {}_{15}q_{60}\right)}\right] \tag{5.13}$$

where $_{15}q_{60}$ is the old-age mortality of the two-input MLT. Subsequently, (5.10) is augmented to the three-input MLT:

$$\log(m_x) = \widehat{a}_x + b_x \cdot \log\left({}_5q_0\right) + c_x \cdot \left[\log\left({}_5q_0\right)\right]^2 + v_x \cdot k, \tag{5.14}$$

$$\widehat{a}_x = \begin{cases} a_x, x < 60, \\ a_x + \log\left[\dfrac{\log\left(1 - {}_{15}\widehat{q}_{60}\right)}{\log\left(1 - {}_{15}q_{60}\right)}\right], x \geq 60, \end{cases} \tag{5.15}$$

which will exactly fit the three inputs: child, adult, and old-age mortality.

5.3 Validations

We use the data of HMD to test whether or not the three-input MLT (with $_5q_0$, $_{45}q_{15}$, and $_{15}q_{60}$) can improve the performance of the two-input MLT with only $_5q_0$ and $_{45}q_{15}$. We choose the periods after 1950 to avoid the irregular effect of World War II, and all the countries or areas except Israel, for which the Census Method could not work because of territory change. In HMD, all 'census' dates are adjusted to January first. Consequently, periods 1950–1959, 1960–1969, . . ., and 2000–2009, and the Census Method with survival model, are chosen to carry out the validations. In real census, there are undercounts. Nonetheless, these undercounts tend to cancel each other in causing the errors of estimating mortality level, as is indicated in appendix B.

We first choose the observed $_5q_0$ and $_{45}q_{15}$ of a certain population in a certain period as the inputs of two-input MLT, which will produce a life table that includes an estimated $_{15}\tilde{q}_{60}$. This $_{15}\tilde{q}_{60}$ will differ from the observed old-age mortality, $_{15}q_{60}$.

We then use the 'census' populations at the two ends of each period to estimate the values of old-age mortality, and use an exponential model to smooth them. The results are denoted as ${}_{15}\widehat{q}_{60}$.

The purpose of two-input MLT is to use the ${}_{5}q_{0}$ and ${}_{45}q_{15}$to best describe the corresponding life table, including particularly the ${}_{15}q_{60}$, using the mortality patterns of the HMD populations. Thus, ${}_{15}\tilde{q}_{60}$ is the best estimated ${}_{15}q_{60}$ that the two-input MLT could provide. We believe that for developing countries ${}_{15}\tilde{q}_{60}$ should also be reasonable to some extent. Therefore, we use

$$ {}_{15}\bar{q}_{60} = \left[w \cdot {}_{15}\widehat{q}_{60} + (1-w) \cdot {}_{15}\tilde{q}_{60}\right] \tag{5.16} $$

as the estimated old-age mortality of the three-input MLT, where the w stands for the weight that can be determined flexibly, and is taken as 0.5 in all the validations here. The values of ${}_{15}\bar{q}_{60}$ are input to the three-input model life tables, which will have the same ${}_{5}q_{0}$ and ${}_{45}q_{15}$ as that of two-input MLT. But the values of old-age mortality of these life tables are ${}_{15}\bar{q}_{60}$, which will differ from the observed ${}_{15}q_{60}$.

For a given population, we use the root-mean-squared error (RMSE) to measure errors. More specifically, we use $RMSE_2$ to indicate the difference between ${}_{15}\tilde{q}_{60}$ and ${}_{15}q_{60}$, and $RMSE_3$ to show the distance between ${}_{15}\bar{q}_{60}$ and ${}_{15}q_{60}$. Let the ith estimates be ${}_{15}\tilde{q}_{60}(i)$ and ${}_{15}q_{60}(i)$, and the total number of periods be n, there are

$$ \begin{aligned} RMSE_2 &= \sqrt{\sum_{i=1}^{n}\left[{}_{15}\tilde{q}_{60}(i) - {}_{15}q_{60}(i)\right]^2/n}, \\ RMSE_3 &= \sqrt{\sum_{i=1}^{n}\left[{}_{15}\bar{q}_{60}(i) - {}_{15}q_{60}(i)\right]^2/n}. \end{aligned} \tag{5.17} $$

If $RMSE_3 < RMSE_2$ for a given population, we conclude that the three-input MLT fits this population better than does the two-input MLT, and vice versa.

The validations use HMD data. If reliable life tables for developing countries were not rare, we would choose them to carry out the validation. For the 37 (excluding Israel) countries' 74 populations by sex in HMD, the results of validation are summarized in Fig. 5.1, in which the position of a population is marked by its $RMSE_2$ on the horizontal axis and $RMSE_3$on the vertical axis. When the three-input MLT improves the performance of two-input MLT for a given population, the position of this population is below the equal line, and vice versa.

We see that the three-input MLT improved the performance of the two-input MLT for most of the populations. To be more specific, the three-input MLT improved the performance of the two-input MLT for 55 of the 74 populations. We also see from Fig. 5.1 that the chance for the improvement to occur is bigger when the $RMSE_2$ is larger. Since the two-input MLT is based on the data of HMD of which the populations are almost exclusively of European origin, we expect that for non--European-origin populations the error of two-input MLT are more likely to be larger and therefore improvements are more likely to occur. This expectation turned to be true within the HMD populations. The errors are reduced by 17% for Chile, 48% for

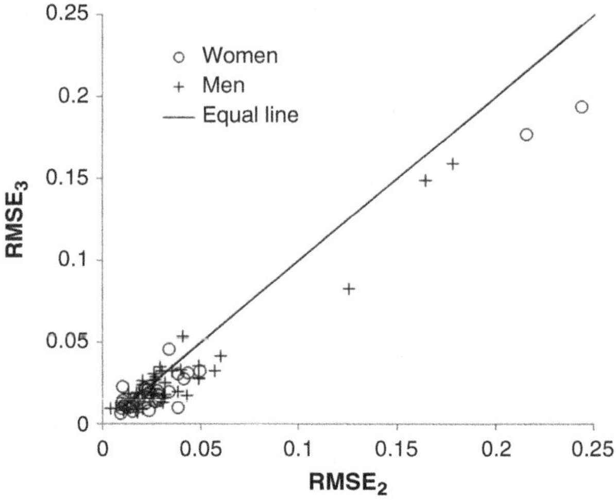

Fig. 5.1 Root-mean-squared errors in predicting ${}_{15}q_{60}$ for the 74 populations by sex in HMD

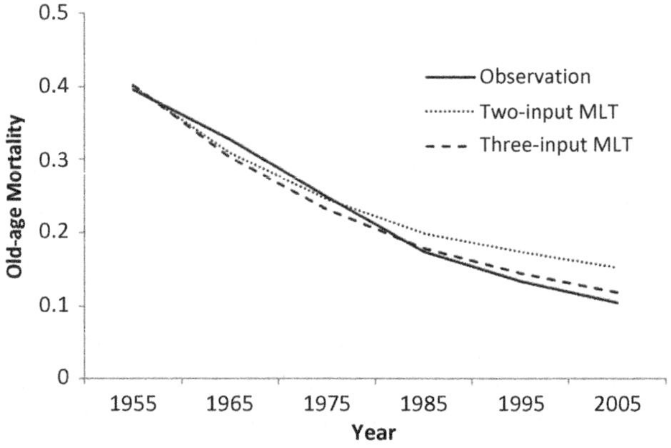

Fig. 5.2 Old-age mortality (${}_{15}q_{60}$) of Japanese women

Japan, and 17% for Taiwan, which are the three non-European-origin populations in HMD. Furthermore, since developing countries are all non-European origin, we expect that the three-input should provide greater improvements than that in the validations.

To see more details of the improvement, we choose Japanese women as an example, and show the fittings of old-age mortality in Fig. 5.2. We see that the three-input MLT performed slightly worse than did the two-input MLT for years before 1980, but remarkably better later. Overall, the three-input MLT reduced the errors of the two-input MLT by 49% (48% for both men and women).

Our final target is not only to better fit ${}_{15}q_{60}$, but to improve the estimates of life tables at old ages. To see how this target is reached, we choose Japanese women in 2000–2009 as an example, and show the result in Fig. 5.3. We see that the three-input MLT remarkably improved the estimates of age-specific death rate at old ages.

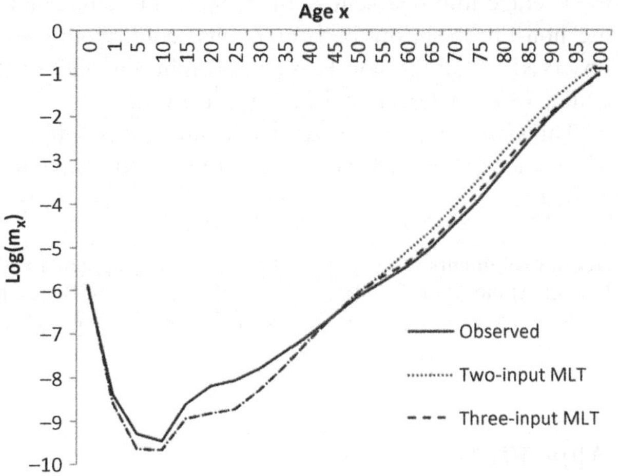

Fig. 5.3 Age-specific death rates of Japanese women, 2000–2009

5.4 Summary

In 2010–2015, for example, the deaths at age 60 and older already reached 60% of all deaths worldwide (UNPD 2015). Compared to the numbers of deaths at child and adult ages, the number of deaths at old ages is the biggest and, ironically, also the least reliable. This is because, for most developing countries, the numbers of old-age deaths are not estimated on the basis of empirical data. They are extrapolations of mortality at younger ages. This reality indicates that improving the estimates of old-age mortality for individual developing countries is not enough, and that establishing a mortality database for all developing countries, which utilizes the improved estimations of old-age mortality, is necessary.

At old ages, migrants are rare comparing to deaths. Thus, census data on population by age and sex could be used to estimate old-age mortality; and such data are available for almost all the countries of the world. For example, among the 233 countries and areas (UNPD 2015), 220 have conducted the 2010-round census between 2005 and 2014 (United Nations Statistics Division 2013b). Moreover, some developing countries had surveys or censuses that collected information on old-age mortality, which can be used as supplementary data to more reliably estimate old-age mortality.

In recent years, new methodological developments have been made to use census population to estimate old-age mortality, and extend one-input model life tables to better utilize existing information. Furthermore, these methods are improved to work better for old ages in recent years. In this paper, we described and organized these methods as the three-input MLT; and we validated performance of the three-input MLT using the HMD data. We found that the three-input MLT could improve the performance of the previous methods for 55 of the 74 populations in HMD, and that the average improvement is 14%. To be more relevant to developing countries that are non-European-origin populations, confirm this suggestion, improvements are observed for all the non-European-origin populations in HMD, which are 17% for Chile, 48% for Japan, and 17% for Taiwan.

This paper indicated that establishing a mortality database for developing countries is necessary, that the methodology is adequate, and that the empirical data are available.

Acknowledgments The work on this paper was supported by the Special Fund of Ministry of Foreign Affairs of the People's Republic of China on The Belt and Road Initiative (2017-2018), and the Key Project of the Social Science of Zhejiang Province (NO. 17NDJC029Z).

Appendices

Appendix A. Adjusting Age Reporting Errors

It is hard to find a proper basis to adjust enumerating errors in a real population, which is affected by historical fertility, mortality and migration. But a stationary population is determined only by mortality. Thus, it is possible to find a proper basis to adjust age errors for stationary populations. According to the United Nations general model life table (United Nations Population Division 1982), there is a common relationship between the survival ratios $S_{60} = \frac{L_{65}}{L_{60}}$ and $S_{65} = \frac{L_{70}}{L_{65}}$ among model life tables, which is

$$S_{65} = -0.29 + 1.27 \cdot S_{60}, R^2 = 0.998. \tag{5.18}$$

This relationship is called the model line. When the observed survival-ratio point, (S_{60}, S_{65}), is above the model line, or when the survival ratio is abnormally rising with age, the difference between the survival-ratio point and the model line is caused mainly by age heaping. Accordingly, assuming that the heaping ratio at age 60 equals to that at age 70, the adjustment is

$$\begin{aligned} \widehat{L}_{60} &= L_{60} - \frac{L_{60}}{L_{70}}\Delta, \\ \widehat{L}_{65} &= L_{65} + \Delta, \\ \widehat{L}_{70} &= L_{70} - \Delta, \end{aligned} \tag{5.19}$$

where

$$
\begin{aligned}
\Delta &= \frac{-B+\sqrt{B^2-4AC}}{2A},\\
A &= b - a\frac{L_{60}}{L_{70}} - \frac{L_{60}}{L_{70}},\\
B &= a\left(L_{60} - \frac{L_{60}}{L_{70}}L_{65}\right) + 2bL_{65} + L_{60} + \frac{L_{60}}{L_{70}}L_{70},\\
C &= L_{65}(aL_{60} + bL_{65}) - L_{60}L_{70},\\
a &= -0.29, b = 1.27.
\end{aligned}
\tag{5.20}
$$

On the other hand, when the survival-ratio point is below the model line, the difference between the survival-ratio point and the model line is caused by nonspecific errors. Accordingly, the adjustment is to move the survival ratio point into the model line through minimal distance as

$$
\begin{aligned}
\widehat{S}_{60} &= \frac{-ab + S_{60} + bS_{65}}{1+b^2},\\
\widehat{S}_{65} &= a + b\widehat{S}_{60}.
\end{aligned}
\tag{5.21}
$$

$$
\begin{aligned}
\widehat{L}_{60} &= w\frac{L_{60} + \widehat{S}_{60}L_{65} + \widehat{S}_{60}\widehat{S}_{65}L_{70}}{1 + \widehat{S}^2_{60} + \widehat{S}^2_{60}\widehat{S}^2_{65}} + (1-w)L_{60},\\
\widehat{L}_{65} &= w\widehat{S}_{60}\frac{L_{60} + \widehat{S}_{60}L_{65} + \widehat{S}_{60}\widehat{S}_{65}L_{70}}{1 + \widehat{S}^2_{60} + \widehat{S}^2_{60}\widehat{S}^2_{65}} + (1-w)L_{65},\\
\widehat{L}_{70} &= w\widehat{S}_{65}\widehat{S}_{60}\frac{L_{60} + \widehat{S}_{60}L_{65} + \widehat{S}_{60}\widehat{S}_{65}L_{70}}{1 + \widehat{S}^2_{60} + \widehat{S}^2_{60}\widehat{S}^2_{65}} + (1-w)L_{70},
\end{aligned}
\tag{5.22}
$$

where $0 \le w \le 1$ is the weight, and is used as 0.5.

Appendix B. The Errors of Estimating Survival Ratio Using Census Population

Let the net undercounting rates be u_1 and u_2 for the first and second censuses, respectively. Neglecting intercensal migration, the estimated survival ratio (*Se*) is:

$$
Se = \frac{p(70-74, t_2)\cdot(1-u_2)}{p(60-64, t_1)\cdot(1-u_1)} = S\frac{(1-u_2)}{(1-u_1)}. \tag{5.23}
$$

Subsequently, the relative error in estimating survival ratio is:

$$
E(u_1, u_2) = \frac{Se - S}{S} = \frac{1-u_2}{1-u_1} - 1 = \frac{u_1 - u_2}{1-u_1}. \tag{5.24}
$$

It can be seen that the estimating error of survival ratio is determined only by census undercounts. In addition, census undercounts tend to cancel each other in causing the errors of estimating survival ratio, which would therefore be small in general.

References

Bennett, N. G., & Horiuchi, S. (1981). Estimating the completeness of death registration in a closed population. *Population Index, 47*(2), 207–221.

Human Mortality Database. (2016). University of California, Berkeley (USA), and Max Planck Institute for Demographic Research (Germany). Available at www.mortality.org or www.humanmortality.de

Li, N. (2014). *Estimating life tables for developing countries*. Technical paper of the United Nations Population Devision 2014/4. Available at http://www.un.org/en/development/desa/population/publications/pdf/technical/TP2014-4.pdf

Li, N., & Gerland, P. (2013). *Using census data to estimate old-age mortality for developing countries*. Paper prepared for session 17–05: Indirect methods of mortality and fertility estimation: New techniques for new realities, in XXVII IUSSP International Population Conference. Busan, Korea. http://iussp.org/en/event/17/programme/paper/1959

Preston, S. H., Heuveline, P., & Guillot, M. (2001). *Demography, measuring and modeling population process*. Oxford: Blackwell Publishers Ltd.

Timæus, I. M. (2013). Estimation of adult mortality from sibling histories. In T. A. Moultrie, R. E. Dorrington, A. G. Hill, K. Hill, I. M. Timæus, & B. Zaba (Eds.), *Tools for demographic estimation*. Paris: International Union for the Scientific Study of Population. http://demographicestimation.iussp.org/content/sibling-histories

United Nations Population Division. (1982). *Model life tables for developing countries*. New York: United Nations.

United Nations Population Division. (2015). *World population prospects: The 2015 revision*. New York: United Nations.

United Nations Statistics Division. (2008). *Principles and recommendations for population and housing censuses* (Revision 2, Statistical papers Series M, Rev. 2nd ed.). New York:United Nations. http://unstats.un.org/unsd/demographic/sources/census/census3.htm

United Nations Statistics Division. (2013a). *Demographic yearbook 2012*. Sixty-third issue. New York: United Nations. https://unstats.un.org/unsd/demographic/products/dyb/2010_round_latest.htm

United Nations Statistics Division. (2013b). Available http://unstats.un.org/unsd/demographic/sources/census/2010_PHC/censusclockmore.htm

Wang, H., Dwyer-Lindgren, L., Lofgren, K. T., Rajaratnam, J. K., Marcus, J. R., Levin-Rector, A., Levitz, C., Lopez, A. D., & Murray, C. J. L. (2012, December 13). Age-specific and sex-specific mortality in 187 countries, 1970–2010: A systematic analysis for the global burden of disease study 2010. *The Lancet, 380*, 2071–2094.

Wilmoth, J., Zureick, S., Canudas-Romo, V., Inoue, V., & Sawyer, C. (2012). A flexible two-dimensional mortality model for use in indirect estimation. *Population Studies, 66*, 1–28.

Chapter 6
A Method for the Evaluation of Health Trends in Greece, 1961–2013

Konstantinos N. Zafeiris and Christos H. Skiadas

6.1 Introduction

The period 1961–2013 is characterized by enormous developments in the economic, political and social characteristics of Greece. After the political instability in the 1960s and the dictatorship of the Colonels (1967–1974), the country progressively underwent a rapid democratization process; thus the progressive political stability and the social and economic growth which occurred caused the rapid modernization of Greece. During that course, the country rejoined NATO and became a full member of the European Union at the beginning of the 1980s. In 2001 the Euro was adopted as a national currency and the country organized the Olympic Games in 2004. However, after 2008 a vast economic crisis afflicted Greece and all the socioeconomic indicators were burdened. Several austerity programs and cuts of the social and health expenses as well as the downgrading of personal income and the GDP of the country, left their clear marks on everyday life (see also Clogg 2002, pp. 166–238 and Eurostat http://ec.europa.eu/eurostat/data/database).

The scope of this paper is to analyze the health trends of the Greek population, separately for each gender during that period. The main question which arises deals with the method which is suitable for that reason.

Of the several methods which have been proposed in the literature the most well-known is that of the World Health Organization. In this method, the results of the

K. N. Zafeiris (✉)
Laboratory of P. Anthropology, Department of History and Ethnology, Democritus University of Thrace, P. Tsaldari 1, Komotini 69100, Rhodopi, Greece
e-mail: kzafiris@he.duth.gr

C. H. Skiadas
ManLab, Technical University of Crete, Chania, Crete, Greece
e-mail: skiadas@cmsim.net

© Springer International Publishing AG, part of Springer Nature 2018
C. H. Skiadas, C. Skiadas (eds.), *Demography and Health Issues*,
The Springer Series on Demographic Methods and Population Analysis 46,
https://doi.org/10.1007/978-3-319-76002-5_6

Global Burden of Disease Study are combined with mortality data (see Murray et al. 2012, 2015) in order to calculate the number of years lost because of disability and consequently the healthy life expectancy (see Vos et al. 2012; WHO 2013, 2014). However, several limitations emanate from this method, among them its extremely high complexity. Others are related to the lack of reliable data on mortality and morbidity for several countries and the lack of comparability of self-reported data from health interviews, which are included in the Global Burden of Disease Study (see also Das and Smarasekera 2013).

Besides this method, Jansen and Skiadas (1995) applied the general theory of dynamic models to life table data in order to evaluate human health. This kind of process is defined by a parent stochastic process, which is the human health being unpredictable, and a boundary, denoted by death (for the first exit time theory see also Ting Lee and Whitmore 2006). Death comes when the human health falls below that boundary. Based on that notion Skiadas and Skiadas (2010, 2012, 2014) and Skiadas (2012a, b) were able to calculate the human health function and based on that, to calculate the years lost either because of severe or because of severe and moderate disabilities using only life table data. The relevant life expectancies were calculated as the difference of life expectancy at birth with the years lost because of the afore mentioned diseases. This method is based on less demanding data than the previous one, though a shortcoming maybe the complexity of the calculations. For that Skiadas has created an EXCEL sheet in order to facilitate the calculations (see http://www.cmsim.net/id31.html).

However, a more parsimonious and less demanding solution was developed quite recently which is based on the force of mortality (Skiadas and Zafeiris 2015). The aim of the method is to express the health state of the population with one main parameter. Thus, a model was proposed containing two parameters with one crucial health parameter and with similar properties of the Gompertz. This model was tested for several European countries against the two previous methods and gave very good results (see Zafeiris and Skiadas 2015), and because of that it will be used in this paper using the mortality data of Greece (1961–2013). If μ_x is the force of mortality in age x, then it comes that:

$$\mu_x = \left(\frac{x}{T}\right)^b \tag{6.1}$$

where T is the age at which $\mu_x = 1$ and b is a parameter expressing the curvature of μ_x.

The main task is to calculate the healthy life years as a fraction of surfaces in a mortality diagram (see Fig. 6.1). This idea, which originates from the First Exit Time Theory and the Health State Function approach, is to estimate the area E_x under the curve OCABO:

$$E_x = \int_0^T \left(\frac{x}{T}\right)^b d_x = \frac{T}{(b+1)}\left(\frac{x}{T}\right)^b$$

where d_x represents the life table's death distribution. The resulting value for E_x in the interval [0, T] is given by:

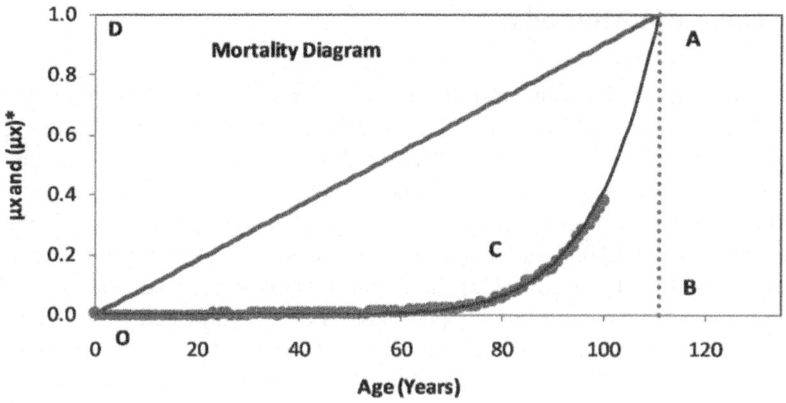

Fig. 6.1 The mortality diagram used in the μ_x based method. μ_x^* values correspond to the fitted ones of μ_x according to formula (6.1)

$$E_{mortality} = \frac{T}{(b+1)}$$

It is also clear that the total area E_{total} for the healthy and mortality part of the life is the area included into the rectangle of length T and height 1, thus $E_{Total} = T$. Then, the healthy area is given by:

$$E_{healthy} = T - E_{mortality} = T - \frac{T}{(b+1)} = \frac{bT}{(b+1)}$$

Obviously:

$$\frac{E_{health}}{E_{mortality}} = b$$

and

$$\frac{E_{total}}{E_{mortality}} = b + 1$$

These two indicators can describe the health status of the population, the second one being compatible with the severe and moderate causes indicator of the health state approach and thus it can be used as an estimator of the loss of healthy life years (LHLY) in the form of:

$$LHLY = \lambda\,(b+1)$$

where λ is a correction multiplier, which for multiple comparisons can be set to be one year. In that way similar results with the World Health Organization approach are found.

6.2 Data and Methods

Data come from the Human Mortality Database (www.mortality.org) for the years 1981–2013. Before 1981, they come from the Eurostat database (http://ec.europa.eu/eurostat/data/database), because the Human Mortality Database has not uploaded any data due to quality reasons (see also Agorastakis et al. 2015). In any case, mortality data of the Greek population become of lower quality towards the past; nevertheless, it should be used in order to examine any long or short term trends. For that reason the Life Tables of males and females were used for the years 1961–1980. However, because the open-ended open interval of the published Life Tables is the 85+ μ_x values were extrapolated until the age of 110 years by applying a cubic spline to the ages 70–84 of the form (see also http://mathworld.wolfram.com/CubicSpline.html):

$$\widehat{q}_i = q_x + a(x_i - x) + b(x_i - x)^2 + c(x_i - x)^3$$

where $x = 70$ and x_i is each age until the 84th year of human life.

Afterwards, the μx based method as described in the previous session was applied. All the calculations were carried out in an EXCEL sheet.

6.3 Results

The results of the analysis indicate that a continuous and rather linear increase of life expectancy at birth is observed in both genders between 1961 and 2014 (Fig. 6.2).

The healthy life expectancy (HLE) increases too, though the fluctuations which are observed before 1981 must be mainly attributed to the quality of data, especially for the older ages. In any case, females live longer and healthier lives than males; however, for the last years of the study any improvements are halted. This could be attributed to the effects of the economic crisis, though it must be stressed that longer times series are needed in order for any effects to be accurately found and evaluated.

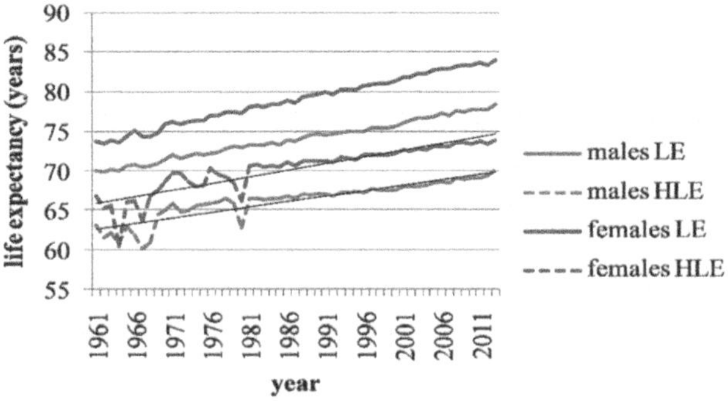

Fig. 6.2 Life expectancy at birth (LE) and healthy life expectancy (HLE). Greece 1961–2013

Fig. 6.3 The between the two genders gap (females-males) in life expectancy at birth (LE) and healthy life expectancy (HLE). Greece 1961–2013

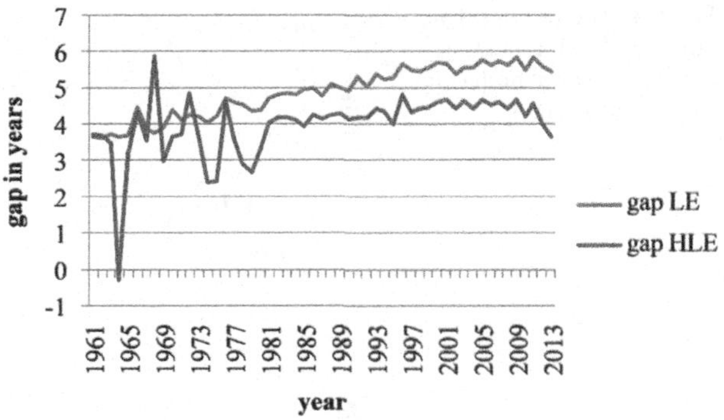

Additionally, the gap of both life expectancy and healthy life expectancy is, with one exception, positive, which means that the relevant values are higher in females (Fig. 6.3). These gaps, despite the large fluctuations observed mainly in HLE until 1981, which have been discussed in the previous paragraph, tend to increase until the onset of the economic crisis. Later on, in both indicators the among the two genders differences tend to become lower. Of course, the gap of life expectancy is always higher than the gap of healthy life expectancy.

Another important finding is seen in the scatter plots of Fig. 6.4. If the period 1961–1980, where several outliers are observed because of the quality of data is omitted, it seems that as life expectancy increases the loss of healthy life years increases too. It is quite obvious then that as long as mortality transition goes on and the longevity of the people becomes higher, the number of years in which these people live in burdened health increases too, a fact which must be taken into consideration in the planning of social and pension systems in the country. It must also be taken into consideration that the relationship between healthy life expectancy and life expectancy at birth is not necessarily linear as is seen in Fig. 6.5, especially in males. In female, after 1981 a more linear trend occurs.

Another, but still open question, is if these results are in accordance with analogous results of other approaches. In Table 6.1 the findings of Murray et al. (2015) concerning Greece are cited in comparison to the results of the analysis undertaken in this paper.

A first observation concerning Murray et al. (2015) analysis is that the published confidence intervals are high concerning the healthy life expectancy (HALE), about 5 years for males and 6 years for females, a fact which indicates the existing high degree of uncertainty. The results of the analysis cited in this paper are within the confidence intervals of Murray et al. (2015), especially the upper one in males while in females they overtook them slightly. However, the temporal trends of healthy life expectancy indentified by the two methods are almost identical. In males, according to Murray et al. (2015) HALE increases between 1990 and 2005 by 1.48 years and 1.1 years between 2005 and 2013. HLE, according to the method used in this paper increased by 1.38 and 1.77 years respectively. In females the analogous figures are

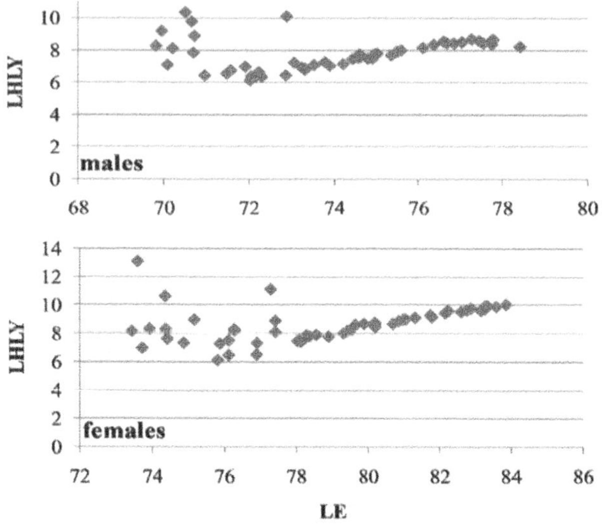

Fig. 6.4 The lost healthy life years (LHLY) and the life expectancy at birth (LE). Greece 1961–2013

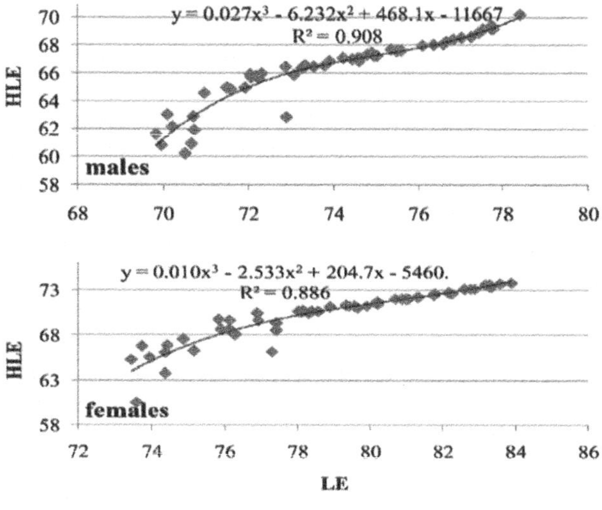

Fig. 6.5 The healthy life expectancy (HLE) and the life expectancy at birth (LE). Greece 1961–2013

+1.8 and +0.53 years according to Murray et al. (2015) and +1.88 and +0.77 years according to the method used in this paper. It seems then that the two methods are in accordance with each other in describing the temporal trends of the healthy life expectancy. The differences they have for each year of study, seem to be acceptable giving the high degree of uncertainty of Murray et al. (2015) method.

Table 6.1 The healthy life expectancy at birth according to Murray et al. (2015) and to the method used in this paper

	Males		Females	
Year	LE	HALE	LE	HALE
Murray et al. (2015)				
1990	74.53 (74.38–74.68)	65.34 (62.70–67.63)	79.44 (79.29–79.59)	68.42 (65.15–71.20)
2005	76.40 (76.26–76.55)	66.82 (64.07–69.25)	81.47 (81.28–81.68)	70.22 (66.93–73.03)
2013	77.41 (76.77–78.07)	67.90 (65.13–70.44)	82.24 (81.67–82.75)	70.75 (67.46–73.67)
This paper				
1990		67.04		71.22
2005		68.42		73.1
2013		70.19		73.87

6.4 Conclusions

The findings of the study can be summarized as follows:

- The loss of healthy life years (LHLY) is always higher for females than for males thus compensating for the extra years for females measured in life expectancy. As we live longer the healthy life years lost are increasing: along with expanding the life span we have to find ways to reduce the number of the healthy life years lost. Also, the simple measures of the social security systems based on the life expectancy should be improved taking the LHLY into serious consideration in the related plans and programs.
- The healthy life expectancy (HLE) is also higher for females than for males and in general in increasing order except for the last years in females. The gap of life expectancy at birth between the two sexes is larger than the gap for the healthy life expectancy.
- It is a challenge for health systems to adapt their support to the growing segment of society which lives above the HLE age.
- By comparing the method of WHO as cited by Murray et al. (2015) with the one cited in this paper similar results are found concerning the temporal trends of healthy life expectancy.
- The method cited here is easier to apply as it is based only on mortality data, thus it can serve positively in the understanding of past and contemporary trends of the health level of a population and in fact in the evaluation of its demographic and epidemiological transition.

References

Agorastakis, M., Jdanov, D., & Grigoriev, P. (2015). *About mortality data for Greece, human mortality database: Background and documentation*. http://www.mortality.org/

Clogg, R. (2002). *A concise history of Greece* (2nd ed.). Cambridge: Cambridge University Press.

Das, P., & Samarasekera, U. (2013). The story of GBD 2010: A "super-human" effort. *The Lancet, 380*(9859), 2067–2070. https://doi.org/10.1016/S0140-6736(12)62174-6.

Janssen, J., & Skiadas, C. H. (1995). Dynamic modeling of life-table data. *Applied Stochastic Models and Data Analysis, 11*(1), 35–49.

Murray, C. J. L., Ezzati, M., et al. (2012). GBD 2010: Design, definitions, and metrics. *The Lancet, 380*, 2063–2066.

Murray, C. J. L., Barber, R. M., et al. (2015). Global, regional, and national disability-adjusted life years (DALYs) for 306 diseases and injuries and healthy life expectancy (HALE) for 188 countries, 1990–2013: Quantifying the epidemiological transition. *The Lancet, 386*, 2145–2191. https://doi.org/10.1016/S0140-6736(15)61340-X.

Skiadas, C. H. (2012a). Life expectancy at birth and forecasts in the Netherlands (females). In C. H. Skiadas & C. Skiadas (Eds.), *The health state function of a population* (1st ed., pp. 47–67). Athens: ISAST.

Skiadas, C. H. (2012b). The health state function, the force of mortality and other characteristics resulting from the first exit time theory applied to life table data. In C. H. Skiadas & C. Skiadas (Eds.), *The health state function of a population* (1st ed., pp. 69–92). Athens: ISAST.

Skiadas, C., & Skiadas, C. H. (2010). Development, simulation and application of first exit time densities to life table data. *Communications in Statistics – Theory and Methods, 39*(3), 444–451.

Skiadas, C. H., & Skiadas, C. (2012). Estimating the healthy life expectancy from the health state function of a population in connection to the life expectancy at birth. In C. H. Skiadas & C. Skiadas (Eds.), *The health state function of a population* (1st ed., pp. 93–109). Athens: ISAST.

Skiadas, C. H., & Skiadas, C. (2014). The first exit time theory applied to life table data: The health state function of a population and other characteristics. *Communications in Statistics-Theory and Methods, 34*, 1585–1600.

Skiadas, C. H., & Zafeiris, K. N. (2015). Population aging and healthy life: Lessons from related studies. In J. Langhamrová, et al. (Eds.), *Proceedings of the RELIK 2015 conference, reproduction of human capital, mutual links and connections* (pp. 289–299). Prague 12–13 Nov. 2015. School of Economics, Prague.

Ting Lee, M.-L., & Whitmore, G. A. (2006). Threshold regression for survival analysis: Modelling event times by a stochastic process reaching a boundary. *Statistical Science, 21*(4), 501–513.

Vos, T. M., Flaxman, A. D., et al. (2012). Years lived with disability (YLDs) for 1160 sequelae of 289 diseases and injuries 1990–2010: A systematic analysis for the Global Burden of Disease Study. *The Lancet, 380*, 2163–2196. https://doi.org/10.1016/S0140-6736(12)61729-2.

WHO, Department of Health Statistics and Information system. (2013). *WHO methods and data sources for the global burden of disease estimates 2000–2011*. Global Health estimates technical paper WHO/HIS/HSI/GHE/2013.4. November, 2013. http://www.who.int/healthinfo/statistics/GlobalDALYmethods_2000_2011.pdf

WHO. (2014). *WHO methods for life expectancy and healthy life expectancy*. Global Health estimates technical paper WHO/HIS/HSI/GHE/2014.5. March, 2014. http://www.who.int/healthinfo/statistics/LT_method.pdf

Zafeiris, K. N., & Skiadas, C. H. (2015). Some methods for the estimation of healthy life expectancy. In: J. Langhamrová, et al. (Eds.), *Proceedings of the RELIK 2015 conference, reproduction of human capital, mutual links and connections* (pp. 406–416). Prague 12-–13 November 2015, School of Economics, Prague.

Chapter 7
A Method for the Forecasting of Mortality

Konstantinos N. Zafeiris

7.1 Introduction

Much effort has been made on mortality projections and forecasting during the last few decades, used for a variety of reasons including social protection programs, pension systems, health research, capital investment, estimation of the future population trends etc. (see Murray and Lopez 1997; Mathers and Loncar 2006; Booth and Tickle 2008; Stoeldraijer et al. 2013; Office of the Chief Actuary 2014; UNPP 2015 etc.).

Booth and Tickle (2008), in their review on mortality forecasting, distinguish three main types of analytical approaches. In the extrapolative approach, which is considered to be the most extensively used, an extrapolation of aggregate measures, like life expectancy at birth, takes place, assuming that the future trends will essentially be a continuation of the past. Several methods have been applied for that reason like the Brass logit transformation (see Pollard 1987) or the Lee-Carter model (1992). In the explanatory approach, structural or epidemiological models of mortality are taken into consideration. These models are about certain causes of death involving disease processes and known risk factors, thus they take into consideration medical knowledge and behavioral and environmental changes. In the third approach (the expectation), forecasts are based on the subjective opinions of the experts involving varying degrees of formality: an assumed forecast or scenario is specified, often accompanied by alternative high and low scenarios (Booth and Trickle 2008).

K. N. Zafeiris (✉)
Laboratory of P. Anthropology, Department of History and Ethnology, Democritus University of Thrace, P. Tsaldari 1, Komotini 69100, Rhodopi, Greece
e-mail: kzafiris@he.duth.gr

© Springer International Publishing AG, part of Springer Nature 2018

C. H. Skiadas, C. Skiadas (eds.), *Demography and Health Issues*,
The Springer Series on Demographic Methods and Population Analysis 46,
https://doi.org/10.1007/978-3-319-76002-5_7

In any case, the measure that will be forecast may depend on the purpose of the forecast and data availability. In most of the cases either the age specific mortality rates or probabilities are forecasted. In others, only the future levels of life expectancy at birth are estimated and the age specific pattern of mortality is applied with the use of an appropriate life table. If the future number of deaths is in question, the analysis is based on the forecasted mortality rates (see Booth 2006).

Quite often, mainly during the last few years, the mortality forecasts have a probabilistic character. Two relevant examples which have been developed recently are those of the United Nations' Population Division and of the Wittgenstein Centre for Population and Global Human Capital (WIC). The United Nations Population Division (UNPP 2015) after estimating the mortality levels in the future (life expectancy at birth) for females, by using a random walk model with drift, apply an autoregressive model in order for life expectancy at birth for males to be estimated. Afterwards an age pattern of mortality, which corresponds to the observed mortality levels, is estimated for five year age groups by applying several methods like an extension of the Lee-Carter method, the method of Andreev et al. (2013) or on the basis of model life tables (see also Raftery et al. 2012, 2013; Li et al. 2013). In the population projections of the Wittgenstein Centre for Population and Global Human Capital (WIC), the future levels of mortality are estimated on the basis of life expectancy at birth by a group of experts followed by several workshops. For each area of the planet a process of σ-convergence (see Sala-I-Martin 1996) is assumed between a country, which is considered to be the model one of that area, and the rest of the surrounding countries (see Torri and Vaupel 2012; Garbero and Sanderson 2014). The future levels of life expectancy at birth are estimated firstly for the females and afterwards for the males on the basis of the differences they had with the other gender in the 2010 revision of the World Population Prospects (Samir et al. 2013). In both of these examples, the life expectancy at birth of females is considered to be the main element of mortality forecasting and afterwards the relevant values for males are estimated and an age pattern of mortality is assigned to each of the genders.

In this paper, an alternative method for forecasting mortality trends will be presented. The analysis will not be focused on the estimation of future age specific mortality rates, for the calculation of which many procedures may be used, as for example seen in the Booth and Trickle publication (2008) and elsewhere. Instead, the procedure which is proposed here, except for infant mortality ${}_1q_0$, is based on the death probabilities of large age groups specifically ${}_9q_1$, ${}_{10}q_{10}$, ${}_{15}q_{20}$, ${}_{30}q_{35}$ and ${}_{20}q_{65}$, where the number on the left of the letter q denotes the size of an age group in years and the number on the right the first age at that group. These probabilities, which will be considered to be known (their future levels are estimated in some way as said before), will be expanded to one year probabilities of death in a full life table by applying Kostaki's relational method (2000, see also Kostaki 1991; Kostaki and Lanke 2000; Kostaki and Panousis 2001). It must be stressed that the original method of Kostaki focuses on the calculation of full life tables on the basis of five years age group abridged ones and actually it was not considered to be a method of forecasting. The use of this method as a tool in the forecasting process is the first innovation of the paper, the second one being the use of large age groups, which facilitates its applicability. Afterwards, the one year probabilities of death will be smoothed by applying a new combination of methods: the Heligman-Pollard (1980) method as modified by Kostaki (1992) will be used up to an age and afterwards three cubic splines will be applied.

However, a question is still open concerning the effectiveness of the method. In order for this question to be answered this procedure will be applied on known data and any discrepancies of the findings, if found, will be examined. The procedure that was followed will be discussed later on in this paper.

7.2 The Relational Method of Kostaki

According to this method (Kostaki 2000, see also Kostaki 1991; Kostaki and Lanke 2000; Kostaki and Panousis 2001) an abridged life table is expanded to a full one in relationship to another and known full life table, which is used as standard and is denoted in the following formulas with the letter *S*. In an abridged life table the one year death probabilities q_{x+i} $(i = 0.\ 1.\ 2\ldots n-1)$ in each of its n years intervals are equal to:

$$1-\left(1-q_{x+i}^{(S)}\right)^{nKx} \tag{7.1}$$

The term nKx equals to:

$$nKx = \frac{\ln(1-nqx)}{\sum_{i=0}^{n-1}\ln\left(1-q_{x+i}^{(S)}\right)} \tag{7.2}$$

Thus, if the values of ${}_nq_x$ of an abridged life table as well as the one year probabilities of death of the full standard life Table (S) are known, first the values of nKx are calculated with 7.2 and afterwards the one year probabilities of death which correspond to the abridged life table are calculated with 7.1. The following property must be fulfilled:

$$1-\prod_{i=1}^{n-1}\left(1-q_{x+i}\right) = nqx$$

7.3 The Modified 9 Parameters Heligman-Pollard Formula and the Cubic Splines

After the estimation of the one year probabilities of death with the previous method, results need to be smoothed and for that the modified 9 parameters Heligman-Pollard formula was used. In its original form (Heligman and Pollard 1980) the formula is as follows:

$$\frac{q_x}{p_x} = A^{(x+B)^C} + De^{-E(lnx-lnF)^2} + GH^x \tag{7.3}$$

where x is the age and A, B, C, D, E, F, G and H are parameters.

The term q_x/p_x is the summation of 3 components (Fig. 7.1). The first component, which includes the parameters A, B, and C, represents the fall in mortality during early childhood as the child adapts to its new environment and gains immunity from diseases from the outside world. The second component includes the parameters D, E and F. It describes the accident hump between ages 10 and 40, which appears either as a distinct hump in the mortality curve or at least as a flattening out of the mortality rates. The third term corresponds to a Gompertz exponential which represents the aging or the deterioration of the body.

Kostaki (1992) observed some systematic variations in the Heligman-Pollard 8 parameters formula concerning the spread of the accident hump. Thus, she proposed that a better fit of the model is achieved if:

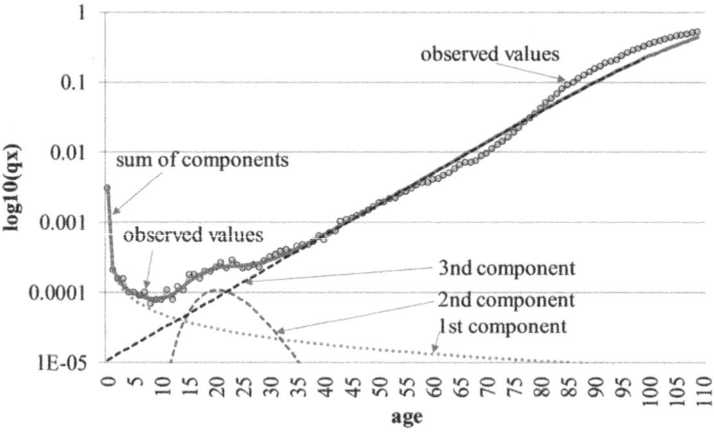

Fig. 7.1 The probabilities of death [*log10(qx)*] and the Heligman-Pollard formula. Greece, females, 2010–2013. (Data Source: Human Mortality Database. www.mortality.org)

$$\frac{q_x}{p_x} = \begin{cases} A^{(x+B)^C} + De^{-E_1(lnx - lnF)^2} + GH^x, & for\ x \leq F \\ A^{(x+B)^C} + \mathrm{D}e^{-E_3(lnx - lnF)^2} + GH^x, & for\ x > F \end{cases} \tag{7.4}$$

She proposed, then, that the parameter E which denotes the spread of the accident hump should be replaced with the relevant E_1 and E_2, representing the spread of the accident hump to the left and right of its top (its location denoted by the parameter F) respectively.

However, the most important deviation is the one observed in the senescent mortality (see Fig. 7.1), which cannot be described with the Gompertz law, at least when it is applied to the modern Greek data. Because of that, an alternative project was applied as follows. First of all, the Heligman-Pollard 9 parameters model (the one with Kostaki's modification) was applied up to the age of 40. After that age 3 cubic polynomials, known as cubic splines were used, each of them for 15 years until the age of 84. These third order polynomials (see also http://mathworld.wolfram.com/CubicSpline.html) were of the type:

$$\widehat{q}_i = \widehat{q}_x + a_k(x_i - x) + b_k(x_i - x)^2 + c_k(x_i - x)^3$$

where $k = 1\ldots3$ the number of spline, and x_i the age and $\widehat{q}_x$ is the fitted value for $x = x_i$. Obviously the end of each spline is the beginning of the next one. After the age of 84 the probabilities of death were extrapolated with the aid of the last spline. EXCEL SOLVER was used in order for the Sum of Squared errors of the fit to be minimized. For the 9 parameters formula the following term was chosen to be minimized, as happened in the original paper of Heligman and Pollard (1980):

$$\sum_x \left(\frac{\widehat{q}_x}{q_x} - 1 \right)^2$$

where $\widehat{q}_x$ is the fitted value for age x and q_x is the observed one. A crude estimation of the fit was given by the R^2 estimator which tended to be 1 in both genders for all of the years studied (see also Zafeiris and Kostaki 2017).

7.4 An Application with the Greek Data

In order to test for the validity and the effectiveness of the method the following procedure was used:

1. The full life tables of the Greek population, separately for each gender, were calculated for the years 2001, 2005, 2010 and 2014 using the Calot and Sardon (2004) procedure (see also Calot and Franco 2001; Calot 1999) and the original software which was developed by Calot himself. The analysis took place in the Laboratory of Demographic and Social Analyses of the University of Thessaly (Department of Regional Planning and Development). The analysis was based on

the most recent available data from the National Statistical Authority of Greece (November, 2015, ELSTAT).

2. For each of the genders the full life tables of the year 2001 were used as standards. The probabilities of death per age of these life tables were smoothed as described in session 3 of this paper and afterwards the life tables were recalculated.
3. The probabilities of death for the large age classes (except of the first one) $_{1}q_{0}$, $_{9}q_{1}$, $_{10}q_{10}$, $_{15}q_{20}$, $_{30}q_{35}$ and $_{20}q_{65}$ were calculated on the basis of the observed data for the years 2005, 2010 and 2014. These probabilities were calculated with the formula:

$$1 - \prod_{i=1}^{n-1} \left(1 - q_{x+i}\right) = nqx$$

as described in Kostaki (2000).

4. The relational method of Kostaki (2000), which is described in the session 2 of this paper was used in order for the large age classes probabilities to be expanded into one year of age probabilities, separately for each gender and year of study.
5. The estimated probability of death distributions were smoothed with the procedure described in session 3 of this paper.
6. The results of the analysis were compared with the observed ones, that is the known full life tables for each of the years 2005, 2010 and 2014.

7.5 The Results of the Analysis

The results of the analysis concerning the probabilities of death are shown in Figs. 7.2 (males) and 7.3 (females). The forecasted probabilities are denoted as "qx expansion" and the observed as "qx observed". The term "qx fitted" denotes the results of the smoothing procedure, as described in session 7.3 of this paper, which has been applied to the observed probabilities of death. In both genders, it can be seen that the method applied gave excellent results and, as a matter of fact, the forecasted probabilities of death coincide with the observed ones in both genders.

Some minor differences which are found mainly at the very old ages for females are not important at all and in fact they do not have an effect on the life expectancies of differences ages as seen in Figs. 7.4 (males) and 7.5 (females). In these figures, where the ex terms are defined in an analogous way with Figs. 7.2 and 7.3, it is seen that life expectancies at all ages practically coincide.

Thus, the method applied here is very efficient in the forecasting of mortality levels, while, at the same time, it is quite parsimonious in terms of calculations, a property which further enhances its applicability.

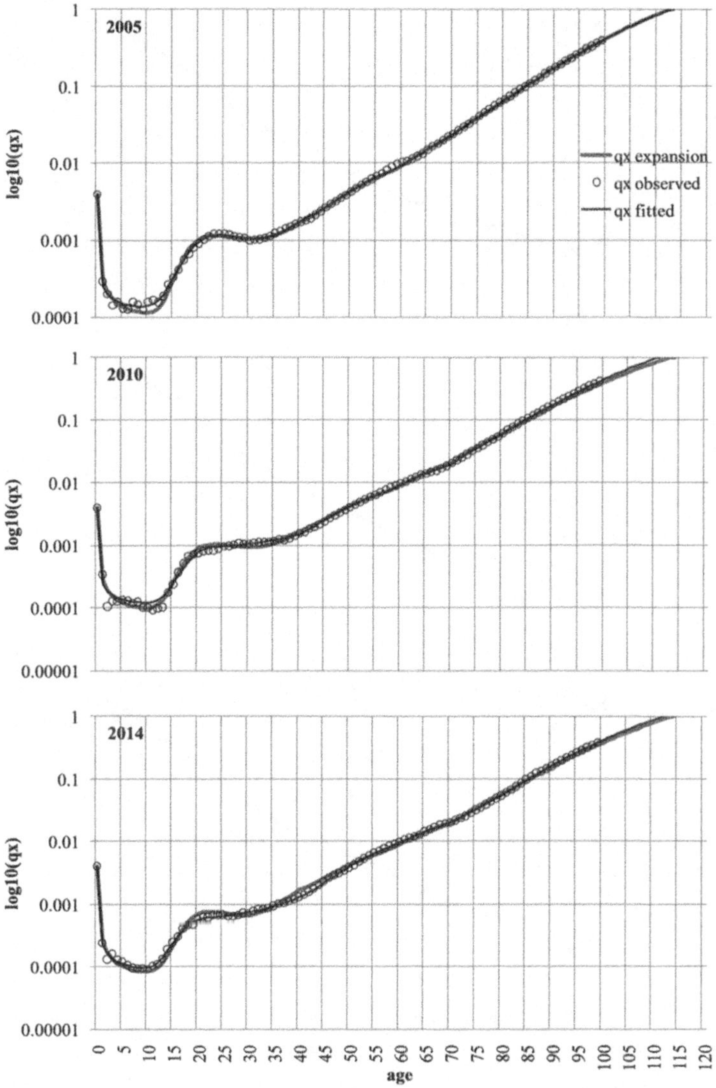

Fig. 7.2 The forecasted probabilities of death [*log10(qx)*] (qx expansion) and the relevant observed values (qx observed and qx fitted). Greece, males 2005, 2010, 2014

7.6 Conclusions

A new method for the forecasting of one year age specific probabilities of death was demonstrated in this paper, with the aid of a relational method which was originally developed by Kostaki (2000) in order for an abridged life table to be expanded into a full one. The probabilities of death for large age groups are used in this paper. These

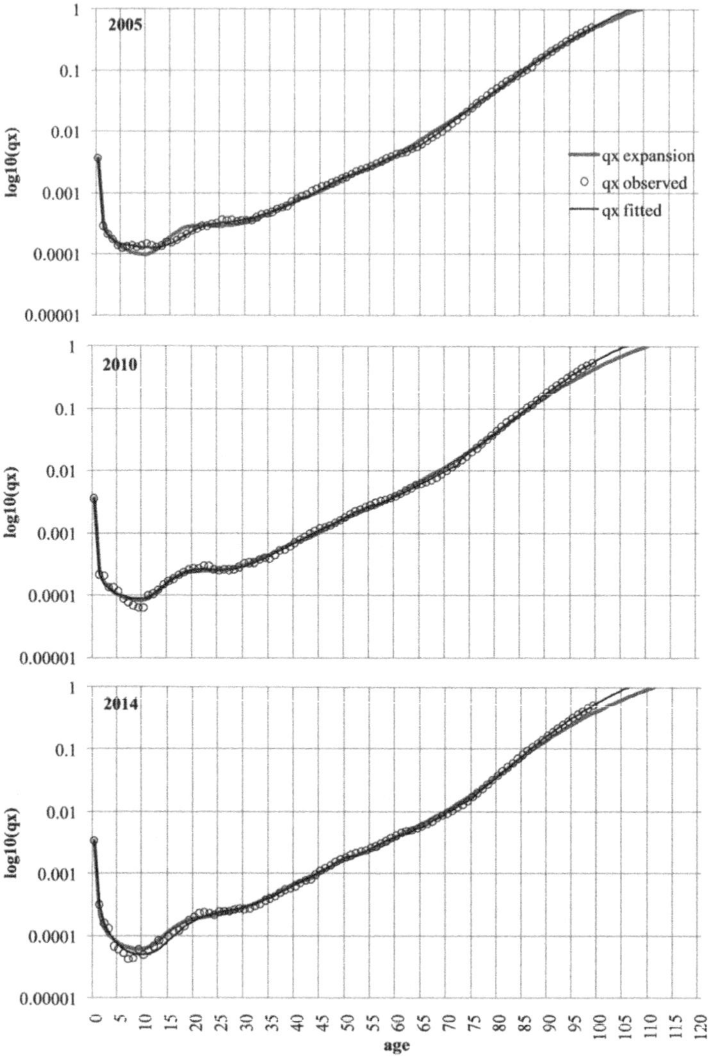

Fig. 7.3 The forecasted probabilities of death [*log10(qx)*] (qx expansion) and the relevant observed values (qx observed and qx fitted). Greece, females 2005, 2010, 2014

probabilities may be assessed with a variety of methods, though this process is not demonstrated here. After the appliance of the relational method the age specific probabilities of death were smoothed with the aid of a combination of the Heligman-Pollard (1980) formula as modified by Kostaki (1992) and three subsequent cubic splines.

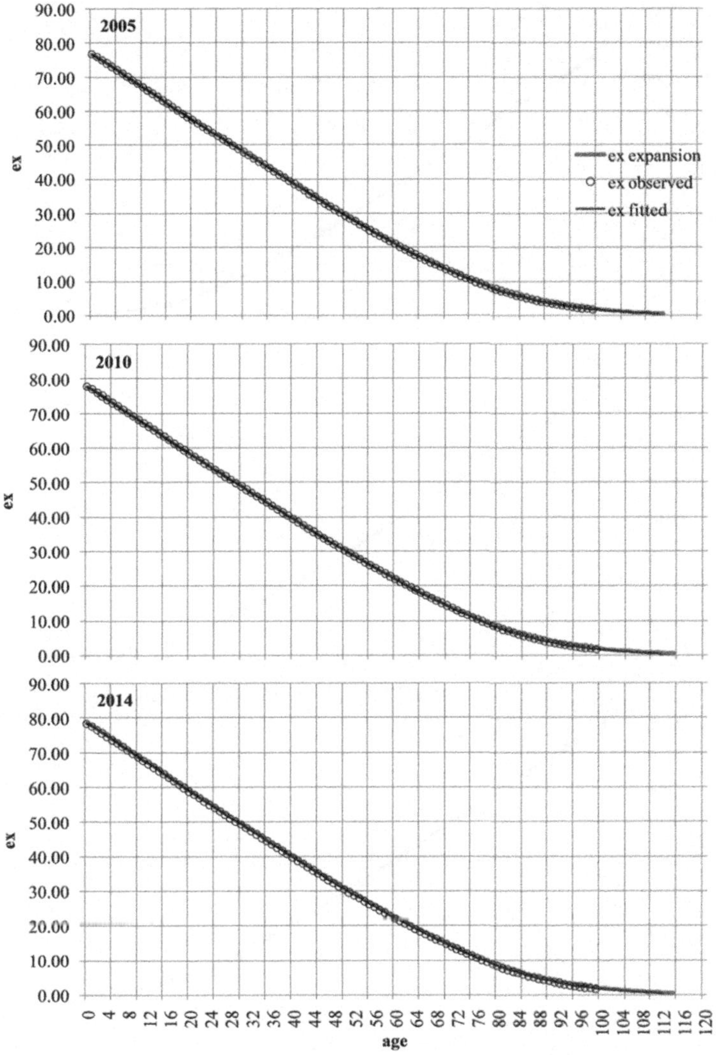

Fig. 7.4 The forecasted life expectancy (ex expansion) and the relevant observed values (ex observed and ex fitted). Greece, males 2005, 2010, 2014

This method, as tested with Greek data, gave excellent results fact which indicates its applicability and effectiveness. One of the advantages of the method used is that it is quite parsimonious in terms of calculations, thus its usefulness is enhanced even more.

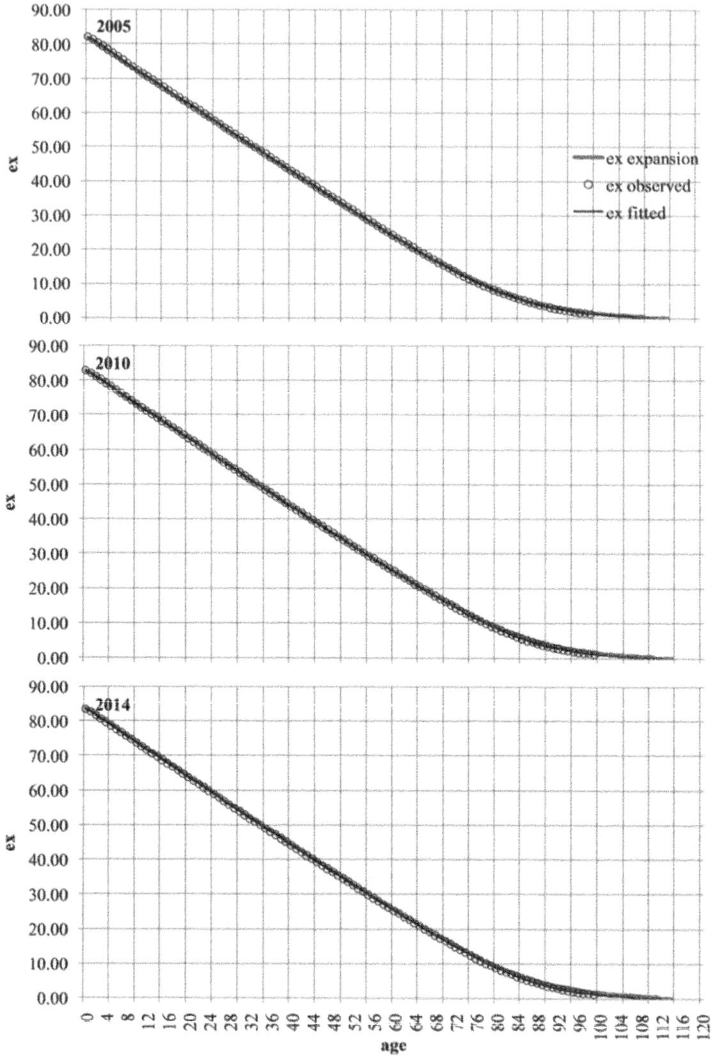

Fig. 7.5 The forecasted life expectancy (ex expansion) and the relevant observed values (ex observed and ex fitted). Greece, females 2005, 2010, 2014

References

Andreev, K., Gu, D., & Gerland, P. (2013). *Patterns of mortality improvement by level of life expectancy at birth*. Paper presented at the annual meeting of the Population Association of America, New Orleans, LA. http://paa2013.princeton.edu/papers/132554

Booth, H. (2006). Demographic forecasting: 1980 to 2005. *International Journal of Forecasting, 22*, 547–581.

Booth, H., & Tickle, L. (2008). Mortality and modeling: A review of methods. *Annals of Actuarial Science, 3*(I/II), 3–43.

Calot, G. (1999). L' analyse démographique conjoncturelle. In A. Kuijsten, H. de Gans, & H. de Feijter (Eds.), *The joy of demography*, édité en l'honneur de D.J. van de Kaa (pp. 295–323). La Haye: NethurD Publications.

Calot, G., & Franco, A. (2001). The construction of life tables. In G. Wunsch, M. Mouchart, & J. Duchêne (Eds.), *Life tables: Data, methods, models* (pp. 31–75). Dordrecht: Kluwer.

Calot, G., & Sardon, J.-P. (2004). *Methodology for the calculation of Eurostat's demographic indicators*. Detailed report for the European Demographic Observatory, Office for Official Publication of the European Communities, Luxemburg.

Garbero, A., & Sanderson, W. (2014). Forecasting mortality convergence up to 2100. In W. Lutz, W. P. Butz, & K. C. Samir (Eds.), *World population and human capital in the 21st century* (pp. 650–665). Oxford: Oxford University Press.

Heligman, L., & Pollard, J. H. (1980). The age pattern of mortality. *Journal of the Institute of Actuaries, 107*, 47–80.

Kostaki, A. (1991). The Heligman – Pollard formula as a tool for expanding an abridged life table. *Journal of Official Statistics, 7*(3), 311–323.

Kostaki, A. (1992). A nine parameter version of the Heligman-Pollard formula. *Mathematical Population Studies, 3*(4), 277–288.

Kostaki, A. (2000). A relational technique for estimating the age – specific mortality pattern from grouped data. *Mathematical Population Studies, 9*(1), 83–95.

Kostaki, A., & Lanke, J. (2000). Degrouping mortality data for the elderly. *Mathematical Population Studies, 7*(4), 331–341.

Kostaki, A., & Panousis, V. (2001). Expanding an abridged life table. *Demographic Research, 5*(1), 1–22.

Lee, R. D., & Carter, L. R. (1992). Modeling and forecasting U.S. mortality. *Journal of the American Statistical Association, 87*(419), 659–671.

Li, N., Lee, R., & Gerland, P. (2013). Extending the Lee-Carter Method to model the rotation of age patterns of mortality decline for long term projection. *Demography, 50*(6), 2037–2051.

Mathers, C. D., & Loncar, D. (2006). Projections of global mortality and burden of disease from 2002 to 2030. *PLoS Medicine, 3*(11), 2011–2030.

Murray, J. L., & Lopez, A. D. (1997). Alternative projections of mortality and disability by cause 1990–2020: Global burden of disease study. *The Lancet, 349*(9064), 1458–1504.

Office of the Chief Actuary. (2014). *Mortality projections for social security programs in Canada*. Actuarial study Nr. 12. Office of the Superintendent of Financial Institutions Canada. Available at: www.osfi-bsif.gc.ca

Pollard, J. H. (1987). Projection of age-specific mortality rates. *Population Bulletin of the United Nations, 21–22*, 55–69.

Raftery, A. E., Lalic, N., & Gerland, P. (2012). *Joint probabilistic projection of female and male life expectancy*. Paper presented at the annual meeting of the Population Association of America, San Francisco, CA.

Raftery, A. E., Chunn, J. L., Gerland, P., & Ševčíková, H. (2013). Bayesian probabilistic projections of life expectancy for all countries. *Demography, 50*, 777–801.

Sala-I-Martin, X. (1996). The classical approach to convergence analysis. *The Economic Journal, 106*, 1019–1036.

Samir, K.C., Potančoková, M., Bauer, R., Goujon, A., & Striessnig, E. (2013). *Summary of data, assumptions and methods for new Wittgenstein Centre for Demography and Global Human Capital (WIC) population projections by age, sex and level of education for 195 countries to 2100* (Interim Report No. IR-13-018). Laxenburg: International Institute for Applied Systems Analysis.

Stoeldraijer, L., van Duin, C., van Wissen, L., & Janssen, F. (2013). Impact of different mortality forecasting methods and explicit assumptions on projected future life expectancy: The case of the Netherlands. *Demographic Research, 29*(13), 323–354.

Torri, T., & Vaupel, J. W. (2012). Forecasting life expectancy in an international context. *International Journal of Forecasting, 28*(2), 519–531.
UNPP, United Nations, Department of Economic and Social Affairs, Population Division. (2015). *World population prospects, the 2015 revision. Methodology of the United Nations population estimates and projections*. New York: United Nations.
Zafeiris, K. N., & Kostaki, A. (2017). Recent mortality trends in Greece. *Communications in Statistics-Theory and Methods*. https://doi.org/10.1080/03610926.2017.1353625.

Chapter 8
Prospective Scenarios on Coverage of Deaths in Brazil

Neir Antunes Paes and Alisson dos Santos Silva

8.1 Introduction

The primary purpose of the projections in demography is to provide an estimate of future population which is used as a common framework for national and regional planning in a number of different fields. Mortality projections are an essential input for projections of population, and also the financial development of pension schemes. Governments and insurance companies all over the world rely on mortality projections for counting its population and for efficient administration of their pension commitments. They also need to have some idea about how patterns of death (mortality) are likely to change so that they can plan for the future. Thus, plausible projections of mortality are of chief importance to informing welfare and public policy planning about future trends in population aging.

Mortality forecast in Brazil is officially produced by the Brazilian government (IBGE 2005), which every single year has the commitment to review such statistics. According to the government in 2042, the number of deaths in Brazil (more than 2.2 million) will exceed for the first time the number of births (2.1 million), and the population (then of 228 million) will decrease.

The demographic models used in projecting mortality are usually based on statistical modeling of historical data. However, mortality projections and its patterns of deaths for the less developed regions are usually very hard to calculate because the

N. A. Paes (✉)
Postgraduate Program in Decision Modelling and Health, Federal University of Paraíba, João Pessoa, Brazil
e-mail: antunes@de.ufpb.br

A. dos Santos Silva
Postgraduate Program in Mathematical and Computational Modelling, Federal University of Paraíba, João Pessoa, Brazil

© Springer International Publishing AG, part of Springer Nature 2018

C. H. Skiadas, C. Skiadas (eds.), *Demography and Health Issues*,
The Springer Series on Demographic Methods and Population Analysis 46,
https://doi.org/10.1007/978-3-319-76002-5_8

uncertainties regarding the coverage of death in these regions. This is especially true for the Northeast region of Brazil with a population of around 57 million in 2016, where little has been known about the completeness of death, particularly in the future.

Knowing about the completeness of death reporting is essential. First we need to know how complete death reporting is so that we can take actions to improve the quality of the original data. Second, when we know how complete death reporting is, we can make the adjustments needed to permit us to use the death rates derived from death registration in such demographic tasks as projecting future populations. The age-and-sex-specific death rates used in these projections may be calculated when registered data on deaths and on the corresponding population by age and sex are available. Even when such data appear to be complete, however, they should not be accepted blindly when being used for such purposes as constructing a life table.

Before doing projections an important question to be answered is: is it the coverage of deaths complete, and if not, what do demographers need to do to estimate the coverage in the future? In another words, when the coverage of deaths will be complete in the case to be incomplete?

Since mathematical methods may be applied for any region or country which death coverage is not complete, the last question was the motivation for doing this work for the Northeast region of Brazil. In this way is hoped to give a contribution to the government, planners and scholars in this field.

8.2 Study Data and Methods

This study has an ecological time-trend design, which geographical unites are the 9 states (provinces) belonging to the Brazilian Northeast region and the region as whole. A year-by-year longitudinal dataset from 1991 to 2011 was created. The data used in this study refers to the coverage of death for both sexes estimated by RIPSA (2012), organization vinculated to the Ministry of Health. Despite the criticism that can be made, this longitudinal dataset is the only one available for the 27 states of the country. The coverage of death values were calculated dividing the observed death data by the estimated one. The calculation of the latter was based on projections of the population made by IBGE (2005).

There are no specific methods for projecting coverage of death. However, the literature provides mathematical models that can be adapted to situations of coverage projections, as long as they do not violate the assumptions and criteria.

Two types of nonlinear modeling were used to estimate the year of full coverage of death for Northeast states: Logistic Growth Model and Gompertz function. In addition, the Holt Exponential Smoothing Model was used, which presupposes linear growth trend of a series of data.

8.2.1 *Logistic Function (Bezerra 2008)*

The logistic curve is part of the so-called saturation curves. It is applied to phenomena in which the growth rate of its accumulated observations grows to a certain value and, from that point, begins to fall with the same intensity of growth, tending to a long-term stationary value. Thus, in the logistic adjustment, it is implicit that the rate of increase in growth rates is equal to that of the decrease, which in the long run hardly happens with the tendency of projections. The equation is given by

$$Y = \frac{\alpha}{1 + e^{-\gamma(x-\beta)}}$$

where:

Y = coverage of deaths;
e = the natural logarithm base;
x = time in years of coverage of deaths;
α = the curve's maximum value (indicating the stabilization value of the dependent variable in relation to time);
β = the x-value of the sigmoid's midpoin (location parameter); and.
γ = the steepness of the curve (curve growth rate measure).
α, β e γ are parameters, where $\alpha > 0$ e $\gamma > 0$.

8.2.2 *Gompertz Function (Souza et al. 2010)*

A Gompertz curve or Gompertz function, named after Benjamin Gompertz, is a sigmoid function. It is a type of mathematical model for a time series, where growth is slowest at the start and end of a time period. The right-hand or future value asymptote of the function is approached much more gradually by the curve than the left-hand or lower valued asymptote, in contrast to the simple logistic function in which both asymptotes are approached by the curve symmetrically. It is a special case of the generalised logistic function. This Gompertz function is defined by

$$Y = \alpha e^{-e^{\gamma(x-\beta)}}$$

where, the meaning of each variable and parameter of the Gompertz function is the same, as specified for the Logistic function.

8.2.3 *Holt Exponential Smoothing Model (Moretin and Toloi 2006)*

Holt (1957) extended simple exponential smoothing to allow forecasting of data with a trend. This method involves a forecast equation considering the level, trend and residual with zero mean and constant variance:

$$Z_t = \mu_t + T_t + a_t, \quad t = 1, \ldots, N,$$

where:

μtt denotes an estimate of the level of the series at time *t*;
Tt denotes an estimate of the trend of the series at time *t*;
at denotes the random error at time *t*.

The level and trend values of the series were estimated by

$$\bar{Z}_t = AZ_t + (1 - A)(\hat{Z}_{t-1} + \hat{T}_{t-1}), 0 < A < 1, t = 2, \ldots, N,$$
$$\hat{T}_t = C(\bar{Z}_t - \bar{Z}_{t-1}) + (1 - C)\hat{T}_{t-1}, 0 < C < 1, t = 2, \ldots, N,$$

A and *C* are the smoothing constants. The prediction of future series values for this procedure is given by:

$$\bar{Z}_t(h) = \bar{Z}_t + h\hat{T}_t, \forall h > 0$$

That is, the forecast is made by adding to the basic value (*Z¯t*) the multiplicative trend by the number of steps ahead that one wishes to predict (*h*).

8.2.4 *Diagnostic and Residual Measures*

In non-linear regression, the analysis of the residuals of a model is done to check the plausibility of the assumptions involved (Thode 2002). For the verification of the assumptions, a graphical analysis of the residues can be used, this being an informal method of analysis that involves the graphs of residues in relation to the independent variables and the predicted values, or through statistical tests. The latter is a more objective way of analyzing the residues by providing a numerical measure for some of the described discrepancies.

The Shapiro-Wilk statistical test was used to verify the normality assumption. To measure the heteroscedasticity of the residues, the Breusch-Pagan test and the graphic inspection of the residues were used against the estimated values to examine whether the error variances are constant. The Durbin-Watson test was used to verify the existence of first order autocorrelation.

The diagnostic measures were used for residue analysis, detection of outliers, influential points, and colinearity. In addition, tests based on statistical hypotheses were carried out to verify the suitability of the Logistic and Gompertz model adjustments (Bezerra 2008; Souza et al. 2010).

Two statistical tests for time series analysis applied to Holt's exponential smoothing model were used: the Dickey-Fuller and Wilcoxon tests (Moretin and Toloi 2006).

The Mean Square Error (MSE) was proposed as criterion for selecting the best model. The MSE is defined by the sum of the squares of the differences between estimated/predicted results and the observations (Keyfitz 1981).

In order to obtain the estimates from the application of the prediction methods and the error measures, the R-3.3.1 free-access software was used.

8.2.5 Criteria for Selection of Full Coverage of Deaths

The year of optimal coverage was chosen for the first year whose estimate was greater than or equal to 99% or when the maximum inflection point of the model curve was reached.

Then, the criteria for selecting the range of forecast of full coverage of deaths were:

1. When the estimates between the models did not exceed four years a range of forecast of full coverage using both values was adopted;
2. In case the difference between forecasts was greater than four years, a four-year forecast interval was considered based on the model with the lowest MSE;
3. The model with estimated full coverage below 2019 was discarded. In this case, a two year interval was considered based on the selected coverage.

8.3 Results and Discussion

Among the nine states that compose this region, coverage of deaths in 2011 ranged from 79% to 94%. In the beginning of the series, in 1991, the coverage ranged from 25% to 70% (Table 8.1).

There is no technique of correction of the coverage of deaths free of assumptions, which are hardly fulfilled for any region of the world, and Brazil. In this way, errors are allowed in any estimate. The greatest errors in RIPSA's estimates (2012) are related to the period from 1991 to 1999 that made use of the projections of deaths which are part of the population projections elaborated by IBGE (2005). From 2000 onwards, the correction factors of the Active Search Project from the Ministry of Health (Szwarcwald et al. 2011) were used which are considered more accurate.

From 1991 to 1999 Brazil had an increase of 8.3% and the Northeast of 10.5% in the coverage of death. During 1999–2000 the increase in coverage of deaths in Brazil was 5.1% and in the Northeast 17.7%. From 2000 to 2011 this difference was of

Table 8.1 Coverage of deaths in Brazil, Northeast and States of Northeast, 1991–2011

Year	BR	NE	MA	PI	CE	RN	PB	PE	AL	SE	BA
1991	77.6	51.4	31.4	25.1	41.1	44.9	53.5	70.0	57.7	64.2	56.9
1992	78.6	51.9	31.2	32.6	41.0	46.2	51.0	68.7	56.7	73.9	57.8
1993	82.9	55.4	31.7	36.3	49.5	53.5	58.5	72.8	57.8	67.9	58.9
1994	83.4	55.2	28.2	35.9	52.7	52.5	56.5	70.6	55.7	68.7	61.3
1995	83.6	55.4	28.5	34.1	51.5	58.7	57.9	68.0	58.1	80.2	60.8
1996	84.6	55.6	27.3	30.7	53.6	57.3	56.1	70.2	55.5	74.0	62.9
1997	83.7	56.8	30.6	35.6	57.2	56.8	55.9	72.6	57.8	70.7	61.0
1998	85.8	60.8	34.6	39.0	58.7	59.9	58.0	77.0	67.5	78.4	65.3
1999	85.9	61.9	32.7	40.7	64.5	61.2	57.0	77.6	58.8	80.3	68.6
2000	91.0	79.6	55.2	73.1	80.6	77.7	82.1	91.7	87.1	88.2	77.7
2001	91.7	82.0	64.0	79.5	83.1	80.4	83.9	92.2	87.8	89.0	78.8
2002	92.5	83.9	69.1	82.7	84.7	81.0	85.8	92.7	89.0	89.7	81.1
2003	92.9	84.9	72.3	84.0	86.4	81.8	87.3	92.8	89.3	90.1	81.6
2004	93.1	85.1	73.5	84.7	86.5	81.5	88.2	92.7	89.2	90.3	81.9
2005	93.2	85.4	74.4	84.8	86.4	80.6	88.2	92.9	88.7	89.9	83.0
2006	93.3	85.5	74.2	85.5	86.1	80.4	88.4	93.0	89.7	89.8	83.2
2007	93.6	86.1	74.4	86.8	86.3	81.8	89.4	93.2	90.2	90.0	84.0
2008	94.0	87.2	76.5	87.3	87.9	84.8	89.8	93.3	91.5	91.8	84.9
2009	94.3	88.1	78.5	87.4	88.7	86.2	90.7	93.6	91.7	92.4	86.2
2010	94.2	88.9	78.8	88.2	90.0	87.9	91.1	93.6	92.3	92.5	87.4
2011	94.2	88.8	79.1	88.1	89.8	87.6	91.2	93.5	92.2	92.7	87.4
Minimum	77.6	51.4	27.3	25.1	41.0	44.9	51.0	68.0	55.5	64.2	56.9
Maximum	94.3	88.9	79.1	88.2	90.0	87.9	91.2	93.6	92.3	92.7	87.4
1991–1999	8.3	10.5	7.3	15.6	23.5	16.3	7.5	9.6	12.0	16.1	11.7
1999–2000	5.1	17.7	22.5	32.4	16.1	16.5	25.1	14.1	28.3	7.9	9.1
2000–2001	3.3	9.3	23.9	15.1	9.4	10.2	9.1	1.9	5.2	4.2	9.7

Note: BR-Brasil, NE-Northeast, MA-Maranhão, PI-Piauí, CE-Ceará, RN-Rio Grande do Norte, PB-Paraíba, PE-Pernambuco, AL-Alagoas, SE-Sergipe e BA-Bahia
Source: Rede Interagencial de Informações para a Saúde no Brasil – IDB, 2012

3.3% in Brazil and 9.3% in the Northeast. However, the change in coverage levels from 1999 to 2000 was not only due to a change in methodology in its estimates, but also to other factors.

The evolution of coverage levels indicates that the year 2000 can be considered as a milestone in time, after which an unprecedented rate of increase in the history of death coverage in the Brazilian Northeast was triggered. The poor quality of coverage before 2000 may be due to the enormous political and economic crisis that directly affected investments in health and basic care in Brazil (Polignano 2004) reinforced by the precarious training of health professionals regarding data collection and manipulation, and non-standardization of these tasks, which led to poor quality and unreliability of information (Paes 2007; Mello Jorge et al. 2007, 2010).

The main factors that contributed to the great increase in coverage in the Northeastern states particularly since the year 2000 were the technological development of

Table 8.2 Estimates of the residual p-value of the Shapiro-Wilk, Breusch-Pagan e Durbin-Watson tests according to Logistic and Gompertz model for Northeast and states of Northeast, Brazil

	Logistic			Gompertz		
State/Region	Shapiro	Breusch-Pagan	Durbin-Watson	Shapiro	Breusch-Pagan	Durbin-Watson
Maranhão	0.52	1.00	0.00	0.37	1.00	0.00
Piauí	0.19	1.00	0.00	0.20	1.00	0.00
Ceará	0.57	1.00	0.00	0.52	1.00	0.00
Rio G. Norte	0.62	1.00	0.00	0.64	1.00	0.00
Paraíba	0.25	1.00	0.00	0.29	1.00	0.00
Pernambuco	0.50	1.00	0.00	0.51	1.00	0.00
Alagoas	0.72	1.00	0.00	0.77	1.00	0.00
Sergipe	0.48	1.00	0.22	0.52	1.00	0.21
Bahia	0.76	1.00	0.00	0.73	1.00	0.00
Northeast	0.30	1.00	0.00	0.28	1.00	0.00

information, which has enabled a considerable leap in quality in the collection and processing of data.

These actions were reinforced by the expansion of coverage of health services through programs such as the Family Health Strategy, monitoring of the Death Verification System (SVO), and increased awareness, supervision and vigilance by physicians. The significant improvement in the quality of death records from the Mortality Information System of the Ministry of Health can be further credited to the addition of the hospitals in the collection of data, previously collected only in civil registries offices (Mello Jorge et al. 2010; Lima and Queiroz 2014).

The standardized residuals versus the adjusted values for the Northeast and all states indicated homogeneity of the variances that can be confirmed by the estimates of the Breusch-Pagan statistic test. In it, the null hypothesis that the residues were homocedastic was not rejected. Verifying the normality assumption the Shapiro-Wilk test with p-values ≥ 0.05 for the Logistic Model and the Gompertz model did not reject the null hypothesis, indicating that the residues followed a normal distribution. The Durbin-Watson test indicated that the residues were independent as desired. The results of the application of these tests are presented in Table 8.2.

According to the estimates of the p-value of the Dickey-Fuller Test, the time series discussed were stationary over time with a significance level of 5%. The Wilcoxon test pointed to the presence of increasing trend and almost stationary behavior in the series of data for all the regions, satisfying the requirements for the application of the Holt model. The results are showed in Table 8.3.

According to Table 8.4 the deviations between the coverages with the use of the EQM showed that the Holt model had the best performance for five states and the Northeast as a whole. The Logistic model presented the smallest errors for four states. These States are highlighted in Table 8.4.

Figures 8.1a and 8.1b show the time series of observed, and estimated death coverage trend for the Northeast as a whole and the adjustment curves for each

Table 8.3 Estimates of the residual p-value of the Dickey-Fuller and Wilcoxon tests for the application of the Hold model for Northeast and states of Northeast, Brazil

State/Region	P-values	
	Dickey-Fuller	Wilcoxon
Maranhão	0.51	6.403E-05
Piauí	0.64	9.537E-05
Ceará	0.94	6.403E-05
Rio Grande do Norte	0.64	6.395E-05
Paraíba	0.60	6.403E-05
Pernambuco	0.73	6.395E-05
Alagoas	0.77	6.403E-05
Sergipe	0.92	9.537E-05
Bahia	0.47	6.403E-05
Northeast	0.65	6.403E-05

Table 8.4 Mean Square Error of estimates with full coverage of deaths, according to the models for Northeast states, Brazil

State/Region	Mean Square Error (MSE)		
	Logistic	Gompertz	Holt
Maranhão	52.28	58.44	*29.37*
Piauí	70.01	80.20	*56.85*
Ceará	17.82	19.91	*16.49*
Rio G. Norte	*14.38*	15.01	15.61
Paraíba	*37.00*	38.24	37.70
Pernambuco	17.53	18.01	*13.14*
Alagoas	*41.97*	43.48	46.04
Sergipe	*10.38*	11.01	29.03
Bahia	7.38	7.69	*4.84*
Nordeste	21.72	22.92	*15.16*

Note: The model with the lowest MSE is italicised

model adopted. The estimated death coverage trend is also showed for all nine states of the Northeast.

In general a better smoothing was observed for the Holt model. The Logistic model and the Gompertz model did not show any differences in plotting the curve. These patterns in the models for the Northeast were practically the same observed for all states, with small variations in the pace for some states as showed in Figs. 8.1a and 8.1b.

Estimates of Northeast coverage up to the year 1999 showed a steady but fluctuating increase, with a sharp fall in the pace between 1999 and 2000. Then, the rate of increase continues, but in a slower way reaching almost constant behavior at the end of the series.

Two trends are evident, before and after this break. Prior to 2000, the pace of increase was lower than the second, for almost all states, and the Northeast as a whole.

Because the Gompertz model had a very similar behavior to the Logistic model (Figs. 8.1a and 8.1b) and provided the worst accuracy errors for most states (Table 8.4), it was discarded as a predictive model.

Table 8.5 shows the projections of the years when the full coverage of deaths for the Northeast and states will be reached, using the Logistic and Holt's model. The final estimates are presented in forecast intervals, according to the established criteria.

It was considered that maximum amplitude of four years in the forecast of the full coverage to be reached by Northeast states is a reasonable variation in the results generated by the models.

Attention is drawn to the fact that the models captured the behavior of the coverage of deaths of a historical series, and that they are mathematical. Although the coverage of deaths in the past is a reflection of the conditions of life in general (Paes 2007; Mello Jorge et al. 2007, 2010) one may not be assured that living conditions will be maintained in the future, and that they reproduce a pace of evolution of the past. Thus, the forecast interval seeks to cover non-measurable constraints, not captured by a mathematical model.

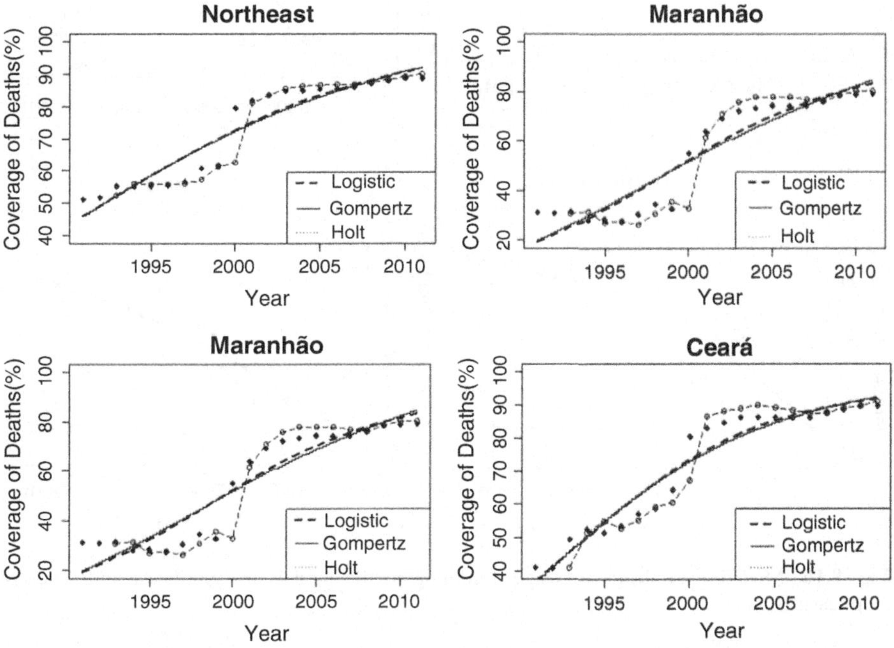

Fig. 8.1a Modeling of death coverage according to the models for Northeast and states of Northeast, Brazil

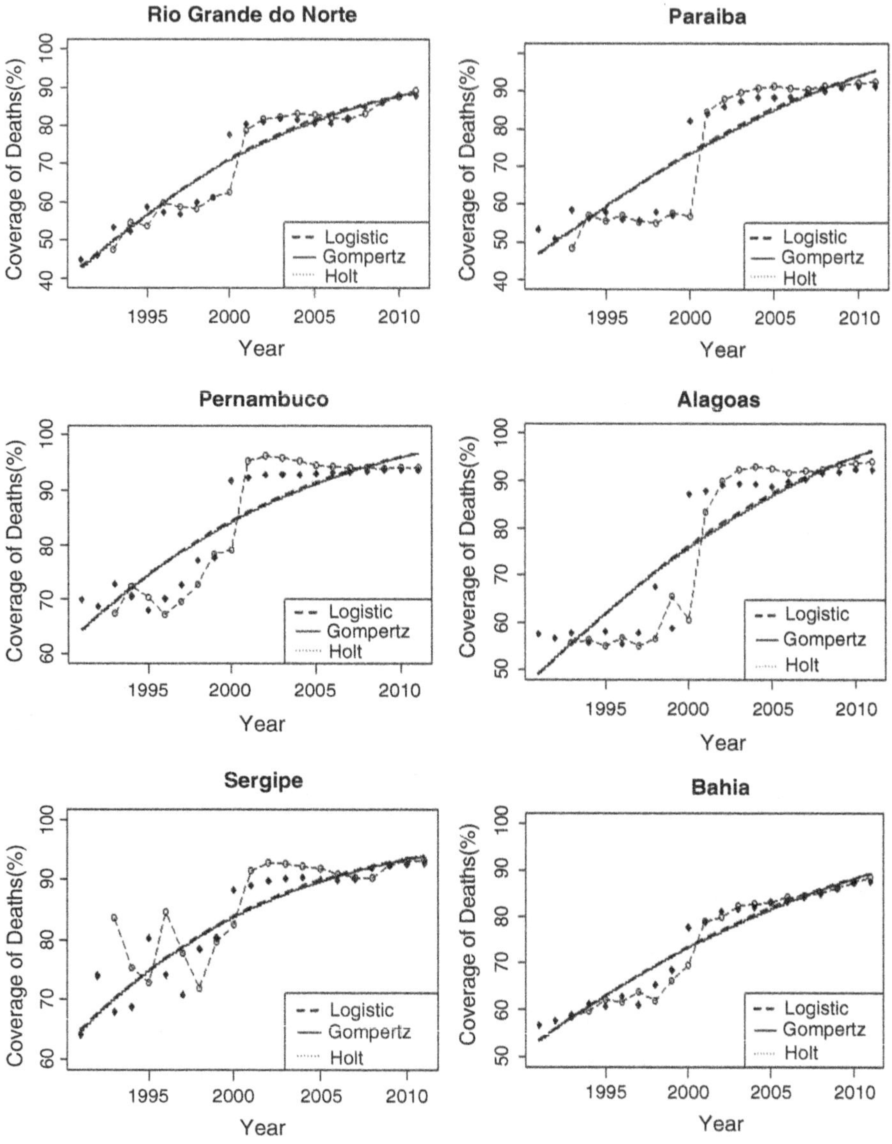

Fig. 8.1b Modeling of death coverage according to the models for Northeast and states of Northeast, Brazil

Table 8.5 Interval of prediction of the year with full coverage of deaths according to Logistic and Holt models for the Northeast and states, Brazil

State/	Model				
Region	Logistic	Holt	Model w/lowest MSE	Criteria	Interval of prediction
Maranhão	2030[a]	2028	Holt	1	2028–2030
Piauí	2032[a]	2016	Holt	[b]	2022–2026
Ceará	2024[a]	2023	Holt	1	2023–2024
Rio G. Norte	2025[a]	2021	Logistic	1	2021–2025
Paraíba	2017	2020	Logistic	3	2020–2022
Pernambuco	2020	2023	Holt	1	2020–2023
Alagoas	2019	2018	Logistic	3	2019–2021
Sergipe	2026[a]	2022	Logistic	1	2022–2026
Bahia	2030	2023	Holt	2	2023–2027
Northeast	2035	2021	Holt	2	2021–2025

[a]Inflection point of the curve below 100%
[b]An interval of two years for plus and minus was considered based on the mean of the two predictions models (2024)

8.4 Conclusions

In view of the established criteria, in general, the Holt model performed better (less deviations in the coverage series) by adhering more to the behavior of the past coverage series.

Obviously, the results should be viewed with caution, since the errors inherent in any prediction must be taken into account. It should be noted that in order to verify the suitability of the models, it is necessary to comply with certain assumptions. One of them referred to the number of points (years) available in the time series, restricted to 21 points. But they are the only ones available in the literature. This restriction may have prevented full use of the application of the models, which should be considered as indicators of the evolution of death coverage.

The final estimates showed three different groups regarding the universalization of coverage of deaths: Alagoas, Paraíba and Pernambuco (2019–2023); these states would be the first to reach full coverage of deaths regarding data quality. In a more distant position were Maranhão and Bahia (2023–2030). And, in an intermediate position, Ceará, Rio Grande do Norte, Sergipe and Piauí (2021–2026). It is estimated that for the Northeast the full coverage of deaths will be reached around 2021–2025.

However, it must be acknowledged that, like any scenario, this outline reflects a possibility considered plausible and that only the future can confirm these scenarios. Nevertheless, it is expected that these scenarios may contribute to the planning strategies, and to the evaluation of managers regarding the actions and policies to be implemented on the performance of death statistics in the Northeast and in the Country.

References

Bezerra, J. (2008). *Population ecology: The logistic curve and population growth* (pp. 1–18). Campinas: NEPAM -UNICAMP.

IBGE, Diretoria de Pesquisas (DPE), Coordenação de População e Indicadores Sociais (COPIS). (2005). *Projections of population of Brazil, large regions and units of Federation, by sex and age for the period 1991–2030*. Rio de Janeiro.

Keyfitz, N. (1981). The limits of populations forecasting. *Population and Development Review, 8*, 579–593.

Lima, E. M. C., & Queiroz, B. L. (2014). The evolution of the mortality registry system in Brazil: Changes in the mortality profile, coverage of the death registry and the ill-defined causes of death. *Cadernos de Saúde Pública, 30*, 1721–1730.

Mello Jorge, M. H. P., Laurenti, R., & Gotlieb, S. L. D. (2007). An analysis of the quality of Brazilian vital statistics: The experience of SIM and SINASC implementation. *Ciencia & Saúde Coletiva, 12*, 643–654.

Mello Jorge, M. H. P., Laurenti, R., & Gotlieb, S. L. D. (2010). Evaluation of health information systems in Brazil. *Cadernos de Saúde Coletiva, 18*, 07–18.

Moretin, P. A., & Toloi, C. M. C. (2006). *Time series analysis* (2nd ed.). São Paulo: Blucher.

Paes, N. A. (2007). Quality of death statistics for unknown causes in Brazilian states. *Revista de Saúde Pública, 41*, 436–445.

Polignano, M. V. (2004). *History of health policies in Brazil – A short review* (pp. 1–35). Ministry of Health of Mato Grosso. Available at http://www.saude.mt.gov.br/ces/arquivo/2165/books. Accessed 25 June 2016.

Rede Interagencial de Informações para a Saúde no Brasil. (2012). Ripsa IDB. Available at http://tabnet.datasus.gov.br/cgi/idb2012/a1801b.htm. Accessed 25 June 2016.

Souza, V. J., Martinez, E. Z., & Nunes, A. A. (2010). Gompertz growth curves for the follow-up of high-risk children. *Revista Brasileira De Biometria, 28*, 39–58.

Szwarcwald, C. L., Neto, O. L. M., Frias, P. G., Junior, P. R. B. S., Escalante, J. C., Lima, R. B., e Viola, R. C. (2011). Active search for deaths and births in the northeast and in the legal Amazon: Estimation of coverage of SIM and SINASC in Brazilian municipalities. In Ministry of Health, organizer. *Health Brazil 2010: An analysis of the health situation and selected evidence of impact of health surveillance actions* (pp. 79–98). Brasília: Ministério da Saúde.

Thode, H. C. (2002). *Testing for normality*. New York: Marcel Dekker.

Part III
Statistical Models and Methods in Biostatistics and Epidemiology

Chapter 9
Applications of the Cumulative Rate to Kidney Cancer Statistics in Australia

Janelle Brennan, K. C. Chan, Rebecca Kippen, C. T. Lenard, T. M. Mills, and Ruth F. G. Williams

9.1 Introduction

We define kidney cancer, which is also known as malignant neoplasm of kidney, as the set of diseases classified as C64 according to the International Statistical Classification of Diseases and Related Health Problems, 10th Revision (ICD10) by Australian Institute of Health and Welfare (2016).

The incidence of kidney cancer is the number of new cases diagnosed each year in a given region, in this case Australia. For each year, the mortality of kidney cancer is the number of deaths for which the primary cause of death is kidney cancer in Australia. Incidence and mortality are whole numbers. Sometimes we may use the terms "incidence" and "mortality" more broadly; we trust that this will not cause confusion.

J. Brennan
Department of Urology, Bendigo Health, Bendigo, Australia

St. Vincent's Hospital Melbourne, Fitzroy, Australia

K. C. Chan
School of Management and Enterprise, University of Southern Queensland, Springfield, Australia
e-mail: ka.chan@latrobe.edu.au

R. Kippen
School of Rural Health, Monash University, Bendigo, Australia
e-mail: rebecca.kippen@monash.edu

C. T. Lenard · T. M. Mills (✉) · R. F. G. Williams
Mathematics and Statistics, La Trobe University, Bendigo, Australia
e-mail: c.lenard@latrobe.edu.au; t.mills@latrobe.edu.au

© Springer International Publishing AG, part of Springer Nature 2018

C. H. Skiadas, C. Skiadas (eds.), *Demography and Health Issues*,
The Springer Series on Demographic Methods and Population Analysis 46,
https://doi.org/10.1007/978-3-319-76002-5_9

The incidence of kidney cancer has been increasing in many parts of the world (De et al. 2014; Li et al. 2015). The reason for this is unknown, especially as there are marked geographic variations, both within the same country and between countries; see, for example, the papers by De et al. (2014), Li et al. (2015) and Znaor et al. (2015). Some of the increase in kidney cancer incidence has been attributed to the increased use of modern diagnostic imaging methods such as ultrasound, computerized tomography and magnetic resonance imaging, resulting in increased detection of renal cell carcinoma (a common type of kidney cancer), and possibly down-ward stage migration. However, over-detection does not entirely explain all of these variations, especially in Europe where there exist variations within a single country with a national health care system; see for example (Li et al. 2015). In addition, the heterogeneity of kidney cancer incidence rates, which is well-known in clinical circles, suggests the existence of modifiable risk factors and potentially unknown genetic, infective, dietary, environmental or behavioural factors that influence prevalence. Detection at an earlier stage of the disease has also been observed in the last two or three decades with more localised tumours being found more recently. According to Tan et al. (2015), "[d]espite the frequent use of aggressive therapy, mortality rates among elderly patients with kidney cancer have remained stagnant over the past quarter century".

It is important for Australia to have an initial framework for understanding the current state of kidney cancer in our society. Examination of the trends in incidence, mortality and survival may allow the identification of modifiable risk factors and also guide future workforce planning. We know, for example, that there is considerable variation in clinical patterns of the disease in Australia (Satasivam et al. 2014). A starting point is to examine the historical Australian data in order to detect patterns that, if they are statistically significant, may help our understanding of the epidemiological differences of kidney cancer. This is particularly important given the increasing incidence rate of kidney cancer with the associated increase in health care costs.

The aim of this paper is to compare the impact of kidney cancer on various sub-populations in Australia through incidence and mortality statistics.

There are two standard methods for making such comparisons. The first is by using age-standardised rates, the second is to use cumulative risks. We have reservations about both these methods.

Calculating age-standardised rates involves introducing an arbitrary, standard population. This allows us to compare the incidence rates in two populations that have different age structures. For example, the Australian Institute of Health and Welfare (AIHW) (2016) provides age-standardised rates based on three, different, standard populations: the Australian 2001 population, the Sergi world standard population, and the WHO standard population and these three rates are quite different from each other. For example, in 2012, the three age-standardised incidence rates for kidney cancer were 12.4, 8.6, and 9.4 per 100,000 persons in Australia respectively. This is confusing for policy makers, the media, and general readers, and we should bear in mind that there is considerable interest in cancer statistics in the community.

Furthermore, if we want to compare the Australian incidence rate with the incidence rate of another country, then we may have to re-calculate the rates for at least one of the countries using a suitable common, standard population.

Finally, it is unlikely that, 100 years from now, we will still be using the Australian 2001 population as a standard, and to make comparisons between then and now will involve re-calculation.

The second standard method for making comparisons is based on the cumulative risk by a certain age. For example, AIHW (2016) reports that the risk of being diagnosed with kidney cancer by age 75 in Australia is 1 in 101. This measure is open to misunderstanding. The model, on which the calculation of this risk or probability is based, contains the assumption that the only cause of death is kidney cancer. This issue has been pointed this out in (Day 1976, p. 443; Lenard et al. 2013) and the underlying mathematical model has been explained in Lenard et al. (2014).

The age-standardised rate and the cumulative risk serve the same purpose: namely, to enable comparing incidence (or mortality) rates in populations with different age-structures. Both methods involve introducing assumptions that may be misleading. The age-standardised rate is based on assuming that the populations have an age-structure that they do not have. The cumulative risk is based on assuming that the disease in question is the only cause of death.

The cumulative rate does not have these deficiencies, as will be explained below. In this paper we compare the incidence and mortality of kidney cancer for various sub-populations in Australia using the cumulative rate.

9.2 Methods

Historical data on the incidence and mortality of kidney cancer were obtained from Australian Institute of Health and Welfare (2016). These data sets contain the incidence of kidney cancer for 1982–2012, the mortality for kidney cancer for 1968–2013, and the population counts for those years. Data are strati ed. by age group and sex. As a note of explanation, incidence data for cancer in Australia have been collected since 1982 whereas mortality data for cancer is available for a much longer period of time. Thus, the two time intervals for incidence and mortality are different. This has no effect on the analysis below. The (estimated) cumulative incidence rate by age 75 is calculated as follows.

$$a(75) = 5 * \sum_{k=1}^{k=15} \frac{x(k)}{n(k)} \tag{9.1}$$

The cumulative incidence rate by age 75 is, essentially, the sum of the age-specific incidence rates for each age from 0 to 75 (if we assume that the age-specific incidence rate is constant throughout any particular 5-year age group). Hence the name “cumulative incidence rate”. Notice that this calculation does not

Table 9.1 Data for calculating cumulative rate by age 75

Group	Age group	Population	Incidence
1	[0;4]	n(1)	x(1)
2	[5;9]	n(2)	x(2)
⋮	⋮	⋮	⋮
k	[5k 5; 5k 1]	n(k)	x(k)
⋮	⋮	⋮	⋮
15	[70;74]	n(15)	x(15)

involve introducing an arbitrary standardised population, and it requires no special assumptions as does the cumulative risk. Note that the cumulative rate and the cumulative risk are approximately equal in value; if y is the cumulative rate by age *t*, then 1 exp(y) is the cumulative risk by age *t* and these are approximately equal if $y > 0$ is small (Lenard et al. 2014) (Table 9.1).

The 95% confidence interval for the cumulative rate by age 75 is given by $a(75) \pm 1{:}96\ s(75)$ where

$$s(75) = 5\sqrt{\sum_{k=1}^{k=15} \frac{x(k)}{n(k)^2}} \tag{9.2}$$

See (Chan et al. 2015; Lenard et al. 2014, 2015) for mathematical details.

9.3 Results

9.3.1 *Incidence and Mortality*

Figure 9.1 shows that the incidence of kidney cancer has been steadily increasing since 1982. In 1982, there were 793 new cases of kidney cancer reported in Australia; by 2012, there were 3082 new cases reported. This increasing incidence leads to increased costs and increased demands on a highly specialised workforce.

Figure 9.2 shows that the mortality associated with kidney cancer has been steadily increasing since 1968: note that the mortality does not necessarily increase from 1 year to the next, but the trend is unmistakable. In 1968, there were 300 deaths from kidney cancer in Australia; by 2013, there were 962 deaths reported.

It is not surprising that incidence and mortality are increasing: after all, the population is increasing, and ageing. So, in the next sub-section, we consider the cumulative rates to age 75. We have chosen the age 75 for several reasons. This upper age limit was proposed by Day (1976) in his original paper. We are trying to isolate the effects of kidney cancer on the population, and health issues become

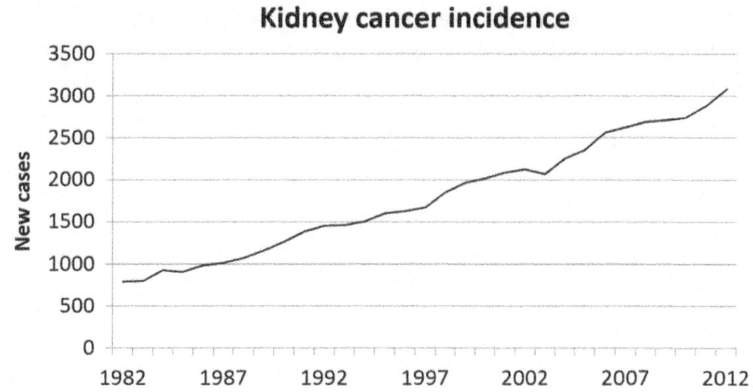

Fig. 9.1 Incidence of kidney cancer in Australia, 1982–2012

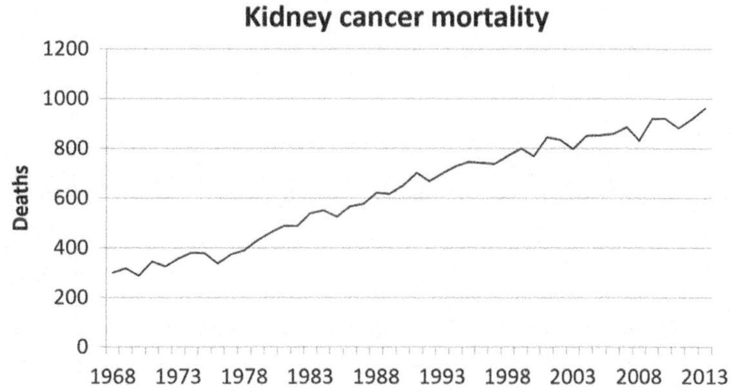

Fig. 9.2 Mortality from kidney cancer in Australia, 1968–2013

complex for people aged over 75. However, in other sections below, we will also consider the cumulative rates for other ages as well, as part of our investigation of the usefulness of cumulative rates.

9.3.2 Cumulative Rates to Age 75

Figure 9.3 shows the cumulative incidence rate of kidney cancer for males and females up to age 75 since 1982 and the corresponding 95% confidence intervals. The rates are increasing, and the rates for males are consistently higher than the rates for females. Thus the increasing incidence of kidney cancer shown in Fig. 9.1 is not simply due to an increasing, ageing population: there are also other forces at work.

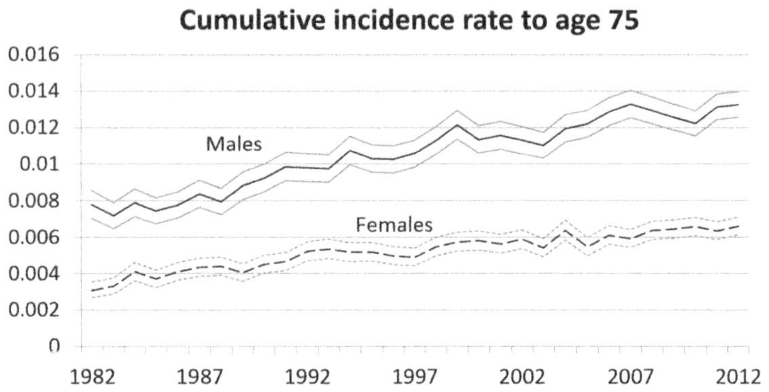

Fig. 9.3 Cumulative incidence by age 75 of kidney cancer in Australia

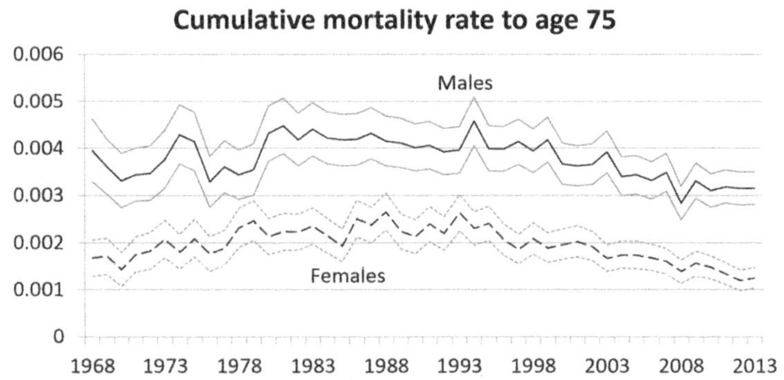

Fig. 9.4 Cumulative mortality by age 75 of kidney cancer in Australia

By contrast, Fig. 9.4 shows the cumulative mortality rate of kidney cancer for males and females up to age 75 since 1968 and the corresponding 95% confidence intervals. Again, the rates for males are consistently higher than the rates for females; however both rates have been decreasing during the last 20 years or so.

9.3.3 Cumulative Rates to Age 40

Kidney cancer affects younger people as well as older people but not to the same extent. We now consider cumulative rates to age 40.

Figure 9.5 shows the cumulative incidence rate of kidney cancer for males and females up to age 40 since 1982 and the corresponding 95% confidence intervals.

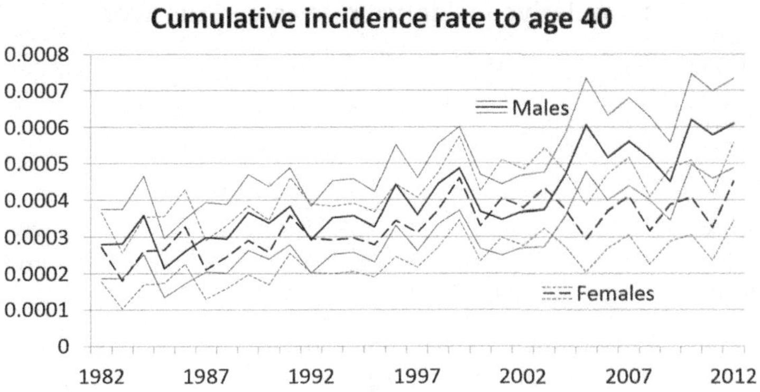

Fig. 9.5 Cumulative incidence by age 40 of kidney cancer in Australia

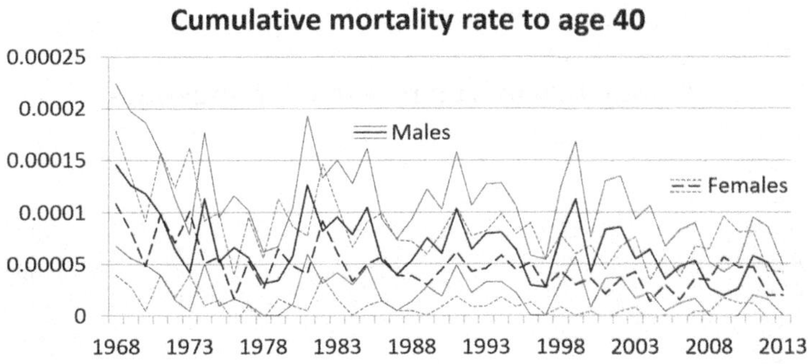

Fig. 9.6 Cumulative mortality by age 40 of kidney cancer in Australia

It is noticeable that, historically, there is no apparent difference between males and females in the cumulative incidence rates to age 40 although Fig. 9.5 suggests that such a difference may be emerging. Only time will tell.

By contrast, Fig. 9.6 shows the cumulative mortality rate of kidney cancer for males and females since 1968 and the corresponding 95% confidence intervals. Again we see that, historically, there is no apparent difference between males and females in the cumulative mortality rates to age 40.

9.3.4 Cumulative Rates to Various Ages

Figure 9.7 shows the cumulative incidence rate of kidney cancer up to various ages for four selected years 1982, 1992, 2002, 2012. The graphs are monotonic with respect to the year. In other words, for just about all ages x, the cumulative incidence rate to age x is monotonic increasing over time. Thus the incidence of kidney cancer

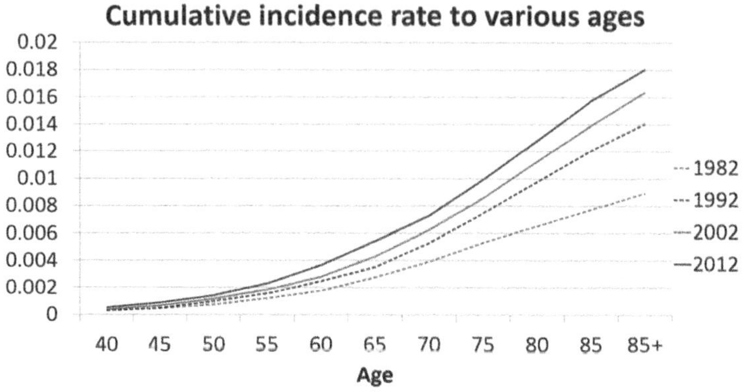

Fig. 9.7 Cumulative incidence rate for various ages of kidney cancer in Australia over several years

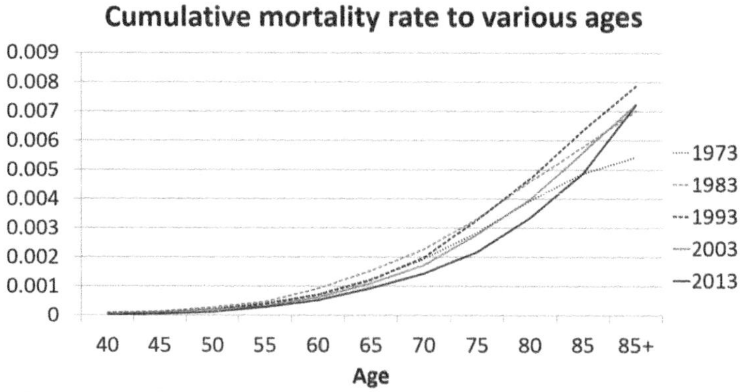

Fig. 9.8 Cumulative mortality rate for various ages of kidney cancer in Australia over several years

is increasing among all age groups. Furthermore, the cumulative incidence rate is considerably higher for higher age limits.

Figure 9.8 shows the cumulative mortality rate of kidney cancer up to various ages for five selected years 1973, 1983, 1993, 2003, 2013. It is surprising that the graphs are not monotonic with respect to the year. In other words, for many ages x, the cumulative mortality rate to age x is not monotonic over time; however, the rate is consistently considerably higher for higher age limits.

9.4 Conclusions

In this paper, we have illustrated the application of the cumulative rate to kidney cancer statistics in Australia. The cumulative rate does not share the disadvantages of the age-standardised rate or the cumulative risk. Furthermore, we have illustrated how the analysis of cancer statistics can raise interesting questions about the disease itself. For example, why is the incidence of kidney cancer higher among men than women? Why are the cumulative mortality rate curves for all ages not monotonic with respect to the year?

The recent clinical literature indicates that there is much to learn about kid-ney cancers. We hope that our work contributes, in a small way, to improving our understanding of kidney cancers, and promotes the use of the cumulative rate in cancer epidemiology.

Acknowledgements We thank the organisers of 4th SMTDA2016 Valletta, Malta, 1–4 June 2016, University of Malta for the opportunity to present our work. Bendigo Health is supported by the government of the state of Victoria in Australia.

References

Australian Institute of Health and Welfare (AIHW). (2016). *Australian Cancer Incidence and Mortality (ACIM) books*. Canberra: AIHW. URL: http://www.aihw.gov.au/acim-books. Viewed on 12 April 2016.

Chan, K. C., Lenard, C. T., Mills, T. M., & Williams, R. F. G. (2015). Bowel cancer demo-graphics. In A. Karagrigoriou, T. Oliveira, & C. H. Skiadas (Eds.), *Statistical, stochastic and data analysis methods and applications*. Athens: International Society for the Advancement of Science and Technology. (to appear).

Day, N. E. (1976). A new measure of age standardized incidence, the cumulative rate. In R. Payne & J. Waterhouse (Eds.), *Cancer incidence in five continents* (Vol. III, pp. 443–452). Lyon: IARC Scienti c Publications, No. 15. International Agency for Research on Cancer.

De, P., Otterstatter, M. C., Semenciw, R., Ellison, L. F., Marrett, L. D., & Dryer, D. (2014). Trends in incidence, mortality, and survival for kidney cancer in Canada, 1986–2007. *Cancer Causes & Control, 25*(10), 1271–1281.

Lenard, C. T., Mills, T. M., & Williams, R. F. G. (2013). The risk of being diagnosed with cancer. *Australian & New Zealand Jounal of Public Health, 37*(5), 489.

Lenard, C. T., Mills, T. M., & Williams, R. F. G. (2014). Cumulative incidence rates of cancer. *The Mathematical Scientist, 39*(2), 83–89.

Lenard, C. T., Mills, T. M., & Williams, R. F. G. (2015). Comparing the cumulative rates of cancer in two populations. In L. Filus, T. Oliveira, & C. H. Skiadas CH (Eds.), *Stochastic modeling, data analysis and statistical applications* (pp. 13–20). Athens: International Society for the Advancement of Science and Technology.

Li, P., Znaor, A., Holcatova, I., Fabianova, E., Mates, D., Wozniak, M. B., Ferlay, J., & Scelo, G. (2015). Regional geographic variations in kidney cancer incidence rates in European countries. *European Urology, 67*(6), 1134–1141.

Satasivam, P., O'Neill, S., Sivarajah, G., Sliwinski, A., Kaiser, C., Niall, O., Goad, J., & Brennan, J. (2014). The dilemma of distance: Patients with kidney cancer from regional Australia present at a more advanced stage. *BJU International, 113*(Suppl 2), 57–63.

Tan, H. J., Filson, C. P., & Litwin, M. S. (2015). Contemporary, age-based trends in the incidence and management of patients with early-stage kidney cancer. *Urologic Oncology, 33*(1), 21.e19–21.e26.

Znaor, A., Lortet-Tieulent, J., Laversanne, M., Jemal, A., & Bray, F. (2015). International variations and trends in renal cell carcinoma incidence and mortality. *European Urology, 67*(3), 519–530.

Chapter 10
To Reliability of Mortality Shifts in Working Population in Russia

Alla Ivanova, Tamara Sabgayda, Viktoria Semyonova, and Elena Zemlyanova

10.1 Introduction

Russian population mortality during last 50 years appears to be widely studied problem both in comparative European context (Shapiro 1995, Shkolnikov et al. 1996, Gavrilova et al. 2008, Semyonova et al. 2012, ets) and in relation to its internal regional variation. Hypotheses regarding the factors determining the long-term negative trends in mortality and its local changes have been repeatedly discussed (Cornia 1996; Leon et al. 1997; Bobak et al. 1998; Brainerd 1998; Walberg et al. 1998; Shkolnikov et al. 2004; Ivanova and Semyonova 2006, ets). The reasons for positive dynamics of mortality in the last decade caused the greatest debate. In this connection, a spectrum of forecasts concerning the future of Russia's mortality and the steps to be taken for positive scenarios is extremely broad (Ivanova and Semyonova 2006; Ivanova and Kondrakova 2008; Nikitina (2008, Demographic prognosis up to 2030, 2012), Andreev et al. (2012) ets).

Working population during several decades occurs to be the key group determining life expectancy level in Russia, its regional variance, trends and projections. Identification of patterns of mortality changes in different age groups of working-age population will help to verify the forecast concerning the future of Russia's mortality.

The aim of the study is to analyze death causes structure of working population (15–59 years) in Russia together with its regularities in ages, causes and gender as well as to define the input of different ages and death causes in changes in life expectancy on various stages of its dynamics.

A. Ivanova (✉) · T. Sabgayda · V. Semyonova · E. Zemlyanova
Department of Health Statistics, Federal Research Institute for Health Organization and Informatics of Ministry of Health of the Russian Federation, Moscow, Russia

© Springer International Publishing AG, part of Springer Nature 2018

C. H. Skiadas, C. Skiadas (eds.), *Demography and Health Issues*,
The Springer Series on Demographic Methods and Population Analysis 46,
https://doi.org/10.1007/978-3-319-76002-5_10

10.2 Methods and Data

The data from the Russian Mortality Database of the Federal State Statistics Service were analyzed. In Russia, all death cases are subject to mandatory registration, so we examine all registered deaths. On the base of official statistics we studies age and gender peculiarities of mortality in working ages; structure of death causes and its shifts at the stages of both negative dynamics and mortality reduction at 50 years period (1965–2016). While dynamics analysis we used indicators recalculated with consideration for population censuses results including 2010 population census. Component analysis was used for determining of age groups and death causes which defined mortality changes during periods of "soviet evolutionary life expectancy reduction" (1965–1980); "opportunistic life expectancy growth as a result of anti-alcohol campaign" (1980–1987); "crisis life expectancy decline at the stage of shock socio-economic reforms" (1987–1994); "opportunistic life expectancy changes during reforms' stagnation" (1994–2005); "life expectancy growth at the background of conduct appropriate policy" (2005–2016).

10.3 Periods of Mortality Dynamics in Russia

Long-term life expectancy dynamics of Russian population is well-known (Andreev and Vishnevsky 2004; Shkolnikov et al. 2004; Semyonova 2005; Millet and Shkolnikov 1996; Ivanova et al. 2009). That's why lets cover the aspects which are important for understanding of periods and their causes.

The middle of 1960s was selected as a starting point of research. At that moment previous positive mortality dynamics which allowed Russia to catch up European countries largely at life expectancy level was depleted (Fig. 10.1). Since the middle of 1960s the negative trend took its shape and it continued till the edge of 1980s. During that period male life expectancy decreased by 2.8 years, female life expectancy – by 0.4 years. The majority of losses (2.5 years in males and 0.35 years in females i.e. about 88% and 92%) were determined by age groups 15–59 years. The causes which determined steady negative dynamics were comprehensively discussed in scientific publications. To resume them briefly – ideological reasons,

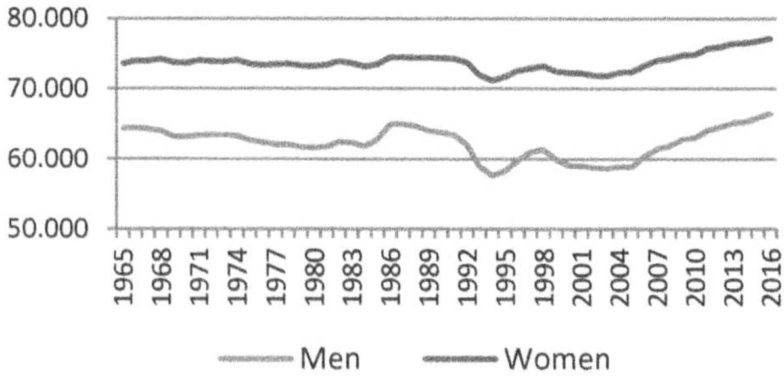

Fig. 10.1 Life expectancy dynamics in Russia, years

which determine the social politics, were principal and first of all – disrespect of life value both at state and individual levels. This is testified by similarity of mortality trends in the majority of socialist countries even levels of mortality could be rather different (TI Zaslavskaya 2004; Savinov et al. 2010; Yastrebov and Krasilova 2012).

The beginning of 1980s was characterized by slight opportunistic fluctuations of life expectancy that transformed into evident positive dynamics with the start of anti-alcohol campaign. It's well known that during the short period of hard-edged antialcoholic measures the life expectancy increased essentially (Mesle and Shkolnikov 1996; Shkolnikov et al. 2004; Andreev and Vishnevskiy 2004; Semyonova 2005; Nemtzov 2011, ets). Up to 1987 losses during previous 15-years period were not only compensated but life expectancy exceeded maximum of 1965 by 0.6 years in males and by 0.9 years in females. During 1980–1987 the share of working population 15–59 years old accounted 2.8 and 0.8 years from 3.4 and 1.3 years in males and females correspondingly, i.e. 82% and 67% of overall life expectancy growth.

Following gradual rejection of hard-edged measures limiting accessibility to alcohol gradual mortality growth upraised and it accelerated since the beginning of 1990s at the background socio-economic reforms that led to sharp impoverishment, losing of social waymarks and perspectives for the majority of Russian population. In total, during 1987–1994 life expectancy losses estimated 7.2 years in males and 3.2 years in females; the share of 15–59 age group was 6.2 and 2.2 years or 80% and 63% in males and females correspondingly.

The period of the second half of 1990s and first half of 2000s was characterized of sharp mortality fluctuations: partial recovery of life expectancy after collapse in the middle of 1990s, new decline after economic crisis in 1998 and gradual way to stabilization in 2002–2005. As a result, the situation with mortality of Russian population occurred to be just slightly better than 10 years before – at the peak of socio-economic crisis. Both in males and females life expectancy was high the level of 1994 by 1.3 years. But this small gain was to minimal extent due to risk groups. Age groups 15–59 years covered only 0.4 and less than 0.1 years in males and females or 29% and 2% correspondingly. In other words, situation with mortality of working population in 2005 was the same sharp as in catastrophic 1994.

New stage of Russian mortality dynamics started since the middle of new decade when positive life expectancy trend developed. It was determined by the whole age range, main death causes and the majority of regions (Demographic prognosis up to 2030, 2012). In general, life expectancy in males increased by 7.6 years, in females – by 4.7 years for 2005–2016; and 5.4 and 2.0 years (or 71.1% and 46.8%) in males and females were due to population in working ages. Thus, a decisive influence of working population on the dynamics of life expectancy in Russia is maintained, but its contribution is lower than in previous decades.

The question about the reasons formatting the positive trend of mortality remains still controversial. Most of authors (Yakunin et al. 2007; Ulumbekova 2010; Kalashnikov et al. 2012; Shamilev 2013) tend to explain the positive trend only by an active policy in the health sector which implemented since 2006. At the same time, the point of view is also told that after 2005 the so-called "recovery growth" of life expectancy started as a part of long-term oscillatory trend, which has not a fundamentally new sources and does not assume the prospects (Vishnevsky 2015). Indeed, to 2014 Russia for the third time almost returned to the levels of life expectancy, already met in its history over the past 50 years: in 1987 and in 1965. In 2014, life expectancy level was higher by only 1.3 years than in 1965 and by 0.9 years than in 1987.

10.4 Age Groups and Death Causes that Determined Life Expectancy Shifts at Stages of Its Growth and Decline

During 15 "soviet" years during 1965–1980 reduction of male life expectancy in working ages was determined by all age groups from 15 to 59 years but one half of all losses was due to 45–59 year-olds (Fig. 10.2).

Among causes the first place was occupied by traumas and poisonings (1.5 years in age interval 15–59 years) and cardio-vascular diseases (0.88 years). It's important that aside from those causes the input into life expectancy losses was made by respiratory diseases (0.2 years); digestive diseases (0.12 years) and partly – neoplasms (0.01 years). Only in class of neoplasms negative dynamics spread to selected age groups (over 45 years). Other causes had determined losses at the whole age range from 15 to 59 years. Only infections in the contrary to other main causes of death didn't participate life expectancy losses in men of working ages in this period.

The situation with women in 1965–1980 was essentially different from men's. First, the losses were formed due to age group over 45 years; in young women mortality trends from the majority of causes and in general were positive. Second, female mortality from neoplasms decreased in all age groups; that's why neoplasms as well as infections didn't participate in life expectancy losses in working ages of females. At the same time, the similarity on formation of life expectancy losses in

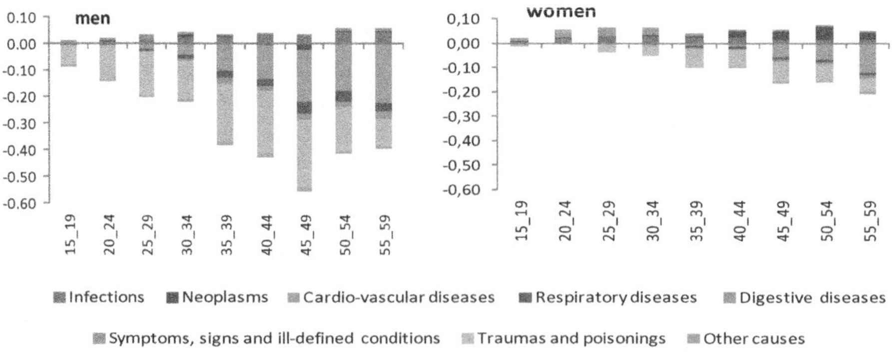

Fig. 10.2 Input of age groups and death causes into life expectancy change in 1965–1980

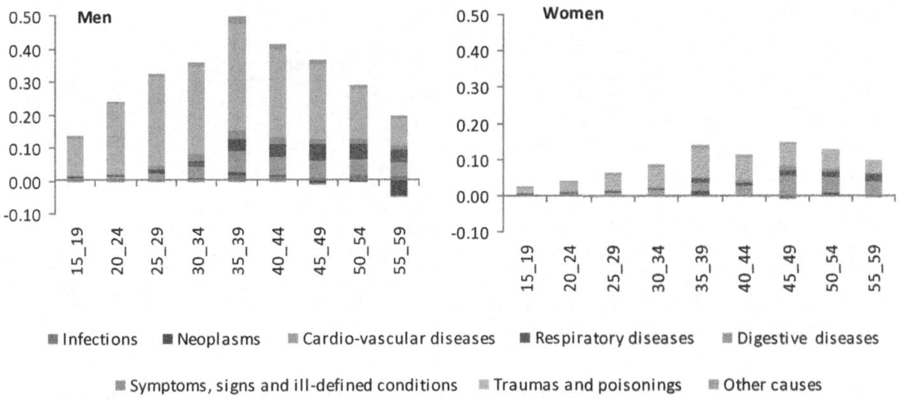

Fig. 10.3 Input of age groups and death causes into life expectancy change in 1980–1987

males and females was in prevalence of external causes and cardio-vascular diseases as well as partial input of respiratory and digestive diseases.

During the period of essential life expectancy growth in 1980–1987 positive dynamics was characteristic to all age groups and main death causes (Fig. 10.3). Both in males and females equal input into life expectancy growth was made by age groups 30–44 years and 45–59 years. That's why the role of external causes in life expectancy gain was critical: 1.91 from 2.8 years of total growth in 15–59 years old males; and 0.42 from 0.84 years in females. In males the role of cardio-vascular and respiratory diseases was relatively comparable (0.32 and 0.25 years); digestive diseases – half as much (0.13 years). In females the role of cardio-vascular diseases was half as much as traumas and poisonings (0.21 years); the role of other causes – negligeable.

The special role as during the previous period was taken by neoplasms. In males neoplasms continued their negative trend apart of sinuosity of anti-alcohol campaign; and it affected ages over 45 years similarly to the previous period. The reduction of female's mortality from neoplasm continued in all age groups.

Life expectancy losses during 1987–1994 formed at the whole range of working ages (Fig. 10.4) but the scales of losses were increasing with age and maximum was observed in the group 45–49 years both in males (2.75 of 6.18 years) and females (1.16 of 2.21 years).

About one half of losses in working ages were due to external causes: 3.31 and 1.0 years in males and females correspondingly; losses due cardio-vascular diseases were twice less – 1.54 and 0.67 years in males and females correspondingly. In contrast to the previous period mortality growth was registered in all death causes and age groups. This emphasizes the universalism of effect of social processes on health and mortality during that period.

The new phenomenon of that period was manifested in increase of mortality in working ages from "Symptoms, signs and ill-defined conditions" which covered life

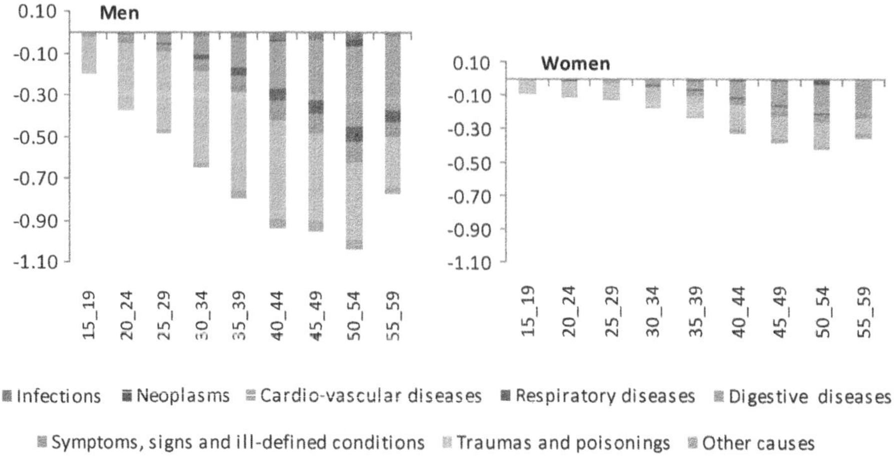

Fig. 10.4 Input of age groups and death causes into life expectancy change in 1987–1994

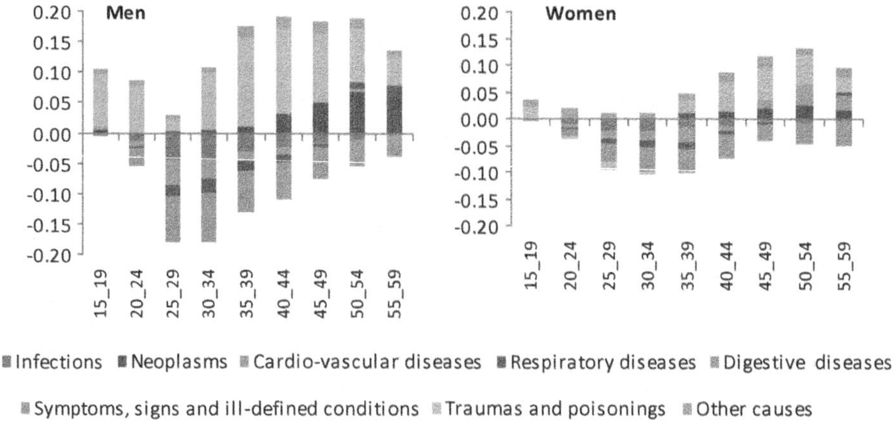

Fig. 10.5 Input of age groups and death causes into life expectancy change in 1994–2000

expectancy losses in working ages comparable to losses from respiratory and digestive diseases and higher than losses from infections.

Since the middle of 1990s till the middle of 2000s mortality dynamics became very diverse; it broke previous uniformity in respect to population response to social changes (Fig. 10.5). In men cumulative results occurred to be positive both for young population groups (15–24 years) and older groups of working ages (35–59 years). But the most active and productive groups (25–34 years) suffered from negative trends. In females gain were achieved only in teenagers (15–19 years) and groups over 40 years. Unfavorable ages covered wider age group than in males: 20–40 year olds.

It is important that slight life expectancy increase during the decade was due to reduction of mortality from traumas and poisonings as well as neoplasms and other diseases apart from 7 main classes of death causes. Mortality from neoplasms declined in all ages providing life expectancy increase in working ages by 0.24 and 0.10 years in males and females correspondingly. Mortality form traumas and poisonings declined in males in all ages, in females – in all ages excluding age group 20–34 years. This provided life expectancy growth in working ages by 0.82 and 0.22 years correspondingly. Mortality from other causes was increasing.

Positive trends in external causes and neoplasms invite some questions but for various reasons. As to external causes, driving forces of mortality reduction have no explanation. There were no evident improvements in living standards of poor population groups in the period under review, there were no implemented measures concerning anti-alcohol policy, there was no special attention to healthy life styles. This is supported by negative dynamics of mortality from causes being markers of these problems – infections and digestive diseases. Characteristically, the mortality from ill-defined conditions continued to rise against decrease in mortality from external causes. It calls into question the progress achieved, as there are substantial grounds for believing that the diagnosis of ill-defined death causes among working-age population is a camouflage of external causes of death (Semyonova et al. 2005; Ivanova et al. 2009; Semyonova and Fedotkina 2010).

In is necessary to make a special reference to neoplasms. Developed positive dynamics of mortality from these causes both in males and females at the whole working age range fell to the most difficult period for Russian health care – protracted reforms at the background of chronic under-financing. It's difficult to find valid explanations for this phenomenon. Several authors pay attention to the problems of diagnosis of cancer as a cause of death, which may explain the underestimation of deaths from malignant neoplasms (Danilova 2003; Petrova et al. 2010; Sabgayda et al. 2010).

The specific feature of that period was the age structure of mortality growth from chronic non-infectious diseases and first of all from cardio-vascular diseases. Both in males and females growth of mortality from cardio-vascular pathology was concentrated in young and middle ages. At the same time there was no growth in males over 45 years and there was even slight reduction in females. It is nonsense from the medical-biological viewpoint. Quite a lot of research dedicated to the phenomenon of rejuvenation of cardiovascular mortality in Russia, where the alcohol played a significant role (Shkolnikov et al. 2002; Leon et al. 2007; Semyonova et al. 2010). The influence of this factor is evident not only in provoking the deaths, but also masking the real cause of death.

Despite of substantial differences of 1994–2005 decade from the previous period it is possible to notice similarity of both decades characteristic to long-running stage of transformation in socio-economic sphere in Russia. This refers to continuous growth of mortality from infections and from "Symptoms, signs and ill-defined conditions" covering whole range of working ages.

Since the middle 2000s we observe the new period of overcoming of negative mortality trends and life expectancy growth in Russia (Fig. 10.6). Life expectancy

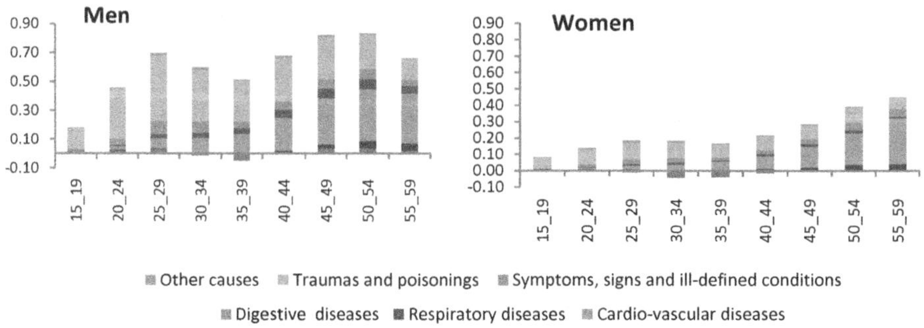

Fig. 10.6 Input of age groups and death causes into life expectancy change in 2005–2016

increase was provided by all age groups with maximal input of ages over 40 years: 3.0 of 5.4 years in men and 1.3 of 2.0 years in women.

Life expectancy growth was provided by all main death causes excluding infections. In males, infections maintained their negative trends in age group 30–39 years but the overall result in working ages was positive (0.091 year). In females, negative trends of infections covered wider age interval 25–49 years and the overall result for working ages occurred to be negative (−0.09 year).

According to younger age profile of life expectancy increase in males the main input into life expectancy growth was made by external causes (2.56 years) and some less by cardiovascular diseases (1.60 years). In females, significance of these causes was almost identical: 0.76 and 0.79 years. The role of all other causes occurred to be less evident.

It is necessary to note that age distribution of external causes input into life expectancy increase in working ages was sufficiently proportional. At the same time, the maximal gain from reduction of mortality from chronic non-infectious diseases, first of all from cardio-vascular diseases was registered in ages over 40 years both in females and males. Thus, cumulated substantial rejuvenation of mortality from chronic non-communicable diseases was not affected yet.

Limitations The assessments of proportions of death causes in mortality for working population may have errors of measurement because namely for this age group the problem of accuracy of death cause establishing is the most urgent in Russia. However, these measurement errors will not affect the resulting conclusions, since they do not exceed 5% (Sabgayda et al. 2010).

10.5 Discussion

Returning to the discussion of hypotheses to explain the causes of a significant increase in life expectancy over the past decade, we must admit that none of the hypotheses does not give a convincing answer.

Table 10.1 Dynamics of Russian mortality in some age groups (per 1000 persons of corresponding sex and age)

	Age groups (years)								
	15–19	20–24	25–29	30–34	35–39	40–44	45–49	50–54	55–59
Males									
2000	2.12	4.95	5.99	7.02	9.12	12.70	17.86	24.42	33.36
2001	1.92	4.35	5.81	7.05	9.42	13.13	18.67	25.73	33.94
2002	1.83	3.96	5.66	7.27	9.87	13.93	19.55	26.91	34.69
2003	1.74	3.90	5.91	7.50	10.19	14.44	20.06	27.91	34.99
2004	1.68	3.91	6.12	7.78	10.21	14.21	19.54	26.78	34.41
2005	1.63	3.80	6.46	8.20	10.30	14.33	19.44	26.90	34.44
Females									
2000	0.80	1.13	1.34	1.73	2.33	3.37	5.08	7.60	11.38
2001	0.75	1.12	1.36	1.81	2.43	3.50	5.33	8.01	11.65
2002	0.71	1.05	1.41	1.94	2.63	3.76	5.54	8.30	11.96
2003	0.69	1.05	1.51	2.05	2.80	3.95	5.74	8.63	12.10
2004	0.68	1.00	1.56	2.13	2.84	3.91	5.57	8.23	11.85
2005	0.69	1.03	1.61	2.21	2.94	4.03	5.56	8.13	11.78

Attempts to explain the success in reducing deaths solely to measures in healthcare are untenable since positive changes among most age groups of working-age population (as it have been shown in the previous section) began in previous period, since 2003 or earlier (Table 10.1).

The increase in mortality among young people aged 15–24 years ended by the year 2000; the growth of mortality among men and women over 40 years old stopped in 2003; and only among the 25–39-year-olds the increasing mortality lasted until 2005. Therefore, in 2006, when the first steps were taken in the framework of priority National project "Health", the positive dynamics among working-age population have been already formed. This does not mean that the policy pursued has not given effect. In fact, it only strengthened the already established positive trend that was initiated by improved living standards, reduction of unemployment, income growth, a sense of positive social change.

The hypothesis of oscillatory dynamics of mortality in Russia based on a multiple return of life expectancy to almost the same it's levels, is also based on a superficial analogy. Similar life expectancy levels in 1965, 1987 and 2014 are based on fundamentally different picture of mortality and, consequently, on its different driving forces and mechanisms.

By 2014 compared to 1987 and especially compared to 1965, the child death rate (especially infant mortality) essentially decreased, which provided an increase in life expectancy of 0.9 and 0.7 years and 1.5 and 1.3 years, respectively, for men and women (Fig. 10.7). The progress in mortality dynamics among men over the age of 60 years and women over 50 years is undeniable. However, the mortality of modern men and women of young and middle ages is above not only in comparison with the

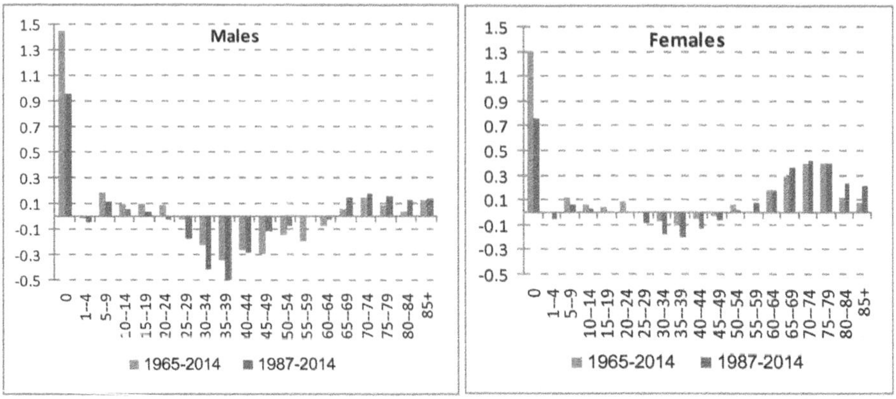

Fig. 10.7 Differences in age patterns of mortality in 1965, 1987, 2014

period of a quarter century ago, but also in comparison with the period of a half century ago.

It must be admitted that in the past decade it has been done much to reduce the loss of life in high-risk groups, but it is premature to even talk about returning to the previously achieved level of population health.

10.6 Conclusions

Summarizing 50-years of history of Russian mortality it is necessary to note several important things.

In 2014 Russia for the third time almost returned to the levels of life expectancy, already met in its history over the past 50 years: in 1987 and in 1965. In 2014, life expectancy level was higher by only 1.3 years than in 1965 and by 0.9 years than in 1987. But this return is illusive as modern life expectancy formed by substantial progress in children and older age groups, while mortality of young and middle age groups is higher than 50 years ago.

The main source of both disadvantages and gains during all stages of nearly half century dynamics is the population of working ages; in males cumulative losses due to population of 15–59 years following the results of 1965–2014 occurred to be 1.2 years of life expectancy, in females – 0.01 years.

The resulting losses during working-life period are combined from 2 age groups: 30–44 year-olds and 45–59 year-olds – in males proportion of those 2 groups was 40% and 60%; in females reverse – 60% and 40%. Input of younger age groups both in males and females occurred small (0.17 and 0.15 year) i.e. levels of mortality in men and women 15–29 years old in 2014 and in 1965 did not differ significantly.

In the ages where resulting mortality during analyzed period didn't change in general, and in ages where it increased the structure of death causes visibly changed:

- as to structure of mortality in young ages, input of respiratory and digestive diseases as well as ill-defined conditions and plus infections and cardio-vascular diseases in males the resulting mortality remained the same as in 1965 only due to reduction of traumas and poisonings and neoplasms;
- as to structure of mortality in working ages over 30 years, input of main somatic diseases (except neoplasms) and external causes increased which determined growth of summarized mortality in these ages.

Altogether, conducted analysis rises following questions:

- reliability of reduction of mortality from external causes that started before improvement of socio-economic situation in the country and implementation of any measures in that sphere (during 1994–2005);
- reliability of growth of cardio-vascular mortality in middle and especially young ages (15–29 years);
- reliability of diagnostics of somatic death causes in general including neoplasms.

After 2014, mortality in Russia continued to decline although the increase in life expectancy by 2016 wasn't not significant: 1.25 years for men and 0.58 years for women. This result was achieved against the backdrop of economic crisis, rising unemployment, falling incomes and reducing investment in the health care system. Apparently, the accumulated positive potential, including in the healthcare system, still provides an inertial reduction in mortality. However, without the resumption of active efforts in the health sector supported by an improvement in socioeconomic status of population, the positive inertia will be exhausted and the increase in mortality may resume.

References

Andreev, E. M., & Vishnevskiy, A. G. (2004). Challenge to high mortality rate. *Narodonaselenie, 3*, 75–84 (in Russian).

Andreev, E. M., Vishnevskiy, A. G., & Trevish, A. I. (2012). *Analytical demographic prognosis up to 2050*. Social problems [Internet]. 2012 [cited 2014 Jun 25]. Available from http://www.socprob.ru/index.php?option=com_content&view=article&id=846:1-----2050--13--lr-&catid=87:2012-03-28-20-08-37 (in Russian).

Bobak, M., Pikhart, H., Hertzman, C., Rose, R., & Marmot, M. (1998). Socioeconomic factors, perceived control and self-reported health in Russia. A cross-sectional survey. *Social Science & Medicine, 47*(2), 269–279.

Brainerd, E. (1998). Market reform and mortality in transition economies. *World Development, 26* (11), 2013–2027.

Cornia, G. A. (1996). Labor market shocks, psychosocial stress and the transition's mortality crisis. *Helsinki: "UNU/WIDER Research in Progress", 4*, 17–19.

Danilova, T. V. (2003). *Health and statistical aspects of registration of cancer patient mortality*. Dr. Med.Sci [dissertation]. Moscow; 174 p (in Russian).

Demographic prognosis up to 2030. (2012). [Интернет]. Rosstat; 2012 [cited 2016 Jen 10]. Available from http://www.gks.ru/free_doc/new_site/population/demo/progn7.htm (in Russian).

Gavrilova, N. S., Semyonova, V. G., Dubrovina, E. V., Evdokushkina, G. N., Ivanova, A. E., & Gavrilov, L. A. (2008). Russian mortality crisis and the quality of vital statistics. *Population Research and Policy Review, 27*, 551–574.

Ivanova, A. E., & Kondrakova, E. V. (2008). *Rationale for the forecast of population life expectancy in the regions of Russia up to 2025*. Sotsial'nye aspekty zdorov'ya naseleniya [serial online]. [cited 2016 Jen 10]; *1*(5). Available from http://vestnik.mednet.ru/content/view/52/30 (in Russian).

Ivanova, A. E., & Semyonova, V. G. (2006). Some criteria for assessing and forecasting the epidemiologic situation in Russia. *Obshchestvennoe zdorov'e i profilaktika zabolevaniy, 6*, 11–21. (in Russian).

Ivanova, A. E., Semyonova, V. G., Kondrakova, E. V., & Mihajlov, A. J. (2009). *The basic tendencies and regional features of death rates among Russian adolescents*. Sotsial'nye aspekty zdorov'ya naseleniya [serial online]. [cited 2016 Jen 10]; 2(10). Available from http://vestnik.mednet.ru/content/view/121/30/lang,ru/ (in Russian).

Yastrebov, G. A., & Krasilova, A. X. (2012). The viability of Russia and other post-socialist societies: The results of 20 years of reform. *Mir Rossii, 21*(1), 40–163 (in Russian).

Kalashnikov, K. N., Shabunova, A. A., & Duganov, M. D. (2012). *Organizational and economic factors for control the regional health care system: A monograph*. Vologda: ISERT RAN. 153 p. ISBN 978-5-93299-194-7 (in Russian).

Leon, D., Chenet, L., Shkolnikov, V. M., Zakharov, S., Shapiro, J., et al. (1997). Huge variation in Russian mortality rates 1984-1994: Artefact, alcohol, or what? *The-Lancet, 350*, 383–388.

Leon, D. A., Saburova, L., Tomkins, S., Andreev, E., Kiryanov, N., McKee, M., & Shkolnikov, V. M. (2007). Hazardous alcohol drinking and premature mortality in Russia: A population based case-control study. *The Lancet, 369*, 2001–2009.

Mille, F., & Shkol'nikov, V. M. (1996). The contemporary tendencies in mortality by causes of death in Russia in 1965–1994. Donnees Statistiques. No 2. 140 p.

Nemtzov, A. (2011). *A contemporary history of alcohol in Russia*. Sodertorns hogskola: Stockholm. 343 p.

Nikitina, S. Yu. (2008). To which extent the previous forecasts have predicted the contemporary dynamics of mortality in Russia? *Demoscop Weekly* [serial online]. [cited 2016 Jen 10]; pp. 321–322. Available from http://demoscope.ru/weekly/2008/0321/analit01.php (in Russian).

Petrova, G. V., Kharchenko, N. V., Gretsova, O. P., Prostov, Yu. I., Prostov, M. Yu., & Privezentseva, L. B. (2010). *Analysis of reliability of the registration documentation of territorial oncological clinics under forms 7 and 35 for 2009*. Sotsial'nye aspekty zdorov'ya naseleniya [serial online]. [cited 2016 Jen 10]; *4*(16). Available from http://vestnik.mednet.ru/content/view/241/30/lang,ru/ (in Russian).

Sabgayda, T. P., Semyonova, V. G., Ivanova, A. E., Sekrieru, Ye. M., & Nikitina, S. Yu. (2010). *Modification of underlying cause of death from diseases of the circulatory system*. Sotsial'nye aspekty zdorov'ya naseleniya [serial online]. [cited 2016 Jen 10]; *4*(38). Available from http://vestnik.mednet.ru/content/view/581/30/lang,ru/ (in Russian).

Savinov, L. I., Kolomasov, E. N., & Romanovskaya, E. S. (2010). *Public health and social policies: A regional perspective*. Scientific notes of Russian State Social University; (11), 23–28 (in Russian).

Semyonova, V. G. (2005). *Reverse epidemiological transition in Russia*. Moscow: Tsentr sotsial'nogo prognozirovaniya. 270 p. (in Russian).

Semyonova, V. G., & Fedotkina, S. A. (2010). Reconstruction of real losses from some socially determined mortality causes in the young population of Krasnoyarsk territory in 2008. *Zdravookhranenie Rossiyskoy Federatsii, 6*, 14–19. (in Russian).

Semyonova, V. G., Dubrovina, E. V., Evdokushkina, G. N., Gavrilova, N. S., & Gavrilov, L. A. (2005). Assessments of real levels of violent mortality in Russia. *Obshchestvennoe zdorov'e i profilaktika zabolevaniy, 3*, 14–23. (in Russian).

Semyonova, V. G., Antonova, O. I., Evdokushkina, G. N., & Gavrilova, N. S. (2010). *Alcohol losses of Russian population in 2000–2008: Scale, structure, and tendencies*. Sotsial'nye aspekty zdorov'ya naseleniya [serial online]. [cited 2016 Jen 10]; *14*(2). Available from http://vestnik.mednet.ru/content/view/188/30 (in Russian).

Semyonova, V. G., Okunev, O. B., Antonyuk, V. V., & Evdokushkina, G. N. (2012). *Age and nosological characteristics of population mortality in Russia in 1990–2009 compared to West European countries*. Sotsial' aspekty zdorov'ya naseleniya [serial online]. [cited 2016 Jen 10]; 26(4). Available from http://vestnik.mednet.ru/content/view/415/27/lang,ru/ (in Russian).

Shamilev, S. R. (2013). *Trends in mortality and the factors of its decline in Russian Federation*. Sovremennie problemi nauki I obrazovania [serial online]. [cited 2016 Jen 10]; (5). Available from http://www.science-education.ru/111-9897 (in Russian).

Shapiro, J. (1995). The Russian mortality crisis and its causes. In A. Aslund (Ed.), *Economic reform at risk* (pp. 149–178). London: Pinter.

Shkolnikov, V., Mesle, F., & Vallin, J. (1996). Health crisis in Russia. *Population, 8*, 123–190.

Shkolnikov, V. M., McKee, M., Chervyakov, V. V., & Kyrianov, N. A. (2002). Is the link between alcohol and cardiovascular death among young Russian men attributable to misclassification of acute alcohol intoxication? Evidence from the city of Izhevsk. *Journal of Epidemiology and Community Health, 56*(3), 171–174.

Shkolnikov, V. M., Andreev, E. M., Leon, D. A., McKee, M., Mesle, F., & Vallin, J. (2004). Mortality reversal in Russia: The story so far. *International Journal of Hygiene and Environmental Health, 4*, 29–80.

Ulumbekova, G. E. (2010). *Health Russia. What to do: The scientific basis "strategy for the development of public health in Russian Federation until 2020". Short version*. GEOTAR Media: Moscow. 96 p. ISBN 978-5-97041-435-4 (in Russian).

Vishnevsky, A. Г. (2015). After the demographic transition: The divergence, convergence or diversity?. *Obchestvevvie nauki i sovremennost*, (2), 112–129 (in Russian).

Walberg, P., McKee, M., Shkolnikov, V. M., Chenet, L., & Leon, D. A. (1998). Economic change, crime, and mortality crisis in Russia: Regional analysis. *British Medical Journal, 317*, 312–318.

Yakunin, V. I., Sulakshin, S. S., & Bagdasarian, V. E.(2007). *State policy of withdrawal of Russia from demographic crisis*. (Ed. S. Sulakshin, 2nd edn.) Moscow: ZAO "Izdatelstvo" "Economica" Scientific Expert. 888 p. ISBN 978-5-91290-007-5 (in Russian).

Zaslavskaya, T. I. (2004). Modern Russian society: Problems and prospects. *Obschestvennie nauki I sovremennost*, (6), 5–18 (in Russian).

Chapter 11
Three-Way Data Analysis Applied to Cause Specific Mortality Trends

Giuseppe Giordano, Steven Haberman, and Maria Russolillo

11.1 Introduction

Mortality forecasts are traditionally based on forecasters' subjective judgements, in light of historical data and expert opinions. We focus on the Lee and Carter (LC) method for modelling and forecasting mortality (Lee and Carter 1992). This method reduces the role of subjective judgement, since takes into account standard diagnostic and modelling procedures for statistical time series analysis. In Kroonenberg et al. (2002) and Russolillo et al. (2011) the authors propose a three-way analysis of mortality data. In the last one, the three-way decomposition is read in the scope of the LC model as a natural extension of the original LC model to a three mode data structure. The three-way LC model (3WLC) allows to enrich the basic LC model by introducing a third mode in the analysis. For instance, the authors propose to consider the death rates aggregated for time, age-groups and Countries. Starting from that paper, we return to the original version of the LC model, but we make use of the exploratory tools of multivariate data analysis to give a new perspective to the demographic analysis supporting the analytical results with a geometrical interpretation and a graphical representation.

The mortality rates are influenced by gender, countries, ethnicity, income, wealth, causes of death and so on. According to the WHO a "right" recognition of the causes of death is important for forecasting more accurately mortality. Aim of this

G. Giordano (✉) · M. Russolillo
Department of Statistics and Economics, University of Salerno, Salerno, Italy
e-mail: ggiordano@unisa.it; mrussolillo@unisa.it

S. Haberman
Faculty of Actuarial Science and Insurance, Cass Business School, City University London, London, UK
e-mail: s.haberman@city.ac.uk

© Springer International Publishing AG, part of Springer Nature 2018
C. H. Skiadas, C. Skiadas (eds.), *Demography and Health Issues*,
The Springer Series on Demographic Methods and Population Analysis 46,
https://doi.org/10.1007/978-3-319-76002-5_11

contribution is to specify the 3WLC model to consider the specific causes of death. The original contribution we propose is to investigate the main causes of death affecting the upcoming human survival, throughout a Multi-dimensional Data Analysis approach to the LC model of mortality trends. In other words, we wish to test the three-way model developed in Russolillo et al. (2011), by looking at the mortality data aggregated according to three criteria: time, age class and causes of death. Specifically, we refer to the Tucker3 decomposition method (Kroonenberg 1983). The remainder of the article is organized as follows. Section 2 introduces the "Mortality by cause of death" issue. In Sect. 3 we present the setting of Multi-dimensional Data Analysis on which we develop the three-way Lee-Carter model. Section 4 shows the numerical application where we furnish a proper interpretation of the model components when the data structure deals with Time × Ages × Causes of death.

11.2 The Framework

The "mortality by cause of death" issue covers areas of particular interest to actuaries. These include the impact of specific causes of death on historical trends in mortality, the use of "by cause" information in mortality projections, the availability and use of data suitable for underwriting, pricing and analysis of life assurance and pensions business products (Ridsdale and Gallop 2010). The twentieth century witnessed longevity improvements in many high-income countries. These improvements were determined especially by the reduction in a few specific major causes of death groups.

In order to obtain good population forecasts, in the last decades a wide variety of models have been proposed for analyzing and projecting mortality for specific groups of causes. Many of these projection methodologies are based on past mortality developments and implicitly make assumptions about the persistence of trends in "by cause" mortality. As it is well known, examination of past trends in causes of death is helpful in understanding the overall mortality improvements in populations. As stated by Gallop (2008), many of the available methodologies can be applied either to aggregate mortality data or data by cause of death. Projecting mortality by cause of death allows for providing insights into the ways in which mortality is changing. However, there are also many drawbacks associated with this approach. One of the most relevant is deaths from specific causes are not always independent. Many models instead assume the independence between the different causes of death. Moreover, the actual cause of death may be difficult to determine or may be misclassified. Last but not least, changes in the diagnosis and classification of causes of deaths can make analysis of trend patterns difficult. The ranking of leading causes of death is affected by a periodic revision that produces structural breaks in the mortality series. These discontinuities lead to a misinterpretation of trends in mortality, problem which should be taken into account in the model considered for projections.

11.3 The Lee-Carter Model and Some Generalizations

Mortality projections depends on several factors among which the most relevant are age, and then gender, geographical region, social class. The LC method is a powerful approach to mortality projections which can be described as follows:

$$\ln\left(y_{ij}\right) = \alpha_j + \kappa_i\beta_j + \varepsilon_{ij} \qquad i = 1, \cdots, I;\; j = 1, \cdots, J \tag{11.1}$$

where $\ln(y_{i,j})$ is the log of a time series of death rates $y_{i,j}$ for each age-specific x; α_j is the age-specific parameter, that is the mean of the $\ln(y_{ij})$ for each j; k_i is the time-varying parameter's vector reflecting the general level of mortality. The vector β_j holds the parameters showing how rapidly or slowly mortality varies at each age-group. The term $\varepsilon_{i,j}$ is the error term assumed to be homoscedastic.

We can state the demographic model also referring to the mean centred log-mortality rates as:

$$\tilde{y}_{ij} = \ln\left(y_{ij}\right) - \alpha_j = \kappa_i\beta_j + \varepsilon_{ij} \qquad i = 1, \cdots, I;\; j = 1, \cdots, J \tag{11.2}$$

11.3.1 The LC Model in the Framework of MDA: Two-Way Data

Following Lee and Carter, the parameters β_j and k_i in eq. 11.2 can be estimated according to the Singular Value Decomposition (SVD) with suitable normality constraints:

$$\sum_j \beta_j^2 = 1; \quad \sum_i k_i = 0 \tag{11.3}$$

Let us notice that the term on the left hand side is shaped as a two-way data matrix:

$$\tilde{\mathbf{Y}} = \begin{pmatrix} \tilde{y}_{11} & \tilde{y}_{12} & \cdots & \tilde{y}_{1J} \\ \tilde{y}_{21} & \tilde{y}_{22} & \cdots & \tilde{y}_{2J} \\ \vdots & \vdots & \tilde{y}_{ij} & \vdots \\ \tilde{y}_{I1} & \tilde{y}_{I2} & \cdots & \tilde{y}_{IJ} \end{pmatrix} \tag{11.4}$$

For major insight on the exploratory reading of the LC model as a two-way decomposition model (see Russolillo et al. 2011).

The SVD of the matrix (4) can be written as the product of three matrices with geometric and statistical interpretation.

In particular, the SVD model is stated as follows:

$$\tilde{\mathbf{Y}}_{(I,J)} = \mathbf{U}_{(I,H)}\mathbf{\Lambda}_{(H,H)}\mathbf{V}_{(H,J)} \qquad H \leq \min\{I, J\} \tag{11.5}$$

The SVD approximation allows a graphical representation in a reduced subspace of both rows and columns of the matrix. The geometric reading of such representation is carried out according to the Biplot graphical display (Gower and Hand 1996). The *biplot* is a low-dimensional display of a rectangular data matrix, where the rows and the columns are represented by points. The interpretation of the biplot is consistent with the scalar products between row and column vectors as defined in the SVD.

The SVD model can be rewritten as:

$$\tilde{\mathbf{Y}} = \sum\nolimits_{m=1}^{n} \lambda_m \mathbf{u}_m \mathbf{v}'_m + \sum\nolimits_{m=n+1}^{H} \lambda_m \mathbf{u}_m \mathbf{v}'_m; \tag{11.6}$$

With $1 \leq n \leq (H-1)$; $H \leq \min\{I, J\}$ and where the second term represents the residual information not captured by the first p components of the SVD approximation. The correspondence of the two models arises by setting $\mathbf{k} = \lambda\mathbf{u}$, $\boldsymbol{\beta} = \mathbf{v}$ and highlighting the role of the first component:

$$\tilde{\mathbf{Y}} = \lambda_1 \mathbf{u}_1 \mathbf{v}'_1 + \sum\nolimits_{m=2}^{H} \lambda_m \mathbf{u}_m \mathbf{v}'_m = \kappa_1 \beta'_1 + E \tag{11.7}$$

Usually, in the actual use of LC-model some aspects are not considered, i.e. there could be meaningful interactions between the elements k and β, which in the basic LC model are not considered. Indeed, further factors could be considered as aggregating criteria: *Country*, *Ethnics* as well as *Causes of Death*, for instance. In order to face with both interactions terms and mortality data arranged according to *Years*, *Age-group* and a further criteria, we introduced the three way extension of the LC model (proposed in Russolillo et al. 2011) in order to describe and interpret the demographic model and give a suitable statistical interpretation.

11.3.2 The Three-Way LC-Model

Sometimes the available data are disaggregated according to different criteria. Let us consider different causes of death, so that the new specification of the LC model can be written as follows:

$$\ln\left(y_{ijl}\right) = \alpha_{jl} + \kappa_i \beta_j \gamma_l + \varepsilon_{ijl} \qquad i = 1, \cdots, I;\ j = 1, \cdots, J;\ l = 1, \ldots, L \tag{11.8}$$

where j is the generic age group, i the generic year and l is the cause-specific death. α_{jl} is the age and cause-specific death parameter independent of time,α_j while β_j and k_i have the same interpretation as in the classical LC model. Finally, γ_l represents the term associated to the causes of death.

We can state the model referring to the mean centered log-mortality rates:

$$\bar{y}_{ijl} = \ln\left(y_{ijl}\right) - \alpha_{jl} = \kappa_i \beta_j \gamma_l + \varepsilon_{ijl} \qquad i = 1, \cdots, I;\ j = 1, \cdots, J;\ l = 1, \ldots, L \tag{11.9}$$

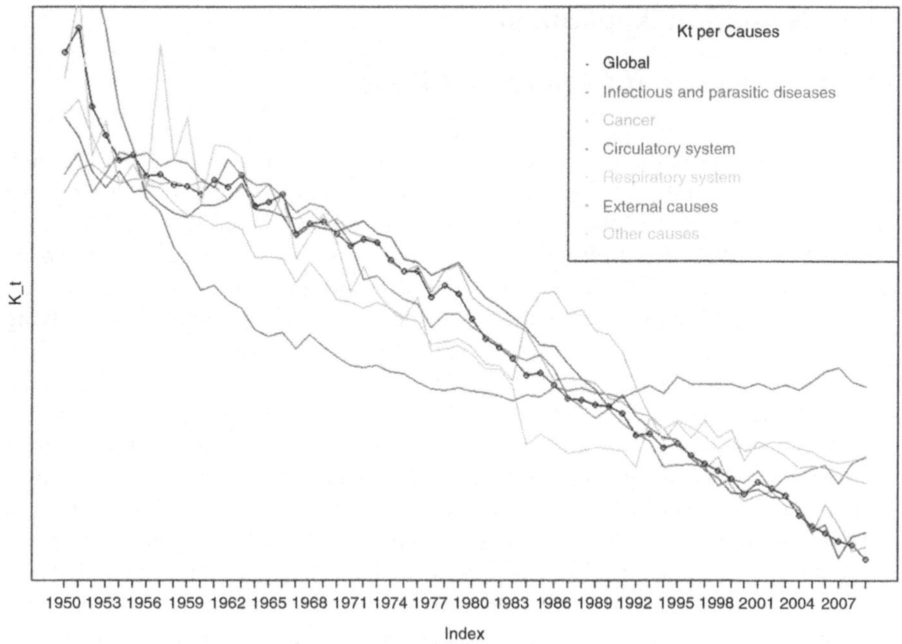

Fig. 11.1 Individual patterns of *Kt* for different causes

The values of α_{jl} are computed by averaging the log-mortality rates across the *n* years, for each age-group $j = 1, 2,\ldots,J$ and for each cause $l = 1,\ldots,L$. Different choices of averaging could be taken into account: we may wish to derive the average pure effect of *Cause of Death*, across *Years* and *Age-groups,* for instance.

In this framework, the singular value decomposition associated to the LC model has to be reformulated to take into account the new data structure. In the literature, to solve the decomposition problem several solutions are proposed which give rise to different statistical methods (Multiple Factorial Analysis, STATIS, Generalized Canonical Analysis, PARAFAC, Tucker's Method). We proposed as natural extension of the SVD in the three-way framework, the *Tucker3* model (Tucker 1964, 1966). This method can be seen as a generalization of the SVD. In the two-way SVD, the singular values are arranged in a diagonal matrix (see eq. 11.5). In the *Tucker 3* model these values form a three-way array – the *core array* – (see Fig.11.1). However, the relationships with the singular values of the various two-way analysis are not so immediate. In Fig. 11.1 is shown the three-way decomposition according to the *Tucker 3* model. The three dimensional array $\tilde{\mathbf{Y}}$ is decomposed into a three-way core array $\mathbf{\Lambda}$ and three matrices (**K**, **B**, **G**).

For further insights on the algorithms for estimating the model see Kroonenberg and De Leeuw (1980).

11.4 Numerical Application

11.4.1 The Case of England and Wales

We discuss the three-way LC model in view of an empirical case study. We consider male central death rates for England and Wales, in 60 years from 1950 up to 2009 divided according to the following six causes of death: *Circulatory system, Cancer, Respiratory system, External causes, Infectious and parasitic diseases and Other causes*. Data are downloaded from the World Health Organization (World Health Organization 2012) and represent the central death rates according to the underlying cause of death for 5 years' age-groups apart for the first two classes which are: 0 and 1—4, then 5—9, 10—14, up to 85—89 for a total of 19 classes. The central death rates are the number of deaths divided by the mid-year population. Mid-year population are used as an approximation to the exposure. The WHO database classifies the causes of death according to the International Classification of Diseases (ICD). The ICD changed three times between 1950 and 2010, from ICD-7 to ICD-10, in order to take into account changes in science and technology and to refine the classification. The ICD is revised periodically. The first draft of ICD-11 was expected in 2010, with publication following by 2014, but the deliverables have not been as ready as expected. Thus our data are related to the ICD-10 adaptation, due to the changes of the classification of the diseases over time.

11.4.2 Discussion of Results

In the present section, we introduce the results obtained by the application of the methodology described in Sect. 3. Different kinds of auxiliary tools are used in interpreting the results. We consider: Joint plots, Component scores and Core matrix elements. With the Joint plots, every pair of components (years and age group) are plotted together for each cause of death onto a factorial subspace. The Component scores allow to give particular attention to the years' score, useful to make forecasts. Finally, the Core matrix elements play almost the same role of singular values in the SVD, so its magnitude helps to understand the importance of each dimension.

In Fig. 11.1 are plotted the six k_t, one for each cause of death and the global one which is derived by the aggregate data. Their patterns are quite different and show idiosyncratic trends. For instance, *Infectious and parasitic cause* k_t trend (red line) shows a sudden decrease till to the end of 70's and then it is stable. However, it is higher than all other trends after 1992.

Peculiar patterns are showed by *Respiratory system* (Cyan line) which is lower in the 80's, and by *Other Causes* which shows some peaks in the same period.

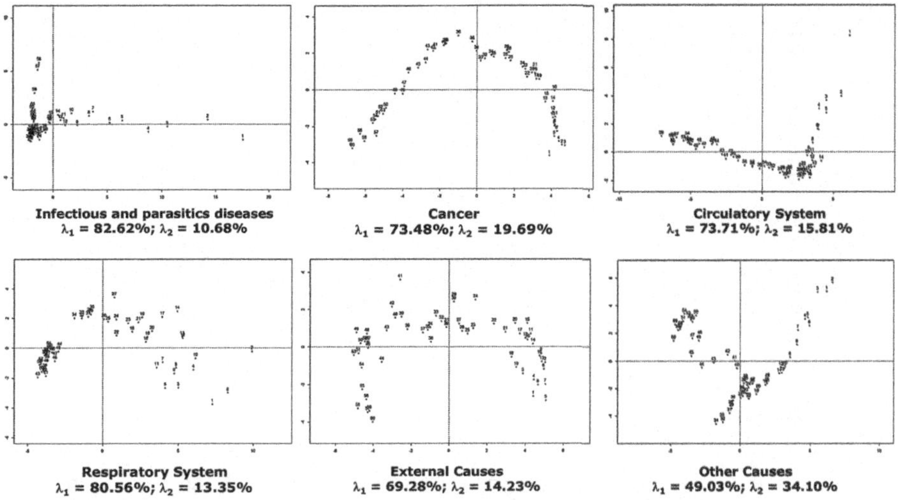

Fig. 11.2 PCA of mortality data table for each Causes of Death: Years Patterns – K_t on the first 2 components of PCA. Clockwise from the top-left: Infectious and parasitic disease, Cancer, Circulatory System, Respiratory system, External Causes, Other Causes

Table 11.1 The core component array

	Age1 × Causes1	Age2 × Causes1	Age1 × Causes2	Age2 × Causes2
Years 1	**0.67**	0.00	0	0.10
Years 2	0.00	0.00	0.16	0.00

This behavior shows as an aggregate estimate can hardly be representative for any causes of death.

An exploratory data analysis has been carried out by decomposing the six mortality tables thorough a Principal Component analysis of each of the 60 per 19 data tables. In Fig. 11.2 are plotted the first two principal components for each cause of death. The points represent the patterns of the k_t all along the 60 years. Once again they show to have very different patterns suggesting that also the analysis in two dimensions reveal the inconsistency of a unique trend extrapolated by aggregated data and just one component.

This lead us to the use of three-way data analysis, looking for a general trend which will be able to take into account all such peculiarities of the single causes of death.

The Tucker3 Analysis of the three-dimensional array (Years per Age-Groups per Causes of Death) give raise to a Core components explaining the 95.23% of the whole amount on variability in the data while retrieving the $2 \times 2 \times 2$ components.

Looking at the core components in Table 11.1 it is evident how the most important elements of the decomposition are the first two components along with

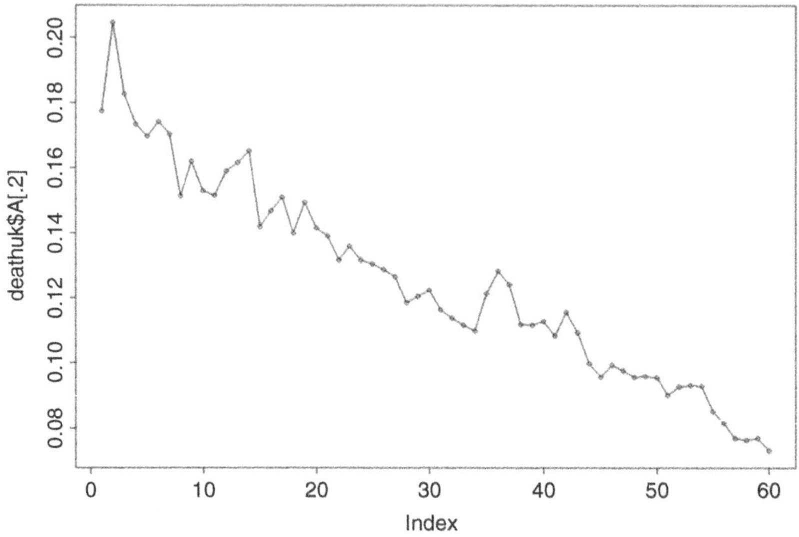

Fig. 11.3 Kt Plot of Tucker-3 model

Years and Causes. On the other side, only the first component of Age-group seems to be relevant. Each entry in the core matrix is used to explain the percentage of explained variance and the three-mode interaction measures.

Since our main interest is in exploring the *Years* component scores, we plot the the K_t first component along the time (Fig. 11.3) and then the first two components of the K_t (Fig. 11.4). Let us notice the peak at the observation index 33 (year 1982) in Fig. 11.3, which shows the perturbation already observed in the Other Causes Components plot (Fig. 11.2). Actually, in the two-dimensional plot it appears a break in the trend for the observation labeled from 1983 to 1992. This is the period already observed in Fig. 11.1 due to same irregularity in the individual patterns of the causes of death and now captured by the three-way model.

Finally, in Fig. 11.5 it is showed the Joint-plot of Causes of Death versus Age-groups. It is evident that the first Axis is correlated with the Age which increases from left to right, so opposing on the left side younger people characterized by External causes and Infectious and parasitic disease as causes of death. On the right side we notice the opposition of Circulatory system and Other causes, both of them are related to elderly people, but combining the information in Fig. 11.4 and in Fig. 11.5, we can now establish that Circulatory system as cause of death characterizes people died in more recent years.

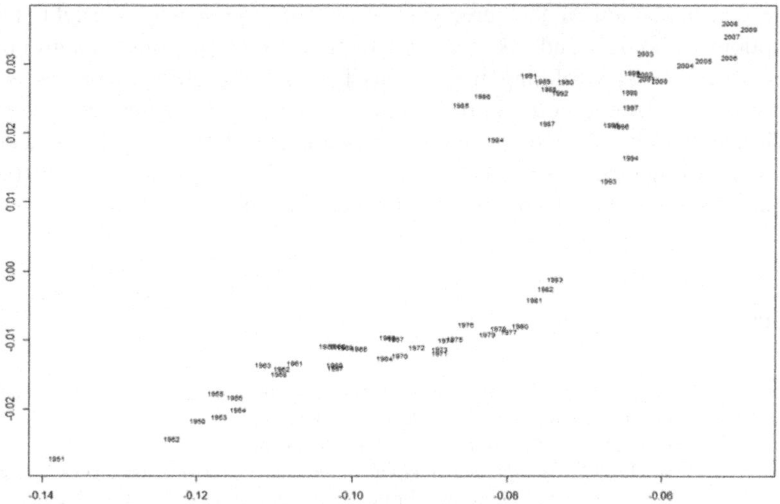

Fig. 11.4 Kt Plot of Tucker-3 model in two dimensions

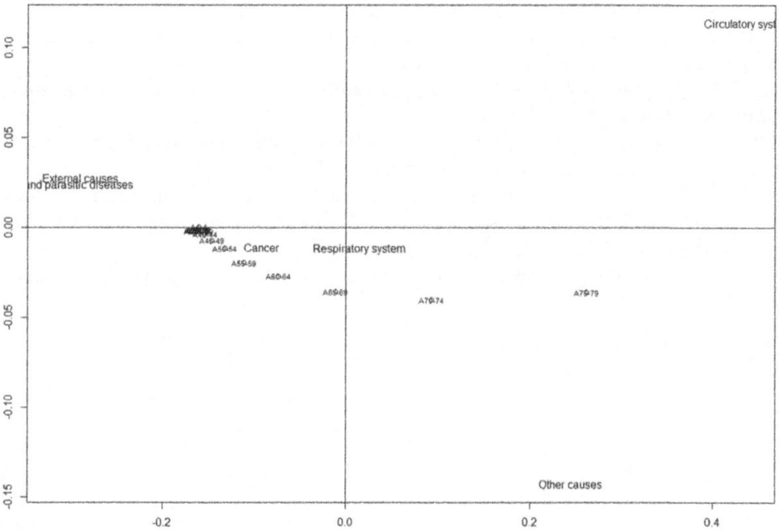

Fig. 11.5 Causes of death Vs/ age-groups

11.5 Conclusions

The LC-model has been extended in order to deal with disaggregated data. The factor we examined are the causes of death, since we wish to explore how different causes could lead to very different mortality patterns along with the years' trend.

The decomposition of the three-way array produces a major insight into the description of the data and about the interactions between years, age-groups and causes of death. By exploring interactions between the different modes we can produce more coherent mortality projections, specific for homogenous age-class or specific causes of death. Also, an aggregate estimate for k_t is derived as result of the three-way decomposition, so it is able to better indulge with idiosyncratic patterns of specific causes of death when they tend to show heterogeneous trends.

References

Gallop, A. (2008). *Mortality projections in the United Kingdom*. Paper presented to the Society of Actuaries Symposium *Living to 100 and Beyond*. Orlando, FL.

Gower, J. C., & Hand, D. J. (1996). *Biplots*. London: Chapman & Hall.

Kroonenberg, P. M. (1983). *Three-mode principal component analysis*. Leiden: DSWO Press.

Kroonenberg, P. M., & De Leeuw, J. (1980). Principal component analysis of three-mode data by means of alternating least squares algorithms. *Psychometrika, 45*, 69–97.

Kroonenberg, P. M., Murakami, T., & Coebergh, J. W. (2002). Added value of three-way methods for the analysis of mortality trends illustrated with worldwide female cancer mortality (1968–1985). *Statistical Methods in Medical Research, 11*(3), 275–292.

Lee, R. D., & Carter, L. R. (1992). Modelling and forecasting U.S. mortality. *Journal of the American Statistical Association, 87*, 659–671.

Ridsdale, & Gallop. (2010). *Mortality by cause of death and by socio-economic and demographic stratification, ICA2010*.

Russolillo, M., Giordano, G., & Haberman, S. (2011). Extending the Lee-Carter model: A three-way decomposition. *Scandinavian Actuarial Journal, 2*, 96–117.

Tucker, L. R. (1964). The extension of factor analysis to three-dimensional matrices. In N. Frederiksen & H. Gulliksen (Eds.), *Contributions to mathematical psychology* (pp. 110–182). New York: Holt, Rinehart & Winston.

Tucker, L. R. (1966). Some mathematical notes on three-mode factor analysis. *Psychometrika, 31*, 279–311.

Part IV
Stochastic and Neuro-Fuzzy Methods

Chapter 12
Measuring Latent Variables in Space and/or Time: A Gender Statistics Exercise

Gaia Bertarelli, Franca Crippa, and Fulvia Mecatti

12.1 Introduction

Composite indicators have the advantage of synthesizing a latent, multidimensional construct in a single number, usually included in the interval (0; 1). They can be derived as a weighted sum of simple indexes, as it is often the case in social statistics, specially when the set of indexes needs to stay unchanged in several geographic areas and/or time periods. In complex settings, the synthetic indicator is conceivable as a latent variable, typically estimated applying Structural Equation Models (SEM) in order to obtain a single measure.

When the latent variable is thought to have a time and-or space dynamic of its own, Multivariate Latent Markov Models (LMMs) may represent a valuable innovation to the construction of composite indicators. LMMs are a particular class of statistical models for the analysis of longitudinal data which assume the existence of a latent process affecting the distribution of the response variables (see Bartolucci et al. (2007); Zucchini and MacDonald (2009) for a general review). The rationale of this methodology considers the latent process as fully explained by the observable behaviour of some items, together with available covariates. The main assumption is conditional independence of the response variables given the latent process, which

G. Bertarelli (✉)
University of Perugia, Perugia, Italy
e-mail: gaia.bertarelli@unipg.it

F. Crippa · F. Mecatti
University of Milano-Bicocca, Milan, Italy
e-mail: franca.crippa@unimib.it; fulvia.mecatti@unimib.it

© Springer International Publishing AG, part of Springer Nature 2018
C. H. Skiadas, C. Skiadas (eds.), *Demography and Health Issues*,
The Springer Series on Demographic Methods and Population Analysis 46,
https://doi.org/10.1007/978-3-319-76002-5_12

follow a first order discrete Markov chain with a finite number of states. The model is composed of two parts, analogously to SEM: the measurement model, concerning the conditional distribution of the response variables given the latent process, and the latent model, pertaining the distribution of the latent process. LMMs can account for measurement errors or unobserved heterogeneity between areas in the analysis. LMMs main advantage is that the unobservable variable is allowed to have its own dynamics and it is not constrained to be time constant. In addition, when the latent states are identified as different subpopulations, LMMs can identify a latent clustering of the population of interest, with areas in the same subpopulation having a common distribution for the response variables. Un-der this respect, a LMM may be seen as an extension of the latent class (LC) model, in which areas are allowed to move between the latent classes during the observational period. Available covariates can be included in the latent model and then they may affect the initial and transition probabilities of the Markov chain. When covariates are included in the measurement model, the latent variables are used to account for the unobserved heterogeneity and the main interest is on a latent variable which is measured through the observable response variables (e.g., health status or gender inequalities) and on the evaluation of this latent variable depending on covariates. We focus on an extended model of the second type, as we are interested in ordinal latent states.

Very recently, Markov models for latent variables have contributed to in-depth investigations in highly specific and therefore narrow topics [?]. Extensive analyses of LMMs, both methodological and applicative, have been performed in the case of small area estimation, taking also into account several points in time (Bertarelli 2015). Our viewpoint aims to adjust the LMMs approach to a wider area of synthetic social indicators in different geographical areas and in time, namely for national gender gap between countries. Gender statistics are de ned as statistics that adequately reflect differences and inequalities in the situation of women and men in all areas of life (United Nation n.d.). Composite gender indicators are usually computed as weighted sum of simple indexes reflecting the multidimensionality of the phenomena and they are periodically released by supranational agencies (see for instance (Mecatti et al. 2012) for a comparative review).

We focus on gender gap as the latent status, since this construct is actually a latent trait, measurable only indirectly through a collection of observable variables and indicators purposively selected as micro-aspects that contribute to the latent macrodimension, aiming to add sensitiveness and discrimination power with respect to current indicators.

12.2 The Proposed Model

In this paper we use an extension of LMM proposed by Bertarelli (2015). The existence of two process is assumed: an observed process ca be expressed as:

$$Y_{jit},\ j = 1, \ldots, J,\ i = 1, \ldots, n \text{ and } t = 1, \ldots, T \tag{12.1}$$

where Y_{itj} denote the response variable j for unit i at time t, and an unobservable finite-state first-order Markov Chain

$$U_{it},\ i = 1, \ldots, n \text{ and } t = 1, \ldots, T \text{ with state space } \{1, \ldots, m\}. \tag{12.2}$$

We assume that the distribution of Y_{jit} depends only on U_{it}; specifically the Y_{jit} are conditionally independent given U_{it}.

We also denote by $\tilde{U}_{it} = \{U_{jt}, j \in \mathcal{G}\rangle\}$, where $_i$ is the set of the neighbours, the latent states realisations in the neighborhood units.

In the measurement model we consider two Gaussian state-dependent distributions:

$$\begin{array}{l} Y_{1it} \mid U_{it} \tilde{} N(\mu_1, \nu_1), \\ Y_{2it} \mid U_{it} \tilde{} N(\mu_2, \nu_2). \end{array} \tag{12.3}$$

The set of parameters of the structural model, corresponding to the latent Markov chain, includes the vector of initial probabilities

$$\pi = (\pi_1, \ldots, \pi_u, \ldots, \pi_m)', \tag{12.4}$$

where

$$\pi_u = P(U_{i1} = u)$$

is the probability of being in state u at the initial time for u = 1;:::; m and the elements of the transition probability matrix

$$\boldsymbol{\Pi} = \{\pi_{u|\bar{u}}, \bar{u}, u = 1, \ldots, m\}, \tag{12.5}$$

where

$$\pi_{u|\bar{u}} = P\left(U_{it} = u | U_{i,t-1} = \bar{u}\right)$$

is the probability that unit i visits state u at time t given that at time t 1 it was in state $\bar{u}$.

Considering spatial dependence is a crucial point in our field of application (Fisher and Naidoo 2016). As in (Bertarelli 2015), we propose to handle spatial dependence introducing a covariate in the structural model based on the information from a neighboring matrix and depending on the latent structure itself. In this way, the influence of spatial structure depends on the latent process, therefore it is not fixed during the observation period.

For each unit i we know the number of neighbouring units, g_i and their corresponding labels which are collected in the sets G_i. Let $\tilde{U}_{it}$ be the vector of latent states at occasion t for the neighbours of unit i. We suppose to handle ordinal latent states in order to model the severity of the gender gap. Let us consider a function ( ) that maps the g_i-dimensional vector $\tilde{U}_{it}$ onto a d-dimensional covariate, the choice of depending on the nature of latent states (ordinal or not). Due to our application context, we decide to work with the mean of neighbourhood latent states. Then, this time-varying covariate affects the initial and transition probabilities through the following multinomial logit parametrization:

$$\log \frac{p(U_{i1} = u | \tilde{U}_{i1} = \tilde{u}_{i1})}{p(U_{i1} = 1 | \tilde{U}_{i1} = \tilde{u}_{i1})} = \beta_{0u} + \eta(\tilde{u}_{i1})' \beta_{1u} \quad \text{for} \quad u \geq 2, \tag{12.6}$$

$$\log \frac{p(U_{it} = u | U_{i,t-1} = \bar{u}, \tilde{U}_{it} = \tilde{u}_{it})}{p(U_{it} = \bar{u} | U_{i,t-1} = \bar{u}, \tilde{U}_{it} = \tilde{u}_{it})} = \gamma_{0u\bar{u}} + \eta(\tilde{u}_{it})' \gamma_{1u\bar{u}}, \quad \text{for } t \geq 2 \text{ and } u \neq \bar{u}, \tag{12.7}$$

where $\beta_u = (\beta_{0u}, \beta'_{1u})'$ and $\gamma_{u\bar{u}} = (\gamma_{0u\bar{u}}, \gamma'_{1u\bar{u}})'$ are vectors of parameters to be estimated. An individual covariate has been introduced, accordingly both the assumptions of local independence and of a first order latent process still hold.

12.3 Estimation and Inference

To estimate the proposed model we adopt the principle of data augmentation Tanner et al. (Tanner and Wong 1987) in which the latent states are introduced as missing data and augmented to the state of the sampler (Germain 2010). In this way we can simplify the process of sampling from the posterior distribution: we can use a Gibbs sampler for the parameters of the measurement model and we can estimate the initial and the transition probabilities by means of a Random Walk Metropolis-Hastings step. We then need to introduce a system of priors for the unknown model parameters. In particular, a system of Dirichlet priors is set on the initial and on the transition probabilities, while for the vectors β_u and $\gamma_{u\bar{u}}$ we assume that they are a priori independent with distribution $N(0, \sigma_\beta^2 \mathrm{I})$ and $N(0, \sigma_\gamma^2 \mathrm{I})$, respectively. The choice for σ_β^2 and σ_γ^2 depends on the context of the application, typically $5 \leq \sigma_\beta^2 = \sigma_\gamma^2 \leq 10$. The prior distribution for the parameters of the measurement model depends on the distribution assumed for the state-dependent distribution. We choose a Gaussian distribution for the priors of μ_1 and μ_2 and inverse gamma distributions for the variances ν_1 and ν_2.

The choice of the number of latent states of the unobserved Markov chain, underlying the observed data, is part of the model selection procedure and is a very important step of the estimation process. We adopt the Bayesian information criterion (BIC) (Schwarz 1978) among a restricted set of models (m = 3; 4; 5).

12.4 LMMs Composite Indicators. A Gender Statistics Exercise

Gender inequality – both in space and time – is indirectly measurable through a collection of observable variables. Gender composite indicators are commonly constructed as statistics indicators, i.e. linear combinations of a collection of simple indexes, such as means and proportions, which represent observable items, aggregated by means of a weighing system. The choice of both indexes and weight introduce a certain level of arbitrariness. Their case-specific technical limitations (Mecatti et al. 2012; Permanyer 2010) often lead to internal inconsistency since the ranking of a single country can vary in relation to the indicator considered. Moreover, few simple indexes, as well as the weighing system, can outweigh the overall results.

LMMs is liable to offer a sound methodology for estimating the latent trait, i.e. the gender gap, in time and in space, resulting in a synthetic indicator. We move from existing source, namely from supranational official statistics, providing different indicators for all nations worldwide. In particular, we take into account the Gender Inequality Index (GII) (United Nations Development Programme 2016) and the Global Gender Gap Index (GGGI) (World Economic Forum 2015). The GII was introduced by UNDP in 2010 and it measures gender inequalities in three aspects of human development: reproductive health, empowerment and economic status. It focus on inequality, therefore a balanced women/man situation is represented by a zero value. The Global Gender Gap Index (GGGI)was introduced by the World Economic Forum in 2006 with the aim of capturing the magnitude of gender-based disparities. It comprises four dimensions: economic participation and opportunity, educational attainment, health and survival, political empowerment. Perfect parity leads to the value 1. Our applicative viewpoint intends to adapt the LMM approach to Gender synthetic index. Gender Inequality Index (GII) and Global Gender Gap Index (GGGI) are composite indicators which aim to capture differences between man and woman in several areas of life. In our case, we focus on gender gap as the latent status, both in space and time. The gap is in fact a latent trait, namely only indirectly measurable through a collection of observable variables and indicators purposively selected as micro-aspects contributing to the latent macro-dimension. To make the interpretation of results easier and more accessible to non-statisticians, we transformed the value of $\beta_u = (\beta_{0u}, \beta'_{1u})'$ and $\gamma_{u\bar{u}} = (\gamma_{0u\bar{u}}, \gamma'_{1u\bar{u}})'$ in order to obtain an unique set of initial and transition probabilities for all the countries and time occasion. That is, our values represent a cross-national, inter-temporal synthesis.

Applying LMMs to n = 30 European countries, with respect to T = 6 time points (from 2010 to 2015), we investigate the unobservable latent gender gap summarizing the GGGI and GII information in a single value and rearranging two distinct and rather different ranking into a single one, as the multivariate latent Markov model identities latent statuses of countries. According to the nature of the proposed indicator, we consider the unit complementary of GGI. The model selects k = 4 latent states, allowing us to organize countries in 4 ordinal latent statuses through the proposed multivariate spatial Latent Markov model with multinomial logit parametrization, where 1 reflects a situation relatively closest to equality and 4 denotes the highest level of Gender Gap severity. The vector of estimated initial probabilities of latent states at the first measurement occasion is

$$\pi = (0.212, 0.483, 0.139, 0.167).$$

These values can be interpreted as sort of relative frequency (Bartholomew 1973) in the first year of observation. On the whole, European countries under consideration are more likely to be in latent status 1 and 2, with a relatively low gender gap, with initial probability status of 0.212 and 0.483 respectively. The higher imparity condition, present in status 3 and 4 is less common, accounting for slightly more than 20%, i.e. 0.139 and 0.167 jointly considered.

The Transition Probabilities matrix for geographical areas is the following, where the identified latent status are denoted S1 S4

	to S1	to S2	to S3	to S4
from S1	0.98	0.02	0	0
from S2	0.1	0.9	0	0
from S3	0	0.14	0.85	0.01
from S4	0	0.3	0.2	0.4

(12.8)

It is noticeable that we obtained a matrix close to diagonality, with more sub-diagonal elements than over-diagonal. Such a matrix implies that on the whole countries did not undergo relevant changes in the ten-year observational periods. Probabilities of improving or worsening with respect to the gender gap are low, except for latent status 4, whose diagonal value is equal to 0.4, meaning that 60% or countries improved their gender gap since 2010. When moving, it is often to a better condition, the probability of joining a worse latent status being limited to the shift from latent status 1–2, with probability 0.02, and from latent status 2 to 3, with probability 0.02. This reflects, on the one side, a relatively high starting point in gender equality, under the constitutional rights perspective and under aspects such as educational opportunities. On the other side, in so called developed countries, gender disparities tend to stay, when not to worsen, even in the most advanced countries. To this respect, some remarks can be posed on the basis of spacial results.

Figure 12.1 shows the geography of latent gap in Europe in 2010 and 2015 (at the beginning and at the end of the observational time period we considered for our exercise). The 4 latent statuses identified by our models are represented in darkening shades of gray from status S1 to S4, meaning a worsened gender gap situation.

In 2010 we obtain the following distribution: (i) Latent status 4: Bulgaria, Greece, Hungary, Italy, Malta, Turkey; (ii) Latent status 3: Ireland, Romania, Spain; (iii) Latent status 2: Austria, Cyprus, Croatia, Czech Republic, Germany, Estonia, France, Latvia, Lithuania, Luxembourg, Poland, Portugal, Slovenia; (iv) Latent status 1: Belgium, Finland, Island, Netherlands, Norway, Sweden, Switzerland, United Kingdom.

Fig. 12.1 Latent Gender Gap Classification in 2010 and 2015

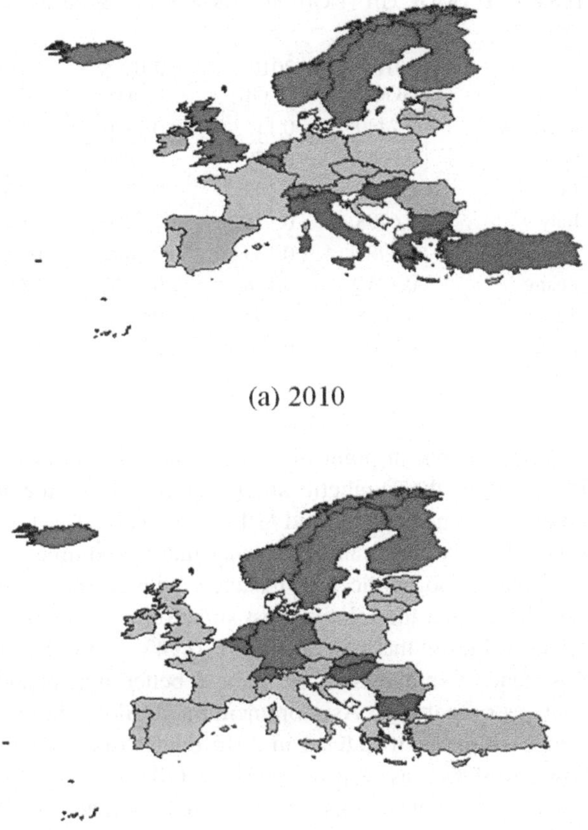

(a) 2010

(b) 2015

Despite the almost diagonal transition matrix, some changes in latent status structure are highlighted in 2015: (i) Latent status 4: Bulgaria, Hungary, Malta; (ii) Latent status 3: Romania, Turkey; (iii) Latent status 2: Austria, Cyprus, Croatia, Czech Republic, Estonia, France, Greece, Ireland, Italy, Latvia, Lithuania, Luxembourg, Poland, Portugal, Spain, United Kingdom; (iv) Latent status 1: Belgium, Finland, Germany, Island, Netherlands, Nor-way, Slovenia, Sweden, Swiss.

Latent status 2 becomes the most crowded. The ten-year span appears to have allowed some countries, like Italy, Greece, Spain, to narrow the gap especially in the educational and, to a lesser extent, in political representation. In the case of Slovenia, the upward shift was impressive. The downward shift experimented by the United Kingdom seems to reflect a general trend in economic conditions that cuts across all European countries, even the ones that are regarded as the most socially fair, like Norway, for instance. The overall change in time signals this aspect in a more concise and sharp form by the transition matrix in time, as discussed below.

Table 12.1 GGGI, GII (1-GII) and latent status for countries with an upward shift in ordinal clustering

Country	2010 GGGI	2010 (1-GII)	2015 GGGI	2015 (1-GII)	2010 status	2015 status
Germany	0,7449	0,117	0,7790	0,073	2	1
Greece	0,6662	0,179	0,6850	0,121	4	2
Ireland	0,7597	0,192	0,8070	0,135	3	2
Italy	0,6798	0,175	0,7260	0,085	4	2
Slovenia	0,6982	0,139	0,7840	0,057	x	1
Spain	0,7345	0,118	0,7420	0,087	3	2
Turkey	0,5828	0,564	0,6240	0,340	4	3
United Kingdom	0,7402	0,206	0,7580	0,149	1	2

Under a spacial point of view, then, a first relevant LMMs contribution can be identified in the synthetic single ranking from the information in two different preexisting ones, GGGI and GII respectively. The LMMs ranking establishes relations of equivalence and order that make a complex situation more accessible and readable to the public. For instance, with reference to 2015, the first latent status establishes that the relative best situation in terms of gender parity is reached with GGGI values in the interval [0:861; 0:947] and GII values in [0:044; 0:076]. Within this general framework, we gain a better understanding of individual countries changes or stability. As aforementioned, Slovenia up-ward shift from latent status 2 in 2010 to latent status 1 in 2015 relates to a remarkable increase in GGGI, from 0.698 to 0.874, as well as in GII (1-GII), from 0.139 to 0.057. Table 12.1 shows values for countries that changed their ordinal clustering ranking in the five-year period.

Official statistics provide the two measure annually. With reference to time latent states, LMMs estimation showed an overall stability of the gender gap in the observational time, since the indicators transitional matrix (8) is almost diagonal. On the first hand, the widespread, general access to education and health has been experimented with different times and speed. Therefore, at the initial time point of our investigation (2010) some countries see slower, if not almost nonexistent, progress rates after 2010. On the other hand, (1-GII) has being decreasing far more slowly since 2010 not only in countries with a longer record of high GII values, like Switzerland, but also for countries that reached these goals more recently, like Greece. Furthermore, GGGI trend is generally very modest (g.2) and it has often come to a halt after 2008 in a specific dimension, Economic Opportunity and Political Empowerment, as signaled by the World Economic Forum's Global Gender Gap Report 2016, that states that the gap in the economic pillar is currently larger since 2008 (World Economic Forum 2016). Besides the disparities in opportunities and salary, a major critical issue is posed by the perspective need for women to acquire Stem (Science, Technology, Engineering and Mathematics) skills, with several implications for everyday social and personal lives (Fig. 12.2).

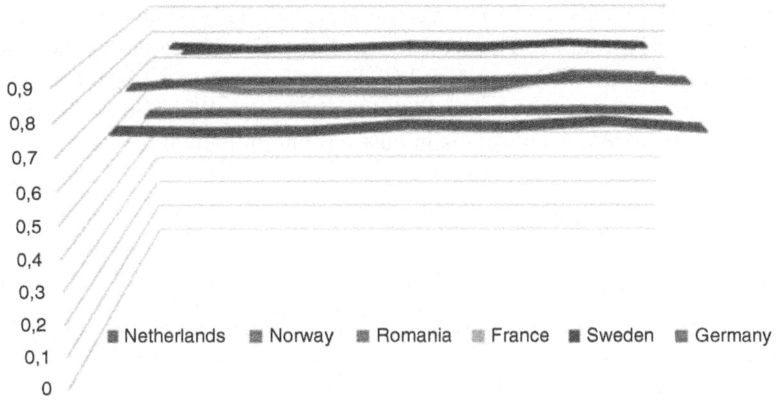

Fig. 12.2 GGGI trend from 2010 to 2016 in some European countries

12.5 Conclusion

LMMS have been recently applied to estimate latent traits in time and/or space in social sciences, mainly to highly specific research areas that did not respond adequately to other techniques. Adapting the model in (Bertarelli 2015) to a wider context of social sciences, our proposal consist in the application of LMMS to a more extensive and explored field, Gender Statistics. By means of an empirical exercise, we showed how these models can provide a relevant contribution, since they produced a latent ordinal classification of gender gap between 30 European countries from 2010 to 2015 using two different social composite indicators. They allowed us to obtain synthetic information from the transition matrix that, when diagonal, expresses absence of change. In our exercise, the matrix was nearly diagonal, with reduced margins of improvement for several countries and in time, especially in the economic sector.

Given the complexity and the multidimensionality of social phenomena, LMMs can contribute highly to a unitarian view. Their latent approach, both in space and in time, can summarise information from different sources. As a matter of fact, both space and time components proved valuable in our application. As far as the former component is concerned, LMMs allowed to identify at a glance areas that are homogeneous or different with respect to gender equality and, in case of differences, permitted to set and order of such a divergence. With respect to the time component, LMMS returned a valuable, concise measure the trend to stagnation that gender parity is experimenting in western countries, due to the rigidness of the economic sector, in particular of the labour market. These models provided also information of national changes in time, i.e. if, how fast and how well some countries were able to set women and men more equal.

Further developments can focus on covariates, especially when expressing opportunities in everyday routines. The persistence of disparities in economic treatment, in fact, can rarely be attributed to explicit law discriminations in western countries, but they can be more often retrieved in availability and in simplification of services to the person and to parenthood, as well as in customs and in mental habits.

References

Bartholomew, D. J. (1973). *Stochastic models for social processes* (2nd ed.). New York: Wiley.

Bartolucci, F., Pennoni, F., & Francis, B. (2007). A latent Markov model for detecting patterns of criminal activity. *Journal of the Royal Statistical Society, Series A, 170*, 151–132.

Bertarelli, G. (2015). *Latent Markov models for aggregate data: application to dis-ease mapping and small area estimation*. Ph.D thesis. https://boa.unimib.it/handle/10281/96252

Fisher, B., & Naidoo, R. (2016). The geography of gender inequality. *PlosOne, 11*(3), 0145778.

Germain, S. H. (2010). *Bayesian spatio-temporal modelling of rainfall through non-homogenous hidden Markov models*. PhD thesis, University of Newcastle Upon Tyne.

Mecatti, F., Crippa, F., & Farina, P. (2012). A special gen(d)re of statistics: Roots, develop-ment and methodological prospects of gender statistics. *International Statistical Review, 80*(3), 452–467.

Permanyer, I. (2010). The measurement of multidimensional gender inequality: Continuing the debate. *Social Indicators Research, 95*(2), 181–198.

Schwarz, G. E. (1978). Estimating the dimension of a model. *Annals of Statistics, 6*(2), 461–464.

Tanner, M. A., & Wong, W. H. (1987). The calculation of posterior distributions by data augmentation. *Journal of the American Statistical Association, 82*, 528–540.

United Nation. What are gender statistics? http://unstats.un.org/unsd/genderstatmanual/What-are-gender-stats.ashx

United Nations Development Programme. (2016). Human development reports. http://hdr.undp.org/en/content/gender-inequality-index-gii/

World Economic Forum. (2015). The global gender index. https://www.weforum.org

World Economic Forum. (2016). The global gender gap report 2016. http://reports.weforum.org/global-gender-gap-report-2016/

Zucchini, W., & MacDonald, I. (2009). *Hidden Markov models for time series*. New York: Springer.

Chapter 13
Stochastic Distance Between Burkitt Lymphoma/Leukemia Strains

Jesús E. García, R. Gholizadeh, and V. A. González López

13.1 Introduction

The Burkitt lymphoma occurs when the chromosome 8 (locus of gene MYC) is broken, which produces a change in the cellular proliferation. The data used in this paper corresponds to the most frequent variant, produced by the translocation between chromosomes 8 and 14. It is known, so far, three variants of Burkitt lymphoma, which are (i) endemic, (ii) sporadic, (iii) produced by immunodeficiency. The first case is observed in children in Equatorial Africa and it is associated with chronic Malaria infections. It does not exist until the moment and according to what we know, a clear notion of the profile of the Burkitt lymphoma's DNA. Considering that it is natural to expect diversity between DNA strains, we will measure the distance between 15 of them. We adopt a distance between the strains which is conditioned to each possible common string s, where s is an element of the state space. That is, suppose that $x_{1,1}^{n_1}$ and $x_{2,1}^{n_2}$ are the concatenations of elements a, c, g and t of the DNA of two patients, say 1 and 2, $d_s(1, 2)$ will be the distance between the sequences in relation to s some string of interest, for instance $s =$ aggc. As there are a variety of possible strings, which we should observe to measure the discrepancy between the strains, we will compute the maximum of all: $\max_s\{d_s(1, 2)\}$, so as to focus on the most extreme situation among them. This notion allows to identify which of these strings can be considered more distant of the majority, and allows us to select the strains which will be used to define the profile of the DNA. To strengthen our conclusions, we compared the model constructed with the selected

J. E. García (✉) · V. A. González López
Department of Statistics, University of Campinas, Campinas, Brazil
e-mail: jg@ime.unicamp.br; veronica@ime.unicamp.br

R. Gholizadeh
University of Campinas, Campinas, Brazil

© Springer International Publishing AG, part of Springer Nature 2018
C. H. Skiadas, C. Skiadas (eds.), *Demography and Health Issues*,
The Springer Series on Demographic Methods and Population Analysis 46,
https://doi.org/10.1007/978-3-319-76002-5_13

strains with the model constructed using the 15 available strains. This work is organized as follows, first we introduce the notion of distance as well as the general notation. Then we will describe the strains of the 15 patients, we will inform their source. In the results we show the values calculated for the maximum distance between strains two to two. We also show the model induced by this strategy.

13.2 Criteria

Let (X_t) be a discrete time (order $o < \infty$) Markov chain on a finite alphabet A. Let us call $\mathcal{S} = A^o$ the state space and denote the string $a_m a_{m+1} \ldots a_n$ by a_m^n, where $a_i \in A$, $m \leq i \leq n$. For each $a \in A$ and $s \in \mathcal{S}$, $P(a|s) = \text{Prob}\left(X_t = a | X_{t-M}^{t-1} = s\right)$. In a given sample x_1^n, coming from the stochastic process, the number of occurrences of s in the sample x_1^n is denoted by $N_n(s)$ and the number of occurrences of s followed by a in the sample x_1^n is denoted by $N_n(s, a)$. In this way $\frac{N_n(s,a)}{N_n(s)}$ is the estimator of $P(a|s)$. In the next paragraph, we give the notion of distance between two processes.

Definition 1 Consider two Markov chains $(X_{1,t})$ and $(X_{2,t})$ of order o, with finite alphabet A and state space $\mathcal{S} = A^o$. With sample $x_{k,1}^{nk}$, for $k = 1, 2$ respectively; for any $s \in \mathcal{S}$,

$$d_s(1,2) = \frac{\alpha}{(|A|-1)\ln(n_1+n_2)} \sum_{a \in A} \left\{ N_{n_1}(s,a) \ln\left(\frac{N_{n_1}(s,a)}{N_{n_1}(s)}\right) + N_{n_2}(s,a) \ln\left(\frac{N_{n_2}(s,a)}{N_{n_2}(s)}\right) - N_{n_1+n_2}(s,a) \ln\left(\frac{N_{n_1+n_2}(s,a)}{N_{n_1+n_2}(s)}\right) \right\}$$

with $N_{n_1+n_2}(s,a) = N_{n_1}(s,a) + N_{n_2}(s,a), N_{n_1+n_2}(s) = N_{n_1}(s) + N_{n_2}(s)$, where N_{n_1} and N_{n_2} are given as usual, computed from the samples $x_{1,1}^{n_1}$ and $x_{2,1}^{n_2}$ respectively, with α real and positive value. In this paper we use $\alpha = 2$, see García and González-López (2017).

The most relevant properties of d are listed below. Both properties are consequence of results derived from concepts introduced in García and González-López (2017):

(i) The function $d_s(1, 2)$ is a distance between the Markov chains relative to the specific string $s \in \mathcal{S}$. If $(X_{i,t})$, $i = 1, 2, 3$ are Markov chains under the assumptions of definition 1, with samples $x_{1,1}^{n_1}$, $i = 1, 2, 3$ respectively,

Table 13.1 Sample sizes n of DNA sequences coming from 15 patients with Burkitt lymphoma/leukemia, AM2871z.1; where z = 39, 40, 41, 46, 50, 52, 57, 58, 59, 61, 62, 65, 76, 81, 87

z	39	40	41	46	50	52	57	
n	3641	2965	4464	2731	5428	2475	3907	
z	58	59	61	62	65	76	81	87
n	3636	4291	2642	3206	2906	2635	3608	3734

$$d_s(1,2) \geq 0 \,\text{with equality} \Leftrightarrow \frac{N_{n_1}(s,a)}{N_{n_1}(s)} = \frac{N_{n_2}(s,a)}{N_{n_2}(s)} \forall a \in A,$$
$$d_s(1,2) = d_s(2,1),$$
$$d_s(1,2) \leq d_s(1,3) + d_s(3,2).$$

(ii) Local behavior of stochastic laws. If the stochastic laws of $(X_{i,\,t})$, $i = 1, 2$ in s are the same, then $d_s(1,2) \underset{\min(n_1,\vec{n_2})\to\infty}{} 0$. Otherwise $d_s(1,2) \underset{\min(n_1,\vec{n_2})\to\infty}{} \infty$.

13.3 DNA Data

The database is composed by 15 DNA sequences, available in the repository: https://www.ncbi.nlm.nih.gov/nuccore/, coming from 15 patients with Burkitt lymphoma/leukemia carrying the t(8;14)(q24;q32) with IgH-MYC fusion, breakpoint in the joining region. The registers (genbank numbers) of the sequences are: AM2871z.1, where z = 39, 40, 41, 46, 50, 52, 57, 58, 59, 61, 62, 65, 76, 81, 87. For each sequence, the concatenation of bases a,c,g,t observed in the code is the realization denoted by x_1^n. The size of each sequence is shown in Table 13.1.

13.4 Results

In Tables 13.2 and 13.3 we expose the dmax values between the DNA sequences, where $dmax(i,j) = \max_{s \in S}\{d_s(i,j)\}$, $i \neq j$, i, j = AM2871z.1 with z = 39, 40, 41, 46, 50, 52, 57, 58, 59, 61, 62, 65, 76, 81, 87. At the end of each column we record the sum of the dmax values that is:

$$S(i) = \sum_j dmax(i,j), \text{for each sequence}\, i = \text{AM2871}z.1,$$

where z = 39, 40, 41, 46, 50, 52, 57, 58, 59, 61, 62, 65, 76, 81, 87. Through d_s we have a criterion to rescue the greatest distance between two DNA sequences. From

Table 13.2 *dmax*(i, j) values, $i \neq j$, $i, j =$ AM2871z.1 where $z = 39, 40, 41, 46, 50, 52, 57, 58, 59, 61, 62, 65, 76, 81, 87$

$j \backslash i$	39	40	41	46	50	52	57
40	0.23625						
41	0.16160	0.25648					
46	0.22578	0.24031	0.21857				
50	0.20218	0.25847	0.17855	0.22644			
52	0.19479	0.17870	0.21143	0.16253	0.33231		
57	0.09777	0.24533	0.13885	0.22058	0.12481	0.19363	
58	0.27729	0.21783	0.30105	0.25156	0.28312	0.23041	0.25738
59	0.12485	0.32050	0.09723	0.24232	0.15545	0.21165	0.09821
61	0.20229	0.10170	0.22626	0.20598	0.30120	0.12572	0.25328
62	0.32556	0.34309	0.35858	0.26633	0.47720	0.24569	0.32362
65	0.22234	0.15183	0.26545	0.15812	0.25339	0.29264	0.27469
76	0.19421	0.24629	0.20804	0.12923	0.23960	0.12786	0.19308
81	0.16363	0.17050	0.19272	0.16614	0.22817	0.17392	0.12994
87	0.26047	0.16796	0.24704	0.25130	0.41112	0.26425	0.22481
$S(i)$	2.8890	3.13523	3.06186	2.96519	3.67203	2.94553	2.77597

Table 13.3 *dmax*(i, j) values, $i \neq j$, $i, j =$ AM2871z.1, where $z = 39, 40, 41, 46, 50, 52, 57, 58, 59, 61, 62, 65, 76, 81, 87$. In bold the lowest value of S, associated to the sequence with $z = 81$

$j \backslash i$	58	59	61	62	65	76	81	87
59	0.30177							
61	0.20284	0.32032						
62	0.27748	0.34112	0.25478					
65	0.25707	0.27412	0.21689	0.30528				
76	0.13397	0.21109	0.13318	0.27990	0.21237			
81	0.25801	0.14463	0.11904	0.23329	0.21155	0.15334		
87	0.23089	0.24762	0.20658	0.37764	0.20689	0.23144	0.19405	
$S(i)$	3.48067	3.09091	2.87007	4.40955	3.30265	2.69363	**2.53891**	3.52205

the magnitudes found, we can affirm that the processes can be considered as coming from the same stochastic law, dmax <1. We also verified the above statement from the dendrograms constructed using the values recorded in Tables 13.2 and 13.3, see Fig. 13.1.

13.4.1 The DNA Profile

The model we will apply in the data is extensively investigated in García and González-López (2017). This is the most general model known to be used in finite order Markov chains on a finite alphabet, since this model includes fixed order Markov chains and the variable length Markov chains (VLMC). Essentially what

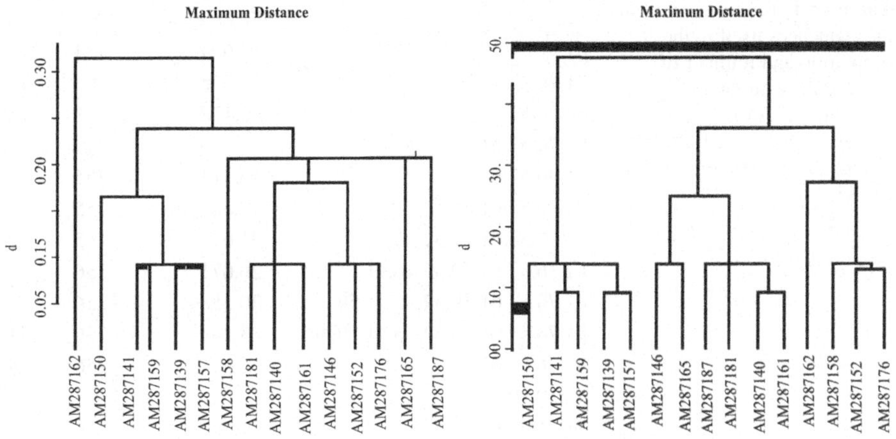

Fig. 13.1 Dendrograms build through the dmax values (Tables 13.2–13.3), agglomeration method: Average, on the left and Complete, on the right

this model proposes is to estimate the transition probabilities that describe the process by identifying a partition $\mathcal{L} = \{L_1, \ldots, L_{|\mathcal{L}|}\}$ in the state space S. The state space is divided into parts L_i, $i = 1, \ldots, |\mathcal{L}|$ which constitute a partition. The strings of each part have in common the characteristic of sharing the same transition probability to any element of the alphabet. In practice, all strings included in the same part of that partition will be used for the computation of the transition probability that identities them. The identification of such partition is done using the Bayesian Information Criterion (BIC), which also is the basis to the concept d_s, previously introduced.

Table 13.4 shows some general characteristics that are observed in the adjustment of the model introduced in García and González-López (2017). We include progressively (from top to bottom) the closest sequences, according to the criterion S. That is, first using the sequence 81, second, using two sequences: 81 and 61 and so on. In other words, we are increasing the sample size from one stage to the next, following as inclusion criterion the magnitude of S. We can not state unequivocally that by increasing the sample sizes we increase the parts of the estimated partition, but it seems to be a trend, as seen in the Table 13.4. But this could also be the result of incorporating in the model gradually the more distant sequences according to criterion S. We apply in all the adjustments the agglomerative method, whose performance is analyzed in García and Gonzalez-Lopez (2017), the memory used in all the adjustments is equal to $4 = \lfloor \log_{|A|}(2475) \rfloor - 1$, with alphabet $A = \{a, c, g, t\}$ where 2475 is the smallest sample size reported in Table 13.1.

We describe in a comparative way the results when applying the model in: (i) the 7 closest sequences according to the criterion S, which are: AM2871z.1, where z = 39, 46, 52, 57, 61, 76, 81 (see Tables 13.5 and 13.6) and (ii) using the 15 sequences (see Tables 13.8 and 13.9). We note (see Table 13.6) that in relation

Table 13.4 Relation between the sequences used in the estimation and number of parts of the estimated partition, for AM2871z.1, where $z = 39, 40, 41, 46, 50, 52, 57, 58, 59, 61, 62, 65, 76, 81, 87$

z	Sample size	$\|S\|$	$\|L\|$
81	3604	134	6
81,76	6235	193	13
81,76,57	10,138	241	18
81,76,57,61	12,776	249	21
81,76,57,61,39	16,413	255	27
81,76,57,61,39,52	18,884	255	28
81,76,57,61,39,52,46	21,611	255	27
81,76,57,61,39,52,46,41	26,071	256	31
81,76,57,61,39,52,46,41,59	30,358	256	33
81,76,57,61,39,52,46,41,59,40	33,319	256	31
81,76,57,61,39,52,46 41,59,40,65	36,221	256	34
81,76,57,61,39,52,46 41,59,40,65,58	39,853	256	37
81,76,57,61,39,52,46 41,59,40,65,58,87	43,583	256	39
81,76,57,61,39,52,46 41,59,40, 65,58,87,50	49,007	256	40
81,76,57,61,39,52,46 41,59,40,65,58,87,50,62	52,209	256	42

to the transition probabilities from part i to the elements of the alphabet, 3 of these parts show their highest values in the transition to a, 10 parts expose their highest values in the transition to c, 9 of those parts show their highest values in the transition to g and 5 of those parts expose their greater probabilities in the transition to t. In Table 13.7 we highlight the composition of the four parts 1, 16, 12 and 26 that show the highest values of transition probability for a, c, g and t respectively. We also emphasize in Table 13.7, the part 14 that joins all those strings whose transition probability to c is zero. We list in Table 13.8 the elements of the partition obtained using all the strains, and then we give their transition probabilities in Table 13.9. According to Table 13.9, 7 parts exhibit their highest transition probability values for the element a, 13 for the element c, 14 for the element g, and 8 for the element t. Note that the parts recorded in the selection given in Table 13.7, where we use only 50% of the nearest strains, are combinations of those listed in Table 13.10 with other parts, in the latter case we use all the strains. We detail the connection in the Table 13.11. We see that the listed parts (to the left of Table 13.11) are dispersed in several parts of the model adjusted with all the sequences. In the case of the last line, the strings listed in part 14 of Table 13.7 occur with nonzero frequencies, when using all the sequences. This last aspect shows evidences of the natural dispersion that is inserted to the model with only 50% of the sequences more near, when we use all the sequences.

Table 13.5 Parts of the partition selected through the Bayesian Information Criterion, using AM2871z.1, where $z = 39, 46, 52, 57, 61, 76, 81$

i of part L_i	Strings
1	acgc, accg, ccag, gacg, acac, gcag, caat, atca
2	ccgc, cggt, cctc, agga, tcac, tagg, acca, gcac
3	gcgc, cgtg, ctat, tctc, cagg, cacc, taag, cgtt, ttct, cccc, ggct, gtca
	ctct, agac, tctt, ctta, tgcc, atgc, gttt, tatc, gctt, cttg, agct
4	tcgc, gaca, tttc, ctgc, ttgt, gata, gtta
5	aggc, aaca, agtc, agca, attc, ttcg, aagt, taca, agcg, cagc, gtcc
6	cggc, cgct, tttg, atac, gccg, caga, ttat, ctaa, tagt, ctca, gaaa
7	gggc, gtct, aatt, ttgg, cctt, ttgc, tgga, ctgt, taat, tgta, ccat
	tcct, ttca, ggaa, ctcg, tgtt, agaa, gtga
8	tggc, atct, gagt, gagc, aatc, tacg, ggcc, ggtt, agtg, cact, ataa
9	gtgc, gatc, catc, aaga, gctc, aaat, aata
10	actc, tgaa, acag, gtat
11	cgtc, tgtc, gtag, aggt, ttag, ttga, gtac, gcct
12	ggtc, gtaa, agtt, caaa, gttc, gaag, atag
13	cttc, taaa, ttta, catt, attt, aaag, ttaa, acat, aagc, cttt, aaac
14	caag, gcca, tgag, gcaa, aacg, acga, ccac
15	tcag, attg, agag, atcc, aact, cgat, cgta, catg, taga, tccc, ttcc, acaa
16	cgag, tccg, tcta, ggta, taac, acgg, gaga, cata
17	ggag, tgtg, tgct, tcca, tctg, tttt, ccca, ccga, ggca, gcgg, gtgg
	tgat, gggg
18	ctag, tcgt, ctgg, aaaa, tcgg, gtgt, gggt, tggt, gatt
19	cacg, aagg, tcaa, cgcg, actg, cgca, tgcg, tcat, ccgt
20	cccg, ctac, atcg, aggg, aatg, ggcg, cggg
21	gtcg, atta, ggat, cgaa, gagg, ggac, tact, tgca, tata, agat, acct
	gcga, tcga
22	ccgg, gatg, caac, cctg, atgg, tatt, tggg, tatg, accc, ggtg, cgac, atgt
	gcta, ggga
23	gctg, gaat, gttg, acgt, tgac, gacc
24	gcat, gact, ccta, gcgt, caca, acta, gaac, ttac
25	atat, cgga, actt, atga, ccct, cagt, aacc, ccaa, agta, ctga
26	tacc
27	gccc, cgcc, ctcc, agcc

13.5 Conclusion

In this paper we show how to use the measure d derived from concepts introduced in García and González-López (2017) to establish a notion of proximity between strains of Burkitt lymphoma/leukemia, over the alphabet $A = \{a, c, g, t\}$ we deal with 15 strains. The state space is formed by strings that are concatenations of size 4 of elements coming from the alphabet, and the DNA sequences are identified with Markov processes of memory 4. From d it is also possible to propose a strategy of

Table 13.6 Transition probabilities P(. | L_i) with $i = 1,...,27$. For each part i listed on the left column (see Table 13.5), we indicate in bold the highest transition probability to the elements of the alphabet

i of part L_i	a	c	g	t
1	**0.52430**	0.24041	0.18670	0.04859
2	0.26705	**0.53977**	0.13636	0.05682
3	**0.31714**	0.25073	0.30718	0.12495
4	0.16245	0.27557	**0.53791**	0.02407
5	**0.47689**	0.07948	0.27542	0.16821
6	0.20235	0.17204	**0.33822**	0.28739
7	0.11628	0.31924	**0.46564**	0.09884
8	0.26162	0.34661	**0.36122**	0.03054
9	0.14495	0.11376	**0.57982**	0.16147
10	0.00487	**0.42336**	0.37226	0.19951
11	0.02754	0.11864	**0.61441**	0.23941
12	0.26225	0.08357	**0.62824**	0.02594
13	0.17198	0.23406	**0.41527**	0.17869
14	0.35484	0.00000	0.18894	**0.45622**
15	0.27907	0.22161	0.12996	**0.36936**
16	0.02667	**0.72800**	0.11200	0.13333
17	0.23476	**0.35264**	0.24390	0.16870
18	0.13996	**0.43050**	0.31757	0.11197
19	0.36605	**0.38650**	0.02658	0.22086
20	0.20380	**0.51813**	0.09845	0.17962
21	0.08753	**0.43885**	0.11631	0.35731
22	0.16603	**0.35227**	0.21136	0.27034
23	0.14469	0.25736	0.23303	**0.36492**
24	0.01155	0.33949	0.22864	**0.42032**
25	0.07393	**0.47471**	0.28664	0.16472
26	0.03922	0.05882	0.03922	**0.86275**
27	0.26437	0.04310	**0.46264**	0.22989

Table 13.7 Selected parts, from Table 13.5, which have the greater (on top)/null (on bottom) transition probabilities to each element of the alphabet {a, c, g, t}

i of part L_i	Strings	Probability
1	acgc, accg, ccag, gacg, acac, gcag, caat, atca	P (a|L_1) = 0.52430
16	cgag, tccg, tcta, ggta, taac, acgg, gaga, cata	P (c|L_{16}) = 0.72800
12	ggtc, gtaa, agtt, caaa, gttc, gaag, atag	P (g|L_{12}) = 0.62824
26	tacc	P (t|L_{26}) = 0.86275
14	caag, gcca, tgag, gcaa, aacg, acga, ccac	P (c|L_{14}) = 0

selection of strains, for the construction of a model that allows to describe the way the elements of the state space are organized. The measure d allows to select the nearest strains to build the model whose represents the majority of the strains. We estimate the transition probability of each string for any element of the alphabet A. By the conception of the model it is possible to classify the strings into 27 categories,

Table 13.8 Parts of the partition selected through the Bayesian Information Criterion, using all the sequences AM2871z.1, where $z = 39, 40, 41, 46, 50, 52, 57, 58, 59, 61, 62, 65, 76, 81, 87$

i of part L_i	Strings
1	acgc, accg
2	ccgc, gagt, acca, gagc, ggcg, cggt
3	gcgc, tacg, cgtg, ccca, gccg, ctat, cacc, ttat, ctaa, caga
4	tcgc, ggtt, aatc, ggcc, atca, agtg, ataa, tggc, atct
5	aggc, agtc, aaca, agca
6	cggc, cgct, tttg, atac
7	gggc, ctcg, gtct, cctt, gaca, tagc
8	atgc, gttt, cttg, tatc, ttgg, cttc, catt, taaa, gctt
9	ctgc, ctgt, gttc, tttc
10	gtgc, ggtc, gaag, atag, agtt, caaa, gtaa
11	ttgc, tgga, taat, aaac, ttca, aaag, ttaa, acat, aagc, ttta, cttt
12	catc, ctcc, gctc, aaga, gccc
13	gatc, aata, aaat, gtac, gtag, ttga, ttag, aggt
14	actc, agaa, cgga, atat, atga
15	cctc, tgcc, ggct, tcca, acac, ggag, tgat, tgtg, tgct, gcac, tctg, tttt, gtca
16	tctc, taag, cccc, cagg, ttct, ctct, tctt
17	cgtc, tgtc, gcct
18	attc, aagt, agct, taca, tagt, ctca, gaaa
19	caag, gcca, ccac
20	acag, gtat, tgaa
21	ccag, agac, agga, gcag, gacg, caat, cgtt
22	tcag, attg, aact, agag, catg, atcc, aatg, cgat, cgta
23	cgag, tccg
24	tgag, acga, gcaa, agcc, cgcc
25	ctag, ggga, accc, gctg, atgt, gaat, acgt, gttg, tgac, gacc
26	aacg, taga, acaa, tccc, ttcc
27	cacg, aagg, tcaa, cgca, actg, cgcg, tagg, tcac
28	cccg, ctac, aggg, atcg, gtcg, atta, cggg
29	agcg, cagc, gtcc, ttcg
30	tgcg, tcat, ccgt, acct
31	gagg, ggac, tgca, gcat, ttac, gact, gaac, caca, tata
32	acgg, agat
33	ccgg, gatg, tact, atgg, cctg, gcta, caac, tggg, tatg, ggtg, tatt, cgac, ggca, ccga
34	gcgg, gtgg, cact, ctta, attt, aaaa, gggg, cgaa
35	tcgg, actt, tggt, gggt, ctgg, tcgt, gatt
36	ccat, ggaa, tgta, tcct, aatt, gata, gtta, gtgt, tgtt, gtga
37	ggat, gcga, gaga, tcga
38	ccct, cagt, aacc, ccta, ccaa, agta, ctga
39	gcgt, acta
40	ttgt
41	cata, tcta, ggta, taac
42	tacc

Table 13.9 Transition probabilities $P(\cdot | L_i)$ with $i = 1,...,42$. For each part i, listed on the left column (see Table 13.8), we indicate in bold the highest transition probability to the elements of the alphabet

i of part L_i	a	c	g	t
1	**0.62162**	0.17568	0.11824	0.08446
2	0.20141	**0.52669**	0.18127	0.09063
3	**0.27795**	0.22742	0.25900	0.23563
4	0.26518	0.31020	**0.37473**	0.04989
5	**0.49296**	0.03873	0.34859	0.11972
6	0.15173	0.17569	**0.36646**	0.30612
7	0.17982	0.28801	**0.44956**	0.08260
8	0.26409	0.22741	**0.38224**	0.12625
9	0.13973	0.20960	**0.58923**	0.06145
10	0.25732	0.09728	**0.57741**	0.06799
11	0.15512	0.23870	**0.42244**	0.18373
12	0.22067	0.08288	**0.50377**	0.19268
13	0.07543	0.16140	**0.58475**	0.17843
14	0.07708	**0.49605**	0.26383	0.16304
15	0.26020	**0.34949**	0.22874	0.16156
16	**0.34054**	0.25250	0.28011	0.12685
17	0.05213	0.06398	**0.55450**	0.32938
18	0.29789	0.14042	**0.34416**	0.21753
19	0.38671	0.04532	0.09970	**0.46828**
20	0.01037	**0.41014**	0.38134	0.19816
21	**0.43774**	0.26038	0.21384	0.08805
22	0.27390	0.29363	0.11684	**0.31563**
23	0.08333	**0.82222**	0.05556	0.03889
24	0.26710	0.05375	**0.35668**	0.32248
25	0.14725	0.28990	0.24258	**0.32027**
26	0.28553	0.14211	0.18027	**0.39211**
27	**0.38189**	0.38091	0.06102	0.17618
28	0.19352	**0.51001**	0.09724	0.19924
29	**0.48899**	0.11006	0.19654	0.20440
30	0.22482	0.37230	0.02698	**0.37590**
31	0.05018	0.35636	0.17236	**0.42109**
32	0.02055	**0.66438**	0.02740	0.28767
33	0.17956	**0.35776**	0.19200	0.27069
34	0.19475	**0.34030**	0.30463	0.16031
35	0.15342	**0.42826**	0.30464	0.11369
36	0.09625	0.36320	**0.44644**	0.09401
37	0.07349	**0.48294**	0.14961	0.29396
38	0.09836	**0.36339**	0.31785	0.22040
39	0.00339	0.35254	0.28136	**0.36271**
40	0.17865	0.31828	**0.49281**	0.01027
41	0.05017	**0.63378**	0.16890	0.14716
42	0.05970	0.10448	0.12687	**0.70896**

Table 13.10 Selected parts, from Tables 13.8 and 13.9, which have the greater transition probabilities to each element of the alphabet {a, c, g, t}

i of part L_i	Strings	Probability
1	acgc, accg	P (a|L_1) = 0.62162
23	cgag, tccg	P (c|L_{23}) = 0.82222
9	ctgc, ctgt, gttc, tttc	P (g|L_9) = 0.58923
42	tacc	P (t|L_{42}) = 0.70896

Table 13.11 Relation between the parts listed in Tables 13.7 and 13.10. On left we display the parts coming from the model using only 50% of the DNA sequences, on right the parts coming from the model using all the DNA strains. In the same line, on the right we list the parts in which are identified the elements into the part on the left

Index of part from Table 13.7	Indices of parts – Table 13.8
1	1,4,15,21
16	23,32,37,41
12	9,10
26	42
14	19,24,26

where each category contains strings with the same transition probability to elements of the alphabet, i.e. within each category, the strings are stochastically equivalent. Comparing the model constructed from the closest strains to the model with all the strains, we noticed that the categories practically double. An open question is to be able to quantify with some level of significance the impact of the inclusion of each strain (DNA sequence) on the model, as the quantity S increases. An answer in that line would allow to classify the different possible models, given the 15 strains.

References

García, J. E., & González-López, V. A. (2015). Detecting regime changes in Markov models. In R. Manca, S. McClean, C. H. Skiadas (Eds) *New trends in stochastic modeling and data analysis*. Chapter 2, 103. ISAST, Athens, Greece (ISBN: 978-618-5180-06-5) .

García, J. E., & González-López, V. A. (2017). Consistent estimation of partition Markov models. *Entropy, 19*(4), 160.

Chapter 14
Monte Carlo Methods Applied in Health Research

J. A. Pereira, L. Mendes, A. Costa, and T. A. Oliveira

14.1 Introduction

The present paper describes an application of Monte Carlo (MC) methods to estimate the sample size under the framework of statistical power (SP) and accuracy in parameter estimation (AIPE), for a multivariate regression analysis on oral health research. The ultimate goal of our research is to create a model to assist in the estimation of the risk of tooth loss due to periodontitis.

Over the past two decades has been established that Monte Carlo method is a very useful tool to sample size planning for multivariate regression analysis in terms of SP and AIPE. With the integration of the structural equation modeling (SEM) approach, together with its implementation in R software language, the estimation of sample size became easier. Muthén and Muthén (2002) showed how researchers can use a Monte Carlo study to decide on sample size and determine power for SEM using the Mplus program. To find sample size according with AIPE, Kelley and Maxewell (2003) undertook a MC study in R/S-PLUS code within the framework of ordinary least squares (OLS) multiple regression. Later on Maxewell et al. (2008) presented

J. A. Pereira (✉)
Faculdade de Medicina Dentária da Universidade do Porto, Departamento de Periodontologia, Porto, Portugal

MBB, Universidade Aberta, Lisboa, Portugal

L. Mendes
Faculdade de Medicina Dentária da Universidade do Porto, Departamento de Periodontologia, Porto, Portugal

A. Costa
Universidad Nacional de Educacion a Distancia, Madrid, Spain

T. A. Oliveira
CEAUL and Universidade Aberta, Lisboa, Portugal

© Springer International Publishing AG, part of Springer Nature 2018
C. H. Skiadas, C. Skiadas (eds.), *Demography and Health Issues*,
The Springer Series on Demographic Methods and Population Analysis 46,
https://doi.org/10.1007/978-3-319-76002-5_14

an extended review on sample size estimation and related topics. In this review specific designs and analyses were considered, including the structural equation modeling (SEM). Afterwards, Beaujean (2014) demonstrated how to use a MC study to decide on sample size for a regression analysis using both power and parameter accuracy perspectives under the SEM framework in R language.

The overall structure of this paper takes the form of three parts. The first provides the medical context of our research and the methods to estimate the sample size and related concepts. The second part describes the application of the statistical methods to the considered data. And finally, the third part provides a brief summary and discussion of the work.

14.2 Medical Context and Statistical Methods

14.2.1 Medical Context

Periodontitis is the most severe form of periodontal disease. It is characterized by the destruction of tooth's supporting tissues such as alveolar bone and periodontal ligament (Fig. 14.1). Together with dental caries, it is the major cause of tooth loss in adults (Hand et al. 1991) and has been shown to be related to adverse effects in systemic health (Kim and Amar 2006). The bone level around the tooth is an estimate of the amount of remaining/destroyed alveolar bone supporting the tooth, reflecting the amount of attachment between tooth and alveolar bone (Yamamoto et al. 2006). The amount of attachment is very important to model the diagnosis and the clinical prognosis (Yamamoto et al. 2006) and it traditionally estimates the percentage of intrabony root. This proportion is calculated from measurements taken on x-ray images along the long axis of the tooth. Since the root shape is approximately conic, the traditional approach seems to be a poor estimate of the dental attachment. Alternatively, the quantification of periodontal destruction through the lateral area of the root surface without bone support seems to be a better

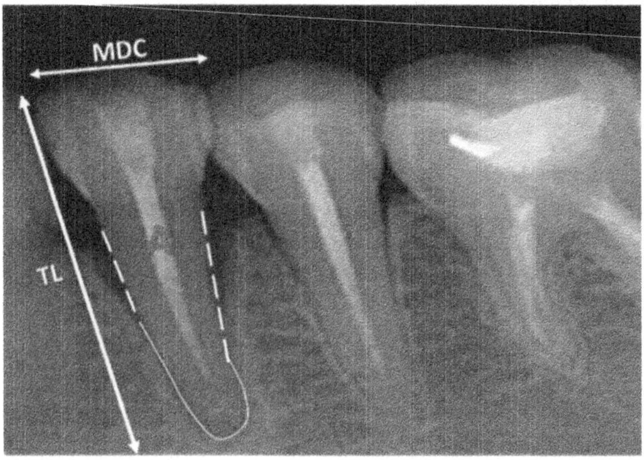

Fig. 14.1 X-ray image of a tooth periodontally affected (A). The portion of the tooth delimited by dashed lines indicates the root portion without bone support. The tooth length and maximum mesio-distal diameter of the crown are represented by TL and MDC respectively

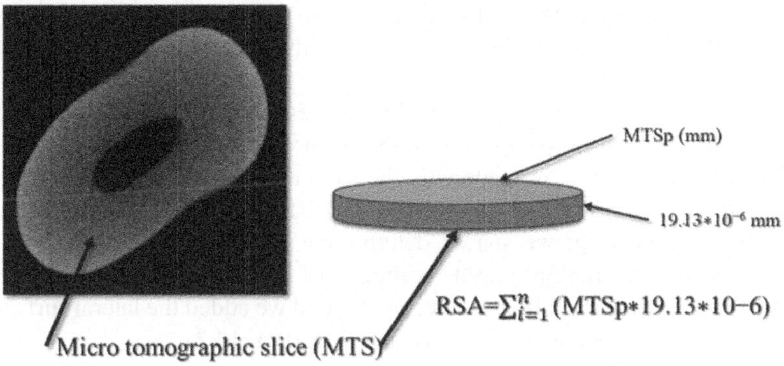

Where: MTSp is the perimeter of MTS and n is the number of MTS

Fig. 14.2 Division planimetry method use to calcule RSA from microtomographic slices

estimate of attachment loss, which can be estimated by subtracting the remaining area of periodontal support to the total lateral area of the root.

In recent years, there is a growing interest in more realistic methods to quantify the periodontal inflammation by the area of the periodontal pocket wall (Nesse et al. 2008). The extension of this concept to periodontal bone support lead us to formulate our research question: "Can we model the total periodontal attachment area from non-invasive measures?". To answer this question we propose to model the total periodontal attachment area by calculating the lateral surface area of the root (RSA) from measures easily obtained in clinical set in a non-invasive way. Accordingly, the tooth length (TL) and the maximum mesio-distal diameter of the crown (MDC) were choosen (Fig. 14.1). The conceptual model assumes that RSA is a linear function of MDC and TL and can be written as:

$$\mathrm{RSA} = \beta_0 + \beta_1 \mathrm{TL} + \beta_2 \mathrm{MDC} + \varepsilon \tag{14.1}$$

The data on RSA is obtained for each tooth by the method of division planimetry applied to microtomographic slices of scanned second mandibular premolars (Fig. 14.2). For each tooth TL and MDC are measured on pictures (Fig. 14.1).

Data Collection and Description

A sample of five second mandibular premolars, extracted for orthodontic treatment purposes, selected at random from 5 Portuguese young adult males. The teeth accomplished with the following selection criteria: absence of lesions of dental hard tissues (carious, abfraction and erosion lesions), restorative dental treatments (dental restorations or fixed prosthesis) and aberrant morphology of the dental roots (incomplete apex and abnormalities of shape or number).

The teeth were scanned individually by an x-ray microtomograph system SkyScan 1072 (SkyScan, Kontich, Belgium) with the resolution set to 19.13 μm voxel size.

Data on tooth length (TL) and maximum mesio-distal diameter of the crown (MDC) were obtained by measuring on the picture taken orthogonally at the scale 1:2. The measurements were made with the software Adobe® Acrobat® 9.0.

The lateral surface area of the dental root (RSA) was estimate by division a planimetry as following: we started determining the lateral surface area of each tomographic slice by multiplying its perimeter of each slice was multiplied by the length of edge of the voxel, in this case, and second we added the lateral surface area of all slices to obtain the total lateral surface area (Fig. 14.2).

14.2.2 Statistical Methods

The first challenge is to determine the minimum sample size to get regression coefficients to operationalize our conceptual model. Thus, the number of teeth to be scanned for estimation of root surface area must be just enough to ensure that β_1 and β_2 are different from zero, considering the true parameters of the population are different from zero, and as close as possible to the respective true values of the population. Thus, the sample size must be estimated within both statistical power and accuracy frameworks.

Sample Size and Statistical Power

From the power analysis perspective the sample size is the number of observations needed to reject the null hypothesis i.e. β be equal to zero (H_0) whereas the alternate state is that β do not conform to the null hypothesis. The power analysis involves four quantities implied in statistical inference: significance level, statistical power, effect size, and sample size, and with any of the three, we can determine the fourth.

The sample size is the unknown number of observations.

The confidence level or type I error (α), also known as "false positive" is the error of rejecting H_0 ($\beta = 0$) when it is actually true or is the error of accepting H_a ($\beta \neq 0$) when the results can be attributed to chance.

The power or one minus type II error which is also known as "false negative" meaning not rejecting the H_0 when H_a is true. That is, this is the error of failing to accept H_a when you do not have adequate power. In this study we decided on type I error of 0.05 and type II error of 0.2 (power = 0.8).

The effect size refers to the magnitude of the effect under H_a and its nature varies with the statistical procedure. In regression analysis it can be defined by the proportion of the variance in the dependent variable that is explained by the regression model and is often represented by R squared (R^2). It needs to be estimated from the correlations, regression coefficients of the variables and variance of the

Table 14.1 Descriptive statistics of data

	n	Mean	SD	Median	Max	Min
TI*	5	23.58	0.78	23.83	24.57	22.54
Mw*	5	7.68	0.46	7.89	8.17	7.04
RSA+	5	283.74	22.18	284.62	315.38	254.09

*measured in mm; + measured in mm^2; Max – maximum value and Min – the minimum

dependent variable (Cohen 1992). Because we have no knowledge from previous studies conducted in this area, the effect size was estimated from data gathered from a pilot study with a sample of 5 teeth. The methodology used to collect the data, and the descriptive statistics are shown below in Table 14.1.

Sample Size and Parameter Accuracy

To know that a parameter is different from zero may be not enough, because do not inform the researcher on its magnitude, which is a limitation of the research results. Therefore, to find an accurate parameter is of the most importance for the researcher.

The accuracy can be defined as the extent that an estimate conforms to the true population value and can be represented by the square root of the mean square error that is expressed by the Eq. (14.2). It indicates how close the estimator is to the true value (Walther and Moore, 2005).

$$REMS = \sqrt{E\left[\left(\widehat{\beta}-\beta\right)^2\right]} = \sqrt{\left(\widehat{\beta}-\left[\widehat{\beta}\right]\right)^2 + \left(E\left[\widehat{\beta}-\beta\right]\right)^2} \qquad (14.2)$$

Where:

β is the true parameter value for the population and $\widehat{\beta}$ is an estimator,
$E\left[\widehat{\beta}-\beta\right]$ is the bias or systematic error
$\left(\widehat{\beta}-\left[\widehat{\beta}\right]\right)$ is the variance or random error which is the inverse of precision.

The bias is the difference between the expected value of the estimator (the mean of the estimates of all possible samples that can be taken from the population) and the true, unknown, population value. The variance is the difference between a sample estimate and the mean of the estimates of all possible samples that can be taken from the population. Thus, when an estimator is unbiased $\left(\left(E\left[\widehat{\beta}-\beta\right]\right)=0\right)$ accuracy coincides with precision.

The precision and likely accuracy is an interval estimate or confidence interval of our $\widehat{\beta}$ and is centered on β and extending a distance w either side of β, where w is called the margin of error, which is based on the standard error (SE). The SE is obtained from the standard deviation (SD) and from the size of the sample (n) being $SE = SD/\sqrt{n}$ and w is the product of SE by the critical value of the t statistic that depends on our chosen value for confidence level (Cumming and Finch 2005).

From the accuracy in parameter estimation (AIPE) perspective, sample size is chosen such that the expected width of the confidence interval will be sufficiently narrow, being the confidence interval defined by an estimated range of values with a given high probability of covering the true population value. It is calculated as described above, i.e. the goal of AIPE is to obtain parameter estimates that accurately correspond to the population value they represent, see (Hays 1973; Kelley and Maxwell 2003).

Monte Carlo Methods

Monte Carlo method consists on generating random data from a population of interest, with plausible parameter values and distributional form. To obtain a sample size an adequate statistical technique is implemented, and the simulation is repeated a large number of times (m) with different sample sizes (n) until the minimum sample size is achieved, where the particular goal is accomplished (Scott Maxwell et al. 2008). In this study we aim to meet the quality criteria for simulated data that was defined by Muthén and Muthén (2002). To estimate the parameters for a multivariate regression, a model is fitted to each one of the numerous drawn samples. Then the averages of the parameters and respective standard errors are calculated over the samples, and the estimate relative parameter bias, relative standard error bias, and coverage are assessed to decide on the sample size (Muthén and Muthén 2002).

The relative parameter estimate bias is defined as:

$$\beta_{\text{bias}} = \frac{\widehat{\beta} - \beta_p}{\beta_p} \tag{14.3}$$

where β_p is a plausible parameter for the population, $\widehat{\beta}$ is the average parameter estimate from the simulated samples.

The relative standard error bias as:

$$\frac{\sigma_{\text{bias}} = \widehat{\sigma}_\beta - \sigma_{\widehat{\beta}}}{\sigma_{\widehat{\beta}}} \tag{14.4}$$

where $\sigma_{\widehat{\beta}}$ is the standard deviation of the parameter estimates and $\widehat{\sigma}_\beta$ is the average of the estimated standard errors for the parameter.

The coverage is the percentage of $(1 - \alpha)\%$ confidence interval that covers parameters underlying the data.

To have a sample with power close to 0.8 the parameter and standard error biases must not exceed 10% for any parameter in the model, the standard error bias for the parameter of interest does not exceed 5% and the coverage should be between 0.91 and 0.98 (Muthén and Muthén 2002).

The power is the proportion of simulated samples for power is the proportion of significant replications when testing whether the parameters are different from zero, according with alpha level (Beaujean 2014).

Structural Equation Modeling Approach

To represent our model and make the simulation we use the structural equation modeling (SEM) approach once SEM framework encompasses the traditional multivariate regression procedures with some advantages, such as the inclusions of means, regression weights and, when visualized by a graphical path diagram, makes evident the correlation between the predictor variables and the residual error (Beaujean 2014). Furthermore, two of the three characteristics of SEM, namely the estimation of multiple and the explanation of the entire set of relationships with the definition of the model (Hair et al. 2012) made this approach more suitable for Monte Carlo studies. Therefore, SEM enables the specification and estimation of more complex path models.

Important aspects of the application of SEM are the following features of data: verified association between the outcome and the predictor variables (Table 14.1), the joint distribution multivariate normal (Table 14.3), and all univariate distributions should be normal (Table 14.4) (Ullman 2006).

14.3 Implementation of the Statistical Methods

The method applied to determine the sample size for a multivariate regression analysis with Monte Carlo study can be described in seven critical steps as described above:

1. **Decide on regression model**

The model to be studied is the conceptual model (Eq. 14.1) to respond to the research question. Another way to state the interrelationship among variables is the path diagram in Fig. 14.3.

2. **Decide on population values for all parameters in the model**, regression coefficients, residual variance (1 – R^2) and covariance among the predictors. Confirm the covariance matrix

The effect size was estimate by the Eq. (14.5) and the standardized regression coefficients by (14.6)

$$\text{Effect size} : \mathrm{R}^2 = \frac{\mathbf{V}_{\mathrm{XX}}\mathbf{b}'_{\mathrm{YX}}\mathbf{b}_{\mathrm{YX}}}{\sigma^2_{\mathrm{Y}}} = \boldsymbol{\rho}'_{\mathrm{YX}}\mathbf{R}^{-1}_{\mathrm{XX}}\boldsymbol{\rho}_{\mathrm{YX}} \tag{14.5}$$

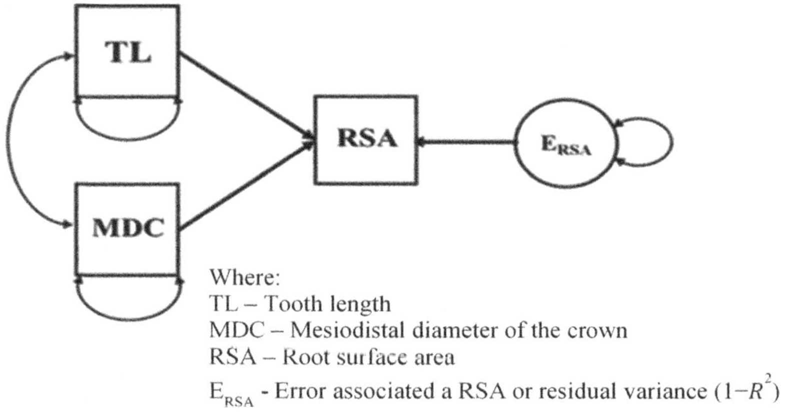

Fig. 14.3 Path diagram for the conceptual model represented by Eq. (14.1)

$$\text{Standardized regression coefficients}: b^* = \mathbf{R}_{XX}^{-1}\boldsymbol{\rho}_{YX} \tag{14.6}$$

where:

$\boldsymbol{\rho}_{YX}$ is the p × 1 vector of correlations between TL, MDC and RSA;
$\mathbf{b}_{YX}$ is the p × 1 column vector of regression coefficients of TL, MW;
$\mathbf{R}_{XX}$ is the p × p correlation matrix of TL and MDC;
$\mathbf{V}_{XX}$ is the p × p covariance matrix of TL and MDC; and
σ_Y^2 is the variance of RSA

The matrices $\boldsymbol{\rho}_{YX}$, $\mathbf{R}_{XX}$, $\mathbf{V}_{XX}$ and σ_Y^2 are obtained with data from Table 14.2 and $\mathbf{b}_{YX}$ was calculated according to Eq. (14.6).

The population estimated values for effect size (R^2) calculated with the Eq. (14.5) is 0.496, the residual variance ($1 - R^2$) is 0.504, standardized coefficients of TL and MDC calculated with Eq. (14.6) are 0.63 and 0.69 respectively. The standardize coefficients were used to annul the intercept of the model.

The conceptual model became the operational model with standardize coefficients. The model was treated as a structural equation model (SEM) (Nachtigall et al. 2003) to include all pertinent information. The data were checked for multivariate and univariate normality (Tables 14.3 and 14.4), being the multivariate normality $\mathbf{X} = [\text{TL}, \text{MDC}, \text{RSA}]^T$ written by $X \tilde{} \mathcal{N}(\boldsymbol{\mu}, \boldsymbol{\Sigma})$,

where μ is the matrix of means $\mu = \begin{bmatrix} 23.58 \\ 7.68 \\ 283.74 \end{bmatrix}$ and Σ is the covariance matrix

$$\Sigma = \begin{bmatrix} 0.61 & -0.16 & 5.73 \\ -0.16 & 0.21 & 4.33 \\ 5.73 & 4.33 & 491.75. \end{bmatrix}$$

Table 14.2 Covariances and correlations between variables

Predictors		TL	MDC	RSA
TL	Covariance	0.61	−0.16	5.73
	Correlation	1	−0.43	0.33
MDC	Covariance	●	0.21	4.33
	Correlation	●	1	0.42
RSA	Covariance	●	●	491.75
	Correlation	●	●	1

Table 14.3 Results of multivariate normality tests

Tests		Statistic	p-value
Mardia	**Skewness**	11.913	0.290
	Kurtosis	10.470	0.355
Henze-Zirkler		0.468	0.320
Royston		0.169	0.981
Mardia		11.913	0.290

Significance level at 5%

Table 14.4 Results of Shapiro-Francia univariate normality test

Predictors	Statistic	p-value
TL	0.963	0.929
MDC	0.930	0.628
RSA	0.960	0.906

Significance level at 5%

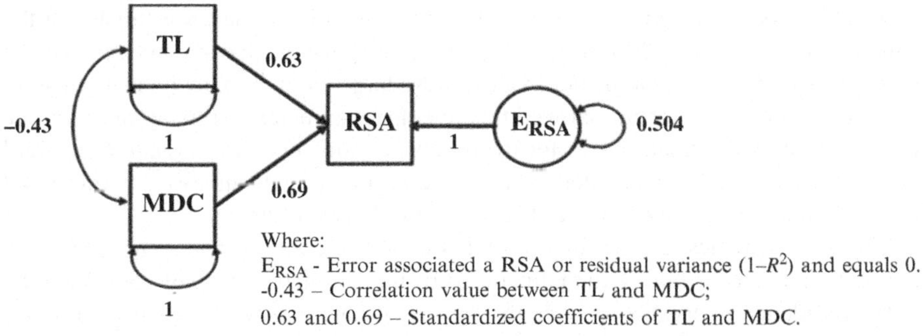

Fig. 14.4 Path diagram with the parameter estimates for the population

The R *lavaan* package (Rosseel 2012) was used to specify the SEM regression model with all the information described in the parameterized path diagram (Fig. 14.4).

3. **Decide on simulation definitions for type 1 error rate (α), power (1 − β); number of samples (m); sample size (n); random seed.**

Table 14.5 Results of Monte Carlo simulation with m = 1000 and n = 300 and seed 565

			Relative Bias				
Predictor (β)	Proposed parameter	Average parameter estimate	Parameter	Standard error	Coverage	Power	95% CI Half-width
TL (β_1)	0.63	0.63	0.003	0.019	0.96	1	0.089
MDC (β_2)	0.69	0.69	0.005	0.020	0.95	1	0.089
Criteria for Monte Carlo data quality*			≤0.1	≤0.1	0.91a0.98	>0.8	

*Values proposed by Muthén and Muthén (2002); Significance level at 5%

The values considered for α, $1 - \beta$, m, n, and randon seed are 0.05, 0.80, 1000, 300 and 565 respectively.

4. **Short algorithm to simulate the m samples of the regression model from Step 2.**

It was considered the simulation ran on *simsem* package (Pornprasertmanit et al. 2012) that accepts *lavaan* specifications. Two models were specified: the first generates the samples and the second estimates the parameters from the replications. The algorithm procedure and respective table of results are:

In the simulated data, check: Relative parameter and standard error biases; Coverage; If the values are acceptable, examine the power or accuracy of the parameters of interest; If the values are not high enough, repeat the simulation with a bigger n.

As it can be observed from Table 14.5, the average parameters estimates in the simulation with m = 1000 and n = 300 equal the plausible parameters for the population, indicating that m and n values were large enough to get convergence. In terms of accuracy the results showed that average parameters estimates are accurate as suggested by the small values for the relative parameters biases, relative standard error biases, and confidence intervals half-widths attaining the quality criteria set out by Muthén and Muthén (2002) and Kelley and Maxwell (2003).

From the statistics, concerning the statistical power, we can realize in Table 14.5 that the coverage (meaning the percentage of the simulated samples for which the 95% confidence intervals) contains the estimated parameters, it was acceptable for all parameters of interest, and in all simulations the parameters estimates were statistically different from zero (Power = 1).

Considering that the results met the quality criteria for the simulated data we then proceed to step 5

5. **Repeat Step 4 using a different random seed**

The step 4 was repeated with a seed of 656 and same values for m and n

6. **Compare results of simulated data from two random seeds**

   Procedure:

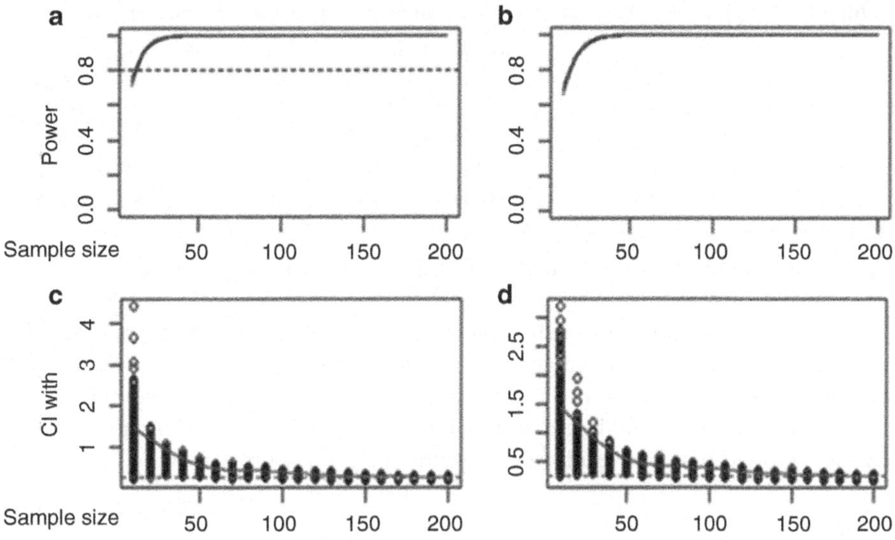

Fig. 14.5 Curves of power and accuracy for the regression coefficients: A and B power curves for β_2 and β_1; and C and D curves of accuracy for β_2 and β_1

If the results converge, no need for further simulations
If the results do not converge, repeat from Step 4 using different random seeds or larger values of m

From the simulations of step 4 and 5 identical results were obtained (not shown) and consequently the quality criteria for data were also met. Since the convergence was observed we found no need to repeat the step 4 with different number of samples.

7. **Finding the sample size**

To select the sample size, the variation of the power and the accuracy was assessed by simulating samples varying from $n = 10$ to 200 in steps of 10 and $m = 1000$.

The Fig. 14.5 provides the graphs presenting the variation of power and confidence intervals half-width (accuracy) with the sample size for the relationships between RSA and TL (β_1) and MDC (β_2). It can be observed that the power of 0.8 is reached with samples above 15, but the confidence intervals are too large to be acceptable. As shown in the graphs, each increment in accuracy implies a much stronger increase on sample sizes below 150 and from that point the confidence intervals width became stable, which makes 150 the best sample size. Considering the high costs of scanning 150 teeth, we decided to estimate the minimum sample size that accomplishes with the quality criteria for simulated data.

From the graph of power we estimate that the maximum power is achieve for samples above ap-proximately 40 and the confidence intervals width around 0.5,

Table 14.6 Results of Monte Carlo simulation with m = 1000 and n = 37 and seed 565

Predictor (β)	Proposed parameter	Average parameter estimate	Relative Bias Parameter	Relative Bias Standard error	Coverage	Power	95% CI Half-width
TL (β_1)	0.63	0.63	0.008	0.088	0.93	0.995	0.253
MDC(β_2)	0.69	0.69	0.002	0.081	0.93	0.995	0.255
Criteria for Monte Carlo data quality*			≤0.1	≤0.1	0.91a0.98	>0.8	

*Values proposed by Muthén and Muthén (2002); Significance level at 5%

however wc do not have information on the estimate relative parameter bias, relative standard error bias, and coverage. To find those values a simulation was ran with m = 1000 and n varying from 35 to 45, and the quality criteria was met for n = 37.

To confirm the last finding a simulation with n = 37, m = 100 and a seed of 565 was carried out. The results are presented in Table 14.6.

14.4 Discussion and Conclusions

The calculation of the number of observations to include in a statistical sample is a step of the research design that can condition the feasibility of the project, its exact calculation assumes increasing importance as the cost, and the time of gathering the data increases. In this study the scanning by x-ray microtomography and the image processing were both costly and time consuming, therefore a method to obtain a precise sample size from the power and accuracy in parameter estimation perspectives was adopted. The methodology to find the sample size, proposed by Beaujean (2014), proved to be useful and simple to apply to our data. The sample of 5 teeth that was used to estimate the population parameters allowed to characterize the joint distribution and the relationships of the variables and to test the applicability of this sample size estimation method to our line of work, serving as a starting point for further research in this field.

The variables selected can be easily obtained in any clinic, MDC can be measured in mouth or in x-ray images, whereas TL is necessarily measured in x-ray images that usually present different grades of distortion, thus the estimates of root length must be pondered for distortion. The RSA was estimated beyond the first cervical 2 mm of root, because, usually, are not periodontal ligament attached in this area.

The second lower pre-molar was selected, because its x-ray images present less distortion and, having only one and approximately conic root, is easier to model than other tooth types.

The number of independent variables was minimal as possible to get a simpler and rational model (Forster 2001).

The simulations were ran with various random seeds and in different occasions and the consistency of the results was verified, although small differences were observed and the rounding of values.

The R software environment showed a great versatility and information to better use the packages of interest and is available online open access.

References

Beaujean, A. A. (2014). Sample size determination for regression models using Monte Carlo methods in R. *Practical Assessment, Research & Evaluation, 19*, 12.

Cohen, J. (1992). A power primer, tutorials in quantitative methods for psychology. *Psychological Bulletin, 112*(I), 155–159.

Cumming, G., & Finch, S. (2005). Inference by eye: Confidence intervals and how to read pictures of data. *American Psychologist, 60*(2), 170–180.

Forster, M. R. (2001). The new science of simplicity. In A. Zellner, H. A. Keuzenkamp, & M. McAleer (Eds.), *Simplicity, inference and modelling: Keeping it sophisticatedly simpley* (pp. 83–119). Cambridge: Cambridge University Press.

Hair, J. F., et al. (2012). *Multivariate data analysis* (6th ed.). Upper Saddle River: Prentice-Hall Inc.

Hand, J. S., Hunt, R. J., & Kohout, F. J. (1991). Five-year incidence of tooth loss in lowans aged 65 and older. *Community Dentistry and Oral Epidemiology, 19*, 48–51.

Hays, W. L. (1973). *Statistics for the social sciences* (2nd ed.). New York: Holt, Rinehart & Winston.

Kelley, K., & Maxwell, S. E. (2003). Sample size for multiple regression: Obtaining regression coefficients that are accurate, not simply significant. *Psychological Methods, 8*(3), 305–321.

Kim, J., & Amar, S. (2006). *Odontology, 94*(1), 10–21.

Muthén, L. K., & Muthén, B. O. (2002). How to use a Monte Carlo study to decide on sample size and determine power. *Structural Equation Modeling: A Multidisciplinary Journal, 9*(4), 599–620.

Nachtigall, C., Kroehne, U., Funke, F., & Steyer, R. (2003). (Why) should we use SEM? Pros and cons of structural equation modeling. *Methods of Psychological Research Online, 8*(2), 1–22.

Nesse, W., Abbas, F., van der Ploeg, I., Spijkervet, F. K. L., Dijkstra, P. U., & Vissink, A. (2008). Periodontal inflamed surface area: Quantifying inflammatory burden. *Journal of Clinical Periodontology, 35*, 668–673.

Pornprasertmanit, S., Miller, P., & Schoemann, A. (2012). *simsem: SIMulated Structural Equation Modeling* [Computer software].

Rosseel, Y. (2012). Lavaan: An R package for structural equation modeling. *Journal of Statistical Software, 48*(2), 1–36.

Scott Maxwell, E., Kelley, K., & Rausch, J. R. (2008). Sample size planning for statistical power and accuracy in parameter estimation. *Annual Review of Psychology, 59*, 537–563.

Ullman, J. B. (2006). Structural equation modeling: Reviewing the basics and moving forward. *Journal of Personality Assessment, 87*(1), 35–50.

Walther, B. A., & Moore, J. L. (2005). The concepts of bias, precision and accuracy, and their use in testing the performance of species richness estimators, with a literature review of estimator performance. *Ecography, 28*, 815–829.

Yamamoto, T., Kinoshita, Y., Tsuneishi, M., Takizawa, H., Umemuraand, O., & Watanabe, T. (2006). Estimation of the remaining periodontal ligament from attachment-level measurements. *Journal of Clinical Periodontology, 33*, 221–225.

Chapter 15
A Neuro-Fuzzy Approach to Measuring Attitudes

Maria Symeonaki, Aggeliki Kazani, and Catherine Michalopoulou

15.1 Introduction

The present paper develops a neuro-fuzzy technique for measuring an attitude. Many definitions have been provided in the literature as to what constitutes an attitude. For example in Hoog and Vaughan (2008) an attitude is defined as 'a relatively enduring organization of beliefs, feelings, and behavioural tendencies towards socially significant objects, groups, events or symbols'. According to Eagly and Chaiken (1993) an attitude is 'a psychological tendency that is expressed by evaluating a particular entity with some degree of favour or disfavour'. In psychology, an attitude is a psychological construct, it is a mental and emotional entity that inheres in, or characterizes a person (Perloff 2016). How to measure attitudes has also been an issue of utmost importance in social sciences and numerous rating scales have been suggested in the past for that reason. The most commonly used rating scale is the Likert scale developed in 1932 (Likert 1932) by the American psychologist Rensis Likert. It is composed of third-person items/questions and it rates the respondents by asking them to place themselves on a scale of favour/disfavour with a neutral midpoint. Therefore a respondent is asked to select between several response categories, indicating various strengths of agreement and disagreement. The response categories are assigned scores and the respondents' attitudes are measured by their total score, which is the sum of the scores of the categories the respondents have chosen for each item-question.

When this traditional type of methodology is used the respondent's attitude is assessed by examining the response categories he/she chooses in a number of items/

M. Symeonaki (✉) · A. Kazani · C. Michalopoulou
Department of Social Policy, School of Political Sciences, Panteion University of Social and Political Sciences, Athens, Greece
e-mail: msymeon@panteion.gr; kmichalop@panteion.gr

© Springer International Publishing AG, part of Springer Nature 2018
C. H. Skiadas, C. Skiadas (eds.), *Demography and Health Issues*,
The Springer Series on Demographic Methods and Population Analysis 46,
https://doi.org/10.1007/978-3-319-76002-5_15

questions. In this study we provide a hybrid expert system that classifies respondents into levels of xenophobia. The focus is on the development of a neuro-fuzzy system that will measure the specific attitude, taking into account a number of important factors such as age, level of education, gender, political and religion beliefs and finally the way each question is answered by the respondent. The proposed system evaluates the answers for each respondent and distinguishes between questionable and non-questionable answers. The intelligent system put forward in the present paper simulates the respondent's final score when the answers are not questionable and takes into account a number of other crucial factors when the answers are questionable so as to classify the respondents into xenophobic levels, reducing therefore the uncertainty.

This approach is an extension of the methodology suggested in Symeonaki and Kazani (2012) and it can be used in every real problem where researchers would like to classify respondents with the aid of Likert scales to different levels of belief, feeling or opinion towards a specific object.

Recently, there have been attempts to combine expert systems with attitude scaling. In Symeonaki et al. (2011) a fuzzy system based on factor analysis is proposed whereas in Symeonaki and Michalopoulou (2011) cluster analysis and fuzzy k-means is used in order to produce a more reliable final scale. Moreover, in Symeonaki et al. (2015) and in Symeonaki and Kazani (2011) a fuzzy system that measures xenophobia in Greece is suggested. In addition, Lalla et al. (2005) proposed a fuzzy system to analyse qualitative ordinal data produced by a course-evaluation questionnaire and Gil and Gil (2012) provided a guideline to design questionnaires allowing free fuzzy-numbered response format.

The paper has been organized in the following way. Section 15.2 provides some information concerning the data and the methodology used in the present study and the respective results. The following Section discusses the validation of the proposed neuro-fuzzy approach, whereas Sect. 15.4 discusses the results and provides concluding remarks and aspects of future work.

15.2 Data, Methodology and Results

The Likert scale studied in the following sections is included in the questionnaire of a large-scale survey conducted under the auspices of the National Centre for Social Research[1] that was designed in order to measure xenophobia in Greece (Michalopoulou et al. 1999). More specifically, the following questions were given (see Symeonaki et al. 2015):

1. Foreigners who live in our country must have equal rights with us.
2. Many of the foreigners who live in our country are responsible for the increase in the crime rate.

[1]www.ekke.gr

3. Foreigners must have lower wages even when they do the same job as we.
4. The foreigners in our country increase unemployment for Greeks.
5. The local authorities must organize events so we get to know the foreigners who live and work here.
6. I would never marry a foreigner.
7. I would never work for a foreigner.
8. We should facilitate foreigners who want to settle in our country.
9. Foreigners who work in our country do harm to our economy.
10. The state must organize programmes of further education to help those foreigners who live in our country.
11. The more foreigners arrive, the lower the wages get.
12. We must create reception departments in our schools for the foreigners' children.
13. Only as tourists should foreigners come.
14. Work permits must be given to foreigners who want to live here.
15. We must close our borders to foreigners who come to work here.

The units had 5 response categories, ranging from total agreement to total disagreement. The sample of the survey was 1200 individuals, aged 18–80 years, residents of Macedonia and Northern Greece during the time of the fieldwork.

Let us now provide a very brief introduction to the theory of Fuzzy Logic presented by L. A. Zadeh (1965) in 1965 and the theory of artificial neural networks.

In fuzzy set theory when A is a fuzzy set and x is a relevant object, the statement, x is a member of A, is not necessarily either true or false, but it may be true only to some degree represented by the membership function of the fuzzy set A, $m_x(A)$. A membership function is a curve that defines how each point in the input space is mapped to a membership value in [0,1]. Fuzzy systems are systems in which variables have as domain fuzzy sets encoding structured, heuristic knowledge in a numerical framework.

Fig. 15.1 Typical form of an artificial neuron

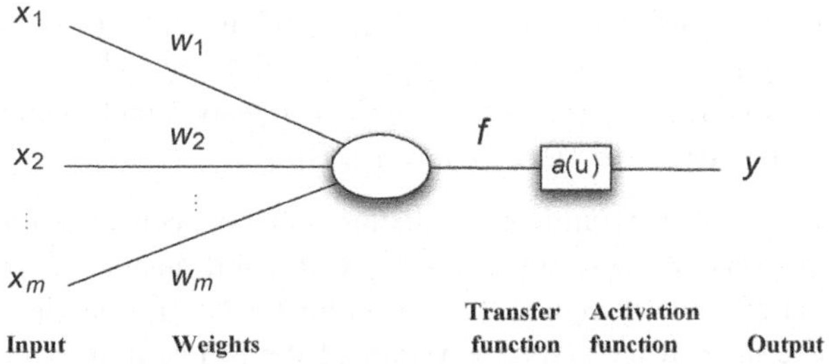

The operation of an artificial neural network is based on a recurrent interconnection of simple processing units, called the neurons. Each neuron receives an input, a vector **x** and produces an output y (Fig. 15.1) through the equations:

$$U = f(\mathbf{x}, \mathbf{w}) - \theta$$
$$y = \alpha(\mathbf{u})$$

where θ represents the activation threshold and $f(\mathbf{x}, \mathbf{w})$ is called the transfer function that relates the input information **x** with the weights **w** that are stored in the neuron. In most cases it is of the form:

$$f(\mathrm{x}, \mathrm{w}) = \sum_{i=1}^{m} w_i x_i$$

The function α is called the activation function and it generally takes values according to:

$$\alpha(\mathbf{u}) = 1, \text{if } \mathbf{u} > \mathbf{0} \text{ and } \alpha(\mathbf{u}) = \mathbf{0}, \text{if } \mathbf{u} < \mathbf{0}.$$

Neural networks are in fact a mass of interconnected simple units and the way the interconnection is carried out defines the network's structure and therefore the way it operates. In order to describe the structure of a network, the nodes (i.e. the neurons) are assumed to be laying in different layers and the basic architecture consists of three types of neuron layers: input, hidden, and output. The nodes that belong to the same layer are being evaluated simultaneously. Another significant matter of artificial neural network modeling is its ability of learning, its ability of adopting and changing its elements in order to simulate a given behaviour.

Our objective here is to develop a neuro-fuzzy system that classifies respondents into xenophobic levels. We denote by:

- m: the number of questions (here $m = 15$)
- Q_j: the j-the question $j = 1,2,\ldots,m$
- $q_j(i)$: the answer of the i-th respondent to the Q_j question, i.e.,
- $q_j(i) = 1,2,3,4$ or 5, $\forall I = 1,2,\ldots,1200$, $\forall j = 1,2,\ldots,m$.
- $\mathbf{x}(i)$: the response vector of the i-th respondent to items-questions $Q_1, Q_2,\ldots, Q_m$, i.e. $\mathbf{x}(i) = [q_1(i), q_2(i),\ldots, q_m(i)]$.

A first step would be to distinguish between questionable and non-questionable answers. We assume that non-questionable answers are those based on which we can classify the respondent to different levels of xenophobia *without uncertainty*. For example, if the response vector of the i-th respondent is $\mathbf{x}(i) = [1,1,\ldots,1]$ then the respondent's score is equal to 15 and he/she is classified into the category denoting a non-xenophobic person, without uncertainty. Let us now examine what could be defined as *questionable answers*. Those answers include a series of responses that lead to a questionable outcome, where the respective respondents cannot be classified to xenophobic levels with certainty. Consider, a respondent that answers that he/she would be willing to marry a foreigner and generally holds a non-xenophobic attitude if one looks at the answers he/she provides, but strongly disagrees with working for a foreigner or believes that only as tourists should foreigners come. His/her response vector would look like $\mathbf{x} = (1,1,1,1,1,1,5,1,1,1,1,1,5,1,1)$ and we could say that there is an ambiguity as to the level of xenophobia that he/she holds. There exist, therefore, certain sets of responses that may lead to an uncertain classification. In those cases there are more factors that need to be taken into account.

Now, for the purpose of this study a statistical analysis was performed on the data with the aid of IBM Statistics SPSS 24.0. The values of all negatively worded items were reversed in order to achieve correspondence between the ordering of the response categories. Summing up the response categories that they have chosen and dividing by the number of the questions estimates the mean scores for each respondent, i.e. $\overline{xen} = \frac{\sum_{i=1}^{m} q_j(i)}{m}$, where m denotes the number of questions.

Definition 2.1 The i-th respondent's answer $\mathbf{x}(i)$ is said to be *questionable at level d* if $\exists j : \left|q_j(i) - \overline{xen}\right| \geq d$.

Definition 2.2 The i-th respondent's answer $\mathbf{x}(i)$ is said to be *non-questionable at level d* if $\nexists j : \left|q_j(i) - \overline{xen}\right| \geq d$.

We denote questionable answers at level d by *QA-d*, whereas *NQA-d* denotes the non-questionable answers at level d. For the purpose of this analysis we consider *QA-3* and *NQA-3* answers. This means that we define questionable answers to be those for which there exists at least one answer (response category chosen by the respondent) whose absolute difference to his/her mean xenophobic score is equal or greater to 3. For example if the i-th respondent's response vector is $\mathbf{x}(i) = [5,1,1,\ldots,1]$, then his/her response vector would be identified as questionable since there exists a $j = 1 : |q_1(i) - \overline{xen}| = |5 - 1.26| = 3.73 \geq$. The sample was split into two categories: respondents providing non-questionable answers ($N = 928$) and respondents providing questionable answers ($N = 160$). The artificial neural network system determines the classification of the respondents in the case of *NQA-3*. For the case of the *QA-3* we develop two fuzzy systems, since there exist several factors that need to be considered and the classification is not ambiguous. The first fuzzy system takes into account a set of rules and determines the *degree of belief (TRUST)* about the xenophobic level of the respondent that will determine the way this answer will be scored. The second fuzzy system determines the *xenophobic level*, considering the *degree of belief (TRUST)*, which is the output of the first fuzzy system and the score of the respondent. Subsequently, a final level is provided for each respondent based on the results (outcomes) of all systems. The neural network that was implemented was a three-layer Back Propagation network (Fig. 15.2). The structure of the proposed intelligent classification system is shown in Fig. 15.3 and a part of the *NQA-3* is revealed in Table 15.1.

For non-questionable answers the Neural Network Toolbox of MATLAB R2014a was used and the xenophobic levels were determined. For validation the

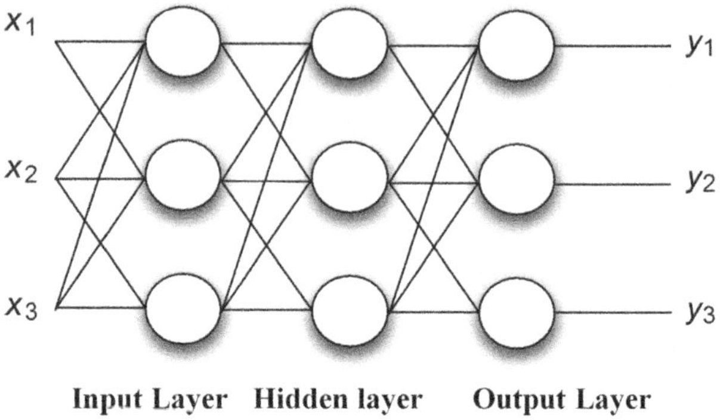

Fig. 15.2 The structure of the implemented artificial neural network

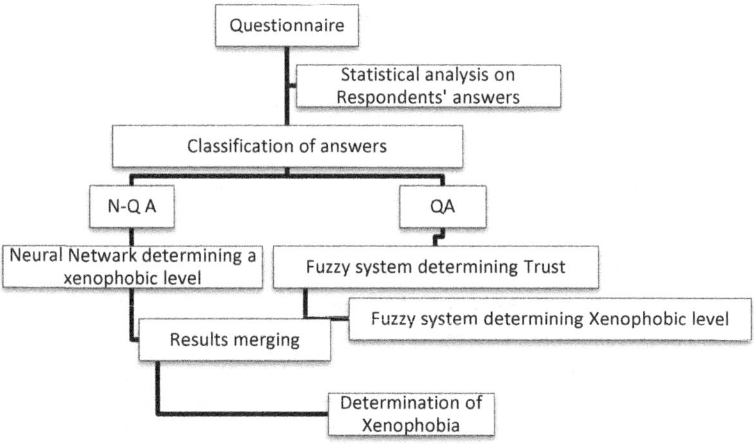

Fig. 15.3 The structure of the proposed system

Table 15.1 An excerpt of non questionable answers and their classifications to levels of xenophobia

Non questionable answers	Level of Xenophobia
$\mathbf{x} = (1, 1, \ldots, 1)$	1
$\mathbf{x} = (2, 1, \ldots, 1)$	1
$\mathbf{x} = (2, 2, \ldots, 2)$	2
$\mathbf{x} = (2, 2, \ldots, 1)$	2
$\mathbf{x} = (3, 3, \ldots, 3)$	3
$\mathbf{x} = (2, 2, \ldots, 3)$	2
$\mathbf{x} = (4, 4, \ldots, 4)$	4
$\mathbf{x} = (4, 4, \ldots, 5)$	4
$\mathbf{x} = (5, 5, \ldots, 5)$	5
$\mathbf{x} = (5, 5, \ldots, 4)$	5

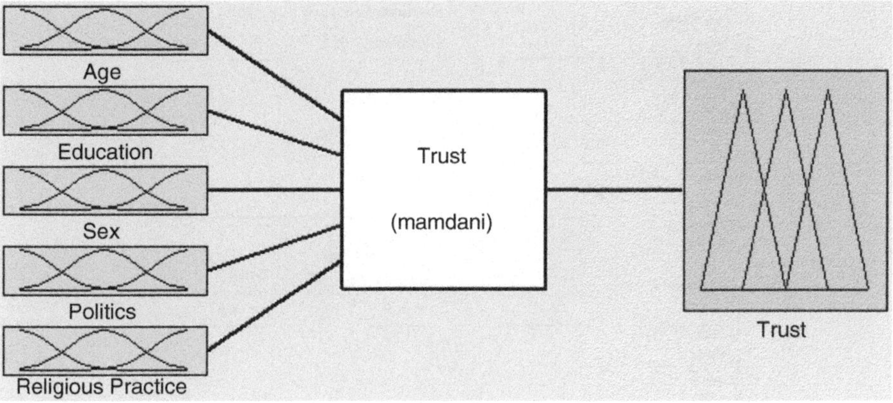

Fig. 15.4 Input and output of the first fuzzy system

analysis was repeated with the Neural Network analysis provided by IBM Statistics SPSS 24.0 and the same results were given as outcomes with very slight differences.

For the questionable answers we firstly develop the following system that has five inputs and one output. The inputs are factors that determine xenophobia: Age, Education, Sex, Politics and Religious Practice. The output is the degree of belief or trust that the specific respondent is of an increased level of xenophobia. Figure 15.4 provides the inputs and output of the first system whereas Fig. 15.5 presents the fuzzy partitioning of Age, Education, Sex, Politics and Religious Practice.

Age is measured in years, Education in one of the categories from 1 = Illiterate/has left primary school to 7 = Postgraduate degree, Gender is either Male (1) or Female (2), Politics is a variable that takes values from 1 (Left wing) to 10 (Right wing) and Religious practice (how often do you go to church) takes values from Every Sunday or more often (1) to Never (5). Therefore, a possible input for the first fuzzy system would be *input* = [23,4,1,4,3]. The fuzzy partition of the output of the first fuzzy system is presented in Fig. 15.6.

An excerpt of the fuzzy rule base for TRUST, which consists of 28 inference rules of the canonical form, i.e. IF-THEN rules, is the following:

1. IF (*Age, Education, Gender, Politics, ReligiousPractice*) IS (Young, High, Male, LeftWing, Rarely), THEN *Trust* IS Low.
2. IF (*Age, Education, Gender, Politics, ReligiousPractice*) IS (Young, High, Female, LeftWing, Rarely), THEN *Trust* IS Low.
3. IF (*Age, Education, Gender, Politics, ReligiousPractice*) IS (Old, Low, Female, RightWing, Frequently), THEN *Trust* IS High, etc.

Table 15.2 provides a selection of the respondents' socio-demographic characteristics (those who provided the questionable answers) and their output (trust in being xenophobic (values from 0 to 1)).

We then proceed with the development of the second system that has two inputs (the respondent's score (RespondentScore) and the degree of belief (Trust)) and

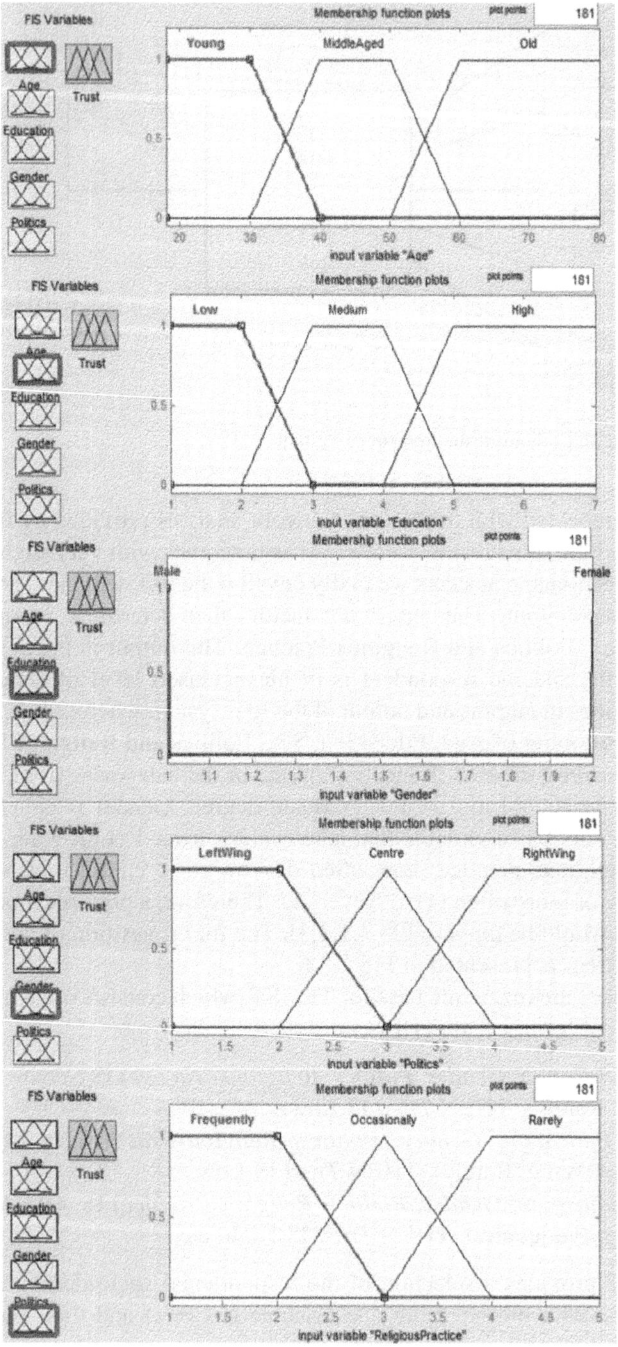

Fig. 15.5 Fuzzy partitioning of age, education, sex, politics and religious practice

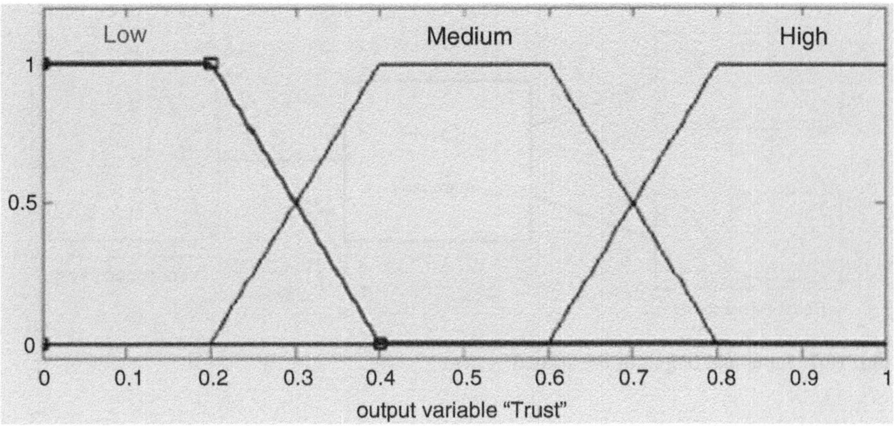

Fig. 15.6 The fuzzy partition of the variable *Trust*

Table 15.2 An excerpt of the respondents' socio-demographic characteristics (*QA-3)* and their output (trust in being xenophobic)

Respondent	Age	Education	Gender	Politics	Religious practice	Degree of belief
4	31	4	1	3	3	0.14
15	30	5	1	3	4	0.15
18	60	3	2	3	1	0.48
24	59	4	1	2	4	0.19
34	32	4	1	5	3	0.61
35	43	1	2	5	2	0.65
37	28	3	2	2	4	0.15
60	36	4	2	1	1	0.17
64	78	4	1	5	3	0.48
65	63	3	1	4	1	0.48

provides as an output the xenophobic level of the respondent (XenophobiaLevel). The inputs and the output of the system are presented in Fig. 15.7.

A possible input for the first fuzzy system would be *input* = [0.52 29]. The fuzzy partition of Trust and Respondent Score can be seen in Fig. 15.8.

An excerpt of the fuzzy rule base for XenophobiaLevel, which consists of IF-THEN inference, is now provided:

1. IF (*Trust, RespondentScore*) IS (Low, Low), THEN *XenophobiaLevel* IS Low.
2. IF (*Trust, RespondentScore*) IS (Medium, Medium), THEN *XenophobiaLevel* IS Medium.
3. IF (*Trust, RespondentScore*) IS (High, High), THEN *XenophobiaLevel* IS High, etc. (Fig. 15.9)

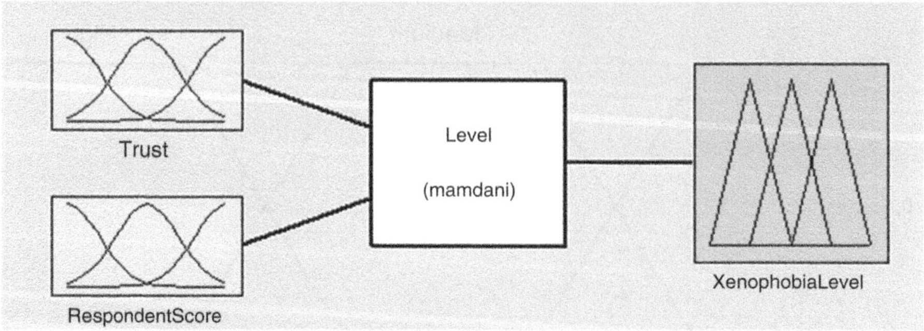

Fig. 15.7 Input and output of the second system

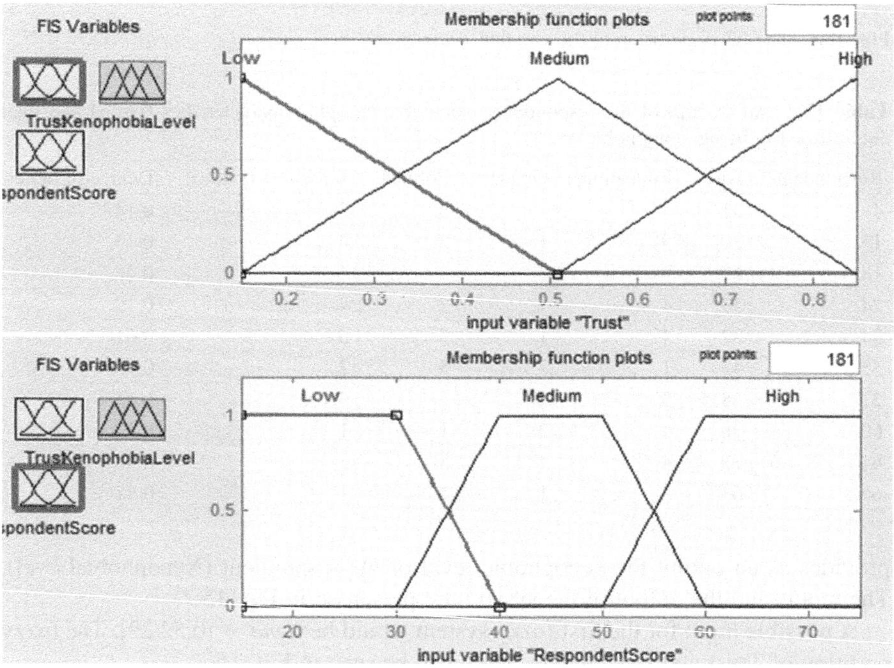

Fig. 15.8 Fuzzy partition of trust and RespondentScore

15.3 Validation

In order to validate the suggested method, the neuro-fuzzy scores were correlated with five single items that are considered in the literature as indicators of xenophobia (Eurobarometer 1989). The same procedure was used in order to validate the proposed method in Symeonaki et al. (2015) where a fuzzy set theory solution to combining Likert items into a single overall scale (or subscales) was presented. A

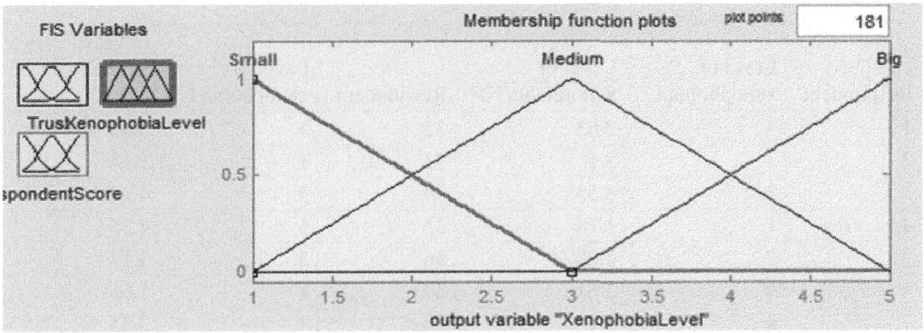

Fig. 15.9 Fuzzy partition of XenophobiaLevel

combination of four of these items was used as an indicator of xenophobia (Michalopoulou et al. 1999). These indicators measure xenophobia based on the perception of the number of 'others' (of another nationality or religion) and the disturbance caused by their presence. Table 15.3 provides the reader with the combined results (*QA-3* and *NQA-3)* for 56 respondents.

The indicators used are given in Table 15.4, whereas Table 15.5 exhibits the correlation analysis results between xenophobia neuro-fuzzy and crisp and all xenophobia indicators. As expected xenophobia crisp and neuro-fuzzy are highly correlated. As shown neuro-fuzzy scores are higher correlated with all xenophobia indicators, thus obviously producing a more accurate measurement of xenophobia (Table 15.6).

15.4 Conclusions

Central to attitude measurement in social survey research is Likert scaling theory. The present paper puts forward an intelligent system that simulates the respondent's final score when the answers are not questionable and takes into account a number of other crucial factors when the answers are questionable in order to classify the respondents into xenophobic levels reducing therefore the uncertainty. The proposed methodology is illustrated using raw data of a survey designed to measure xenophobia but it can be applied in Likert scaling in general. The presented methodology, moreover suggests that semantic information, usually available by the experts of the attitude domain, must also be taken into account, together with results of the statistical analysis produced by the current or previous studies and therefore can handle the uncertainty introduced to attitude measurement in social survey research. The findings show that the measurement of xenophobia levels produced is valid and more accurate since correlation analysis revealed that (a) xenophobia scores (neuro-fuzzy and crisp) are highly correlated and more importantly, (b) neuro-fuzzy scores are higher correlated with a number of xenophobia indicators.

Table 15.3 Levels of xenophobia (classical (C) and Neuro-fuzzy approach (NF)) for 56 respondents

Respondent	Level of xenophobia C	Level of xenophobia NF	Respondent	Level of xenophobia C	Level of xenophobia NF
1	3	2.63	32	3	3.03
2	3	3.1	33	1	1.14
3	3	3.53	34	5	4.35
4	1	1.78	35	5	4.35
5	2	2.08	36	3	3.17
6	4	3.61	37	1	1.65
7	4	4.1	38	4	3.55
8	4	4.41	40	2	1.59
9	4	3.72	41	2	1.82
10	3	3.29	44	1	1.22
11	3	3.12	45	3	2.91
12	2	2.11	46	1	1.17
13	2	2.35	47	3	2.88
15	1	1.65	49	2	2.24
16	2	2.17	51	2	2.23
18	5	4.12	52	4	3.99
19	3	2.57	54	3	3.3
20	3	3.46	55	2	2.19
21	2	1.62	56	1	1.14
22	2	2.19	57	2	2.26
24	1	1.65	60	1	1.65
25	1	1.19	61	1	1.22
26	3	2.87	62	2	2.03
27	3	3.26	63	3	3.26
28	4	3.53	64	4	4.12
29	2	2.48	65	5	4.12
30	5	4.91	66	2	2.13
31	2	2.25	67	4	3.97

Table 15.4 Indicators of xenophobia

Indicator	Question
1	During the last years individuals from other countries which are not members of the European Union have come to live and work in Greece. According to your opinion, these foreigners who live today in Greece are too many, many but not too many, not too many.
2	How do you feel about the presence of individuals of another nationality? Disturbing or not disturbing?
3	How do you feel about the presence of individuals of another religion? Disturbing or not disturbing?
4	In your opinion these individuals of another nationality are too many, many but not too many or not too many.
5	In your opinion these individuals of another religion are too many, many but not too many or not too many
6	Combination of indicators 2–5

Table 15.5 Pearson's correlation coefficients, Xenophobia (classical (C) and neuro-fuzzy approach (NF))

	Xenophobia (NF)	Xenophobia (C)
Xenophobia (NF)		0,936
Xenophobia (C)	0,936	

**Note:* N = 1088, $p < 0.001$

Table 15.6 Spearman's rho correlation coefficients

Indicator	Xenophobia (NF)	Xenophobia (C)
1	−0,239	−0,238
2	−0,438	−0,434
3	−0,384	−0,367
4	−0,219	−0,215
5	−0,218	−0,204
6	0,456	0,434

**Note:* N = 1088, $p < 0.001$

References

Eagly, A., & Chaiken, S. (1993). *The psychology of attitudes*. Fort Worth: Harcourt Brace Jovanovich College Publishers.

Gil, M. A., & Gil, G. -R. (2012). Fuzzy vs. Likert scale in statistics. *Combining Experimentation and Theory Studies in Fuzziness and Soft Computing, 271*, 407–420.

Hogg, M., & Vaughan, G. (2008). *Social psychology*. New York: Prentice Hall.

Lalla, M., Facchinetti, G., & Mastroleo, G. (2005). Ordinal scales and fuzzy set systems to measure agreement: An application to the evaluation of teaching activity. *Quality and Quantity, 38*, 577–601.

Likert, R. (1932). A technique for the measurement of attitudes. *Archiv für Psychologie, 140*, 1–55.

Michalopoulou, A., Tsartas, P., Giannisopoulou, M., Kafetzis, P., & Manologlou, E. (1999). *Macedonia and the Balkans: xenophobia and development*. Alexandria: National Centre of Social Research. (Abridged English edition), Athens, Greece.

Perloff, R. M. (2016). *The dynamics of persuasion: Communication and attitudes in the twenty-first century*. New York: Routledge.

Symeonaki, M., & Kazani, A. (2011). *Developing a fuzzy Likert scale for measuring xenophobia in Greece*. ASMDA, Rome, Italy, 7–10 June, 2011.

Symeonaki, M., & Kazani, A. (2012). *Measuring xenophobia in Greece using neural network and fuzzy techniques*. SMTDA, Chania, Greece, 5–8 June, 2012.

Symeonaki, M., & Michalopoulou, C. (2011). *Measuring xenophobia in Greece: A cluster analysis approach*. ASMDA, Rome, Italy, 7–10 June, 2011.

Symeonaki, M., Kazani, A., & Michalopoulou, C. (2011). *Fuzzifying Likert scales with factor analysis techniques*. ERCIM, London, UK, 15–17 December, 2011.

Symeonaki, M., Michalopoulou, C., & Kazani, A. (2015). A fuzzy set theory solution to combining Likert items into a single overall scale (or subscales). *Quality and Quantity, 49*(2), 739–762.

Zadeh, L. (1965). Fuzzy sets. *Information and Control, 8*, 3.

Part V
Data Analysis in Demography

Chapter 16
Differences in Life Expectancy by Marital Status in the Czech Republic After 1990 and Their Decomposition by Age

Tomas Fiala and Jitka Langhamrova

16.1 Introduction

Demographic studies usually analyze mortality by age and gender. However, mortality also depends on many other factors. One such factor is marital status, which is also one of the very important demographic criteria determining the demographic behavior of the population. Single people have different demographic behavior than married, divorced or widowed people. Therefore, marital status is considered an important social indicator that differentiates the population based on their link to family and marriage. Changes in marital status (marriage, divorce, widowhood) are considered very important demographic events. Marital status also provides indirect information about the lifestyle and status of an individual in society. Social status can sometimes depend on, or be partly determined by, marital status. There is a statistical correlation between marital status and death rate.

The mortality of married people is lower than that of single, divorced or widowed people. This is what William Farr, an epidemiologist, physician and statistician of the General Register Office for England and Wales, (mostly known as the founder of medical statistics and the first classification of death causes) already claimed in the nineteenth century (1858). Based on the analysis of specific mortality rates by age, he showed that the mortality of single people is considerably higher than the mortality of married people of the same age and that the mortality of widowed people is even higher (Parker-Pope 2010).

The differences in mortality by marital status were confirmed by many other studies. Their explanation is based on many theories and hypotheses that can be

T. Fiala (✉) · J. Langhamrova
Department of Demography, Faculty of Informatics and Statistics, University of Economics, Prague, Czech Republic
e-mail: fiala@vse.cz; langhamj@vse.cz

© Springer International Publishing AG, part of Springer Nature 2018
C. H. Skiadas, C. Skiadas (eds.), *Demography and Health Issues*,
The Springer Series on Demographic Methods and Population Analysis 46,
https://doi.org/10.1007/978-3-319-76002-5_16

divided into two basic groups. The first one, the so-called causality theory (protection theory), is based on the hypothesis of a "protective" effect of marriage and its positive influence on health and a longer life. On the other hand, the second theory, the so-called selection theory, is based on the hypothesis that those who get married are healthier on average, and thus their mortality is lower.

The causality theory emphasizes that marriage is an important social institution. Based on this theory, a better quality of life in wedlock stems from the fact that the spouses support each other emotionally and socially. They overcome life problems better and more easily and usually have more social contacts and thus can find necessary support or help from friends more easily in case of any problems. The causality theory also points out the fact that life in wedlock promotes a healthier lifestyle, married people have fewer bad habits, such an excessive alcohol consumption and smoking, and suffer from depression and anxiety less often. Married couples also usually keep track of each other's health condition and thus are more likely to see a physician earlier in case of any medical problem. Women in particular make sure that all family members have preventive checkups and take care of their spouse if he becomes seriously ill. Married people also have a better financial situation and usually a higher standard of living since they have joint funds and share some expenses. If one of the spouses loses work, the other spouse can financially support him or her as long as necessary. According to the causality theory, the longer a marriage lasts, the more benefits it provides (Hamplová 2012, pp. 738–739).

The question is whether marriage is as beneficial for men as for women, or whether marriage provides more advantages to men or women. This issue was researched by Jessie Bernardová, who concluded that marriage provided more advantages to men than to women. According to her, married women are not actually happier, but adjust their answers in different surveys to expected social norms that assume that married women are happier (Hamplová 2009, p. 133).

An interesting question is whether marriage positively affects men about the same as women, or whether men or women benefit from marriage more. Based on some studies, marriage has a bigger impact on men because the differences in mortality between single and married men are bigger than those between single and married women. However, other studies show that women benefit from marriage more than men, or that men and women benefit from marriage about the same but in different areas. Marriage has a positive impact on men by protecting them against depression and on women by protecting them against alcoholism. It is pointed out that men have better psychological health regardless of marital status than women. A life crisis, such as divorce or widowhood, affects men and women differently. These crises affect men much more than women.

On the other hand, the selection theory assumes that people marry or do not marry, or remain in wedlock for a shorter or longer period of time, mostly based on their personality traits. According to this theory, the mortality of married men and women is not lower because they are married. This theory stresses a favorable selective impact of marriage on mortality, e.g. people with a serious illness or a physical handicap usually do not marry, and also assumes that people with certain personality traits, e.g. temperament, optimism, etc., are better preconditioned for creating and maintaining long-term relationships, which is also positively reflected in their lower mortality. On the other hand, people suffering from depression, ill people or alcoholics, etc. (i.e. people whose mortality exceeds the average) have less chance to marry and their risk of divorce is higher.

Nevertheless, Hamplová (2009, pp. 131–132), mentions three reasons why the selection theory has been called into question lately. The first reason is that the measurements of physical and psychological health either do not confirm the selectivity effect or show only a very weak selectivity effect. The second reason is that the mortality of the widowed (who were married for a rather long time) is higher than that of people who are still married, i.e. marriage decreases mortality. The third fact that calls the selection theory into question is based on the conclusions of medical research confirming that single people die more often due to their different lifestyle rather than due to their genetically conditioned illness.

The number of marriages in the Czech Republic and many European countries has currently gone down and more and more couples live together out of wedlock. This fact should also be analyzed and researched to see whether or not living out of wedlock has the same positive impact on mortality as marriage. However, the problem is that there are usually no reliable data about the number, gender and age of people living together out of wedlock and mostly that this fact is not investigated in the deceased.

16.2 Differences in Mortality by Marital Status in the Czech Republic

Pechholdová and Šamanová (2013) provide a very detailed analysis of the correlation between mortality and marital status in the Czech Republic for the years the population census was carried out starting in 1960. In all analyzed years, the life expectancy of married men and women aged 30 is higher than the life expectancy of unmarried men and women, and the difference is higher in men than in women.

The trends during the socialist regime (1961–1990) and the post-socialist era were quite different. The differences in the mortality of the married and the unmarried doubled and even tripled during the 1960s, 1970s and 1980s as compared to the year 1961 (Srb and Boris 1990). During the entire analyzed time period, the mortality of single women was the highest and the mortality of widows the lowest from among unmarried women, although the mortality of divorced and widowed women gradually approximated. In the case of men, the situation was different at first. In the years 1961, 1971 and 1981, the mortality of divorced men was the highest and the mortality of single men the lowest from among unmarried men. This trend changed in 1991 where (similarly to women) the mortality of single men was the highest and the mortality of widowers the lowest (Table 16.1).

Table 16.1 Differences in life expectancy at birth by marital status
Reference category: married

Year	1961	1970	1980	1991	2001	2010
Males						
Single	−3.08	−5.11	−6.59	−9.15	−8.76	−9.58
Divorced	−3.63	−5.58	−7.34	−8.24	−7.47	−7.65
Widowed	−3.54	−5.39	−7.44	−7.16	−7.24	−5.73
Females						
Single	−3.26	−4.67	−5.50	−6.65	−7.57	−7.70
Divorced	−2.46	−3.12	−3.49	−4.77	−4.67	−4.99
Widowed	−1.31	−1.64	−2.39	−3.21	−4.04	−4.69

Source: Pechholdová and Šamanová (2013), Tab. 1

In her analysis of comparative indexes of mortality in individual years during 1982–1993, Rychtaříková (1998) shows that the mortality of single men practically did not change, while mortality in other marital status categories decreased, in particular in married men. The mortality of women in all marital status categories decreased, but considerably less in single women.

16.3 Trends of Life Expectancy Development by Marital Status in 1990–2014

After the year 1989, the behavior of the Czech population in terms of marriage rather considerably changed. People got married at an older age, the marriage rates dropped and the percentage of children born out of wedlock went up. For instance, while almost 79% of men and over 83% of women were married at the age of 30–39 in the year 1991, only about 50% of men and slightly over 60% of women were married at the same age in the year 2010 (Pechholdová and Šamanová 2013, Tab. 2).

This chapter provides the results of the analysis of the trend in the mortality of men and women by marital status and analyzes life expectancy at birth by marital status. This life expectancy was calculated in a usual way based on complete mortality tables by marital status, using the Czech Statistical Office's data containing the number of the deceased and the number of population in the individual years of the analyzed time period classified by gender, age unit and marital status.

Specific death rates for people under the age of 16, when it is not possible to marry, were considered to be the same for all marital status categories (equal to death rates regardless of marital status). Death rates were differentiated based on marital status after the age of 16, but only if the mid-period population of the given age and marital status was higher than 100. In the case that the mid-period population of the

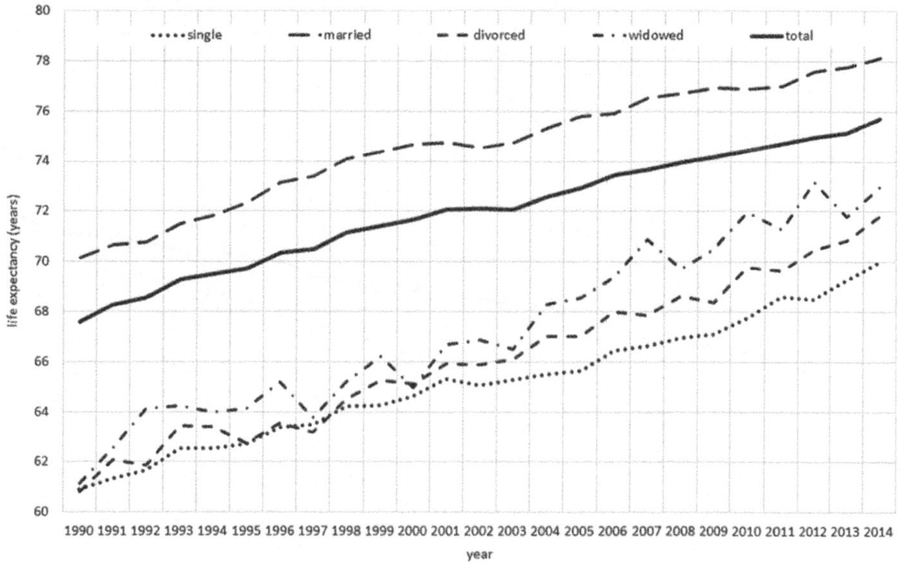

Source: data Czech Statistical Office, authors' calculation

Fig. 16.1 Life expectancy at birth by marital status – males

given age and marital status was lower, the mortality of all people of the given age was used, regardless of marital status.

The life expectancy of men and women kept going up more or less linearly during the entire analyzed time period (Fig. 16.1). The life expectancy of all men went up (regardless of their marital status) from not quite 67.6 years to 75.7 years, i.e. by 3.9 months a year. The increase in the life expectancy of married men was slightly lower (by 3.8 months), but higher in the case of other categories of men (the average increase in the life expectancy of single men was 4.4 months a year, of divorced men 5.3 months a year and of widowers 5.7 months a year). Therefore, the differences of married and unmarried men lessened, while the differences of widowed, divorced and single men increased.

The increase in the life expectancy of women, regardless of marital status, was lower (by 3 months a year on average), from 75.5 in the year 1990 to 81.7 in the year 2014 (Fig. 16.2). When taking into consideration marital status, the increase was also lower in women than in men. The life expectancy of married women during the analyzed time period went up by 2.4 months a year on average, while the life expectancy of single women went up by 3.1 months a year, of divorced women by 3.3 months a year and of widows by 3.2 months a year. Similarly to men, the differences in the life expectancy of married and unmarried women lessened.

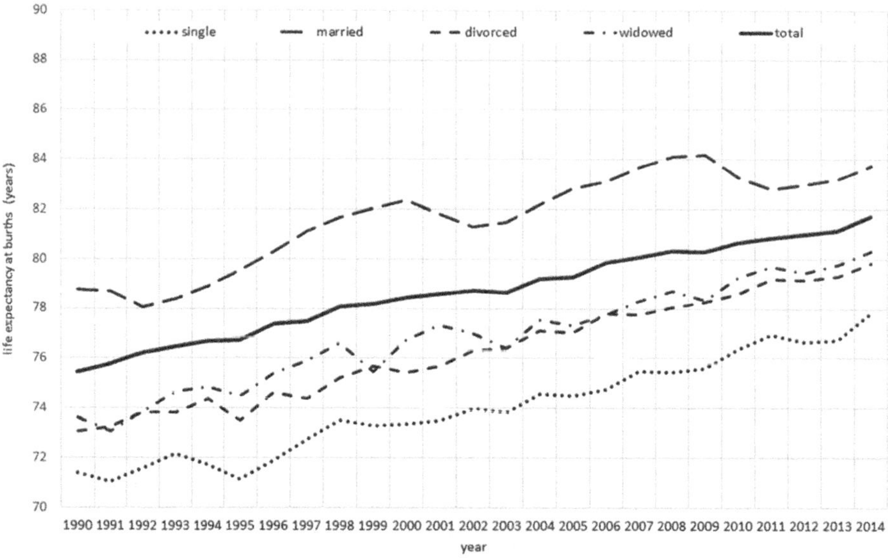

Source: data Czech Statistical Office, authors' calculation

Fig. 16.2 Life expectancy at birth by marital status – females

The trend in life expectancy, taking into account marital status, shows much bigger random deviations from the linear trend since especially the number of people of a certain marital status is very low in particular in some age groups. In order to eliminate these deviations, life expectancy for the individual five-year periods of 1990–1994, 1995–1999, . . ., 2010–2014 were calculated as well. Since the goal of the trend analysis is not really the trend in life expectancy but rather the trend in life expectancy differences by marital status, married men and women were chosen as a reference category and the differences in life expectancy in this reference category and in the individual categories of unmarried people (i.e. single, divorced and widowed people) were analyzed.

The basic trends are the same for both men and women (Figs. 16.3 and 16.4). In all analyzed time periods, the life expectancy of single people differed from the life expectancy of married people the most, while the life expectancy of widowed people differed the least. The difference for females was approximately 1 to 4 years less than in the relevant category of men during the same time period.

While all differences were bigger during 1995–1999 than in the previous time period, they started lessening after 2000 and were smaller in the last analyzed time

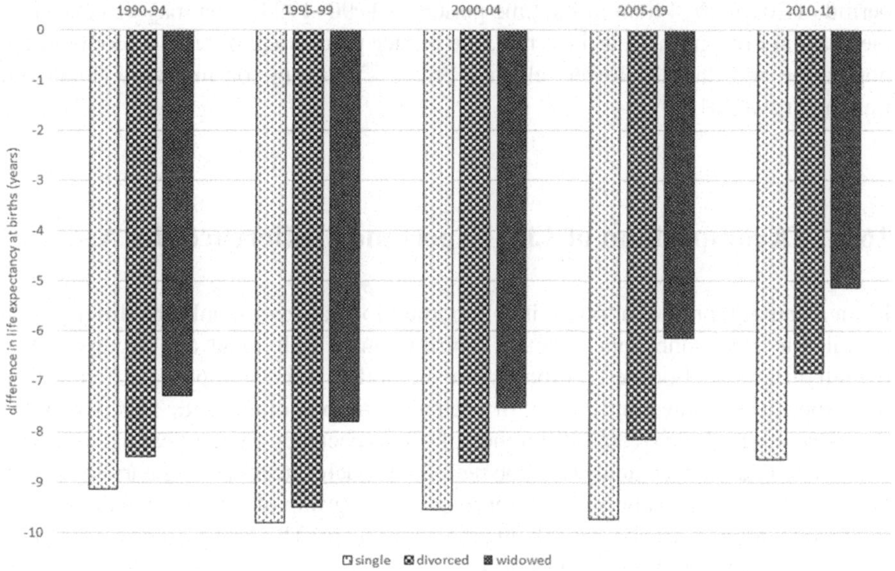

Source: data Czech Statistical Office, authors' calculation

Fig. 16.3 Differences in life expectancy at birth by marital status – males (reference category – married)

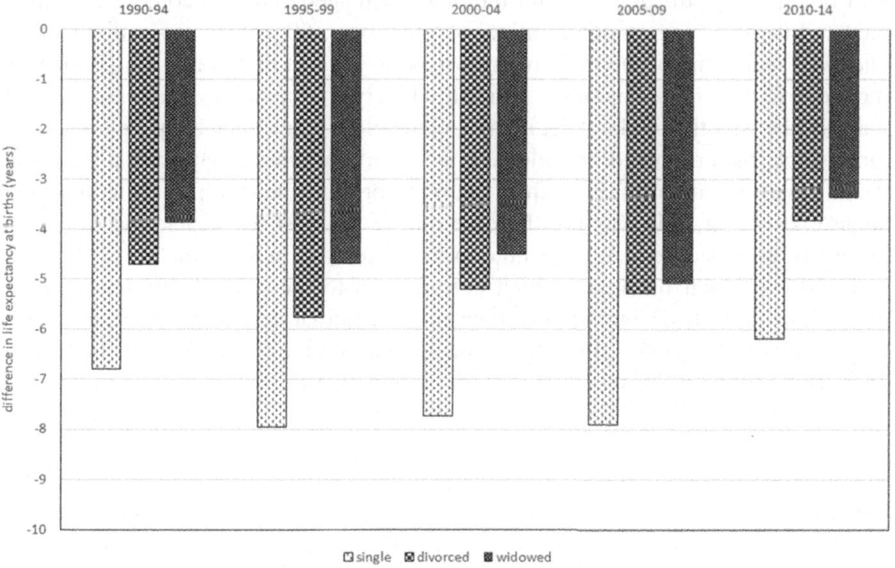

Source: data Czech Statistical Office, authors' calculation

Fig. 16.4 Differences in life expectancy at birth by marital status – females (reference category – married) period of 2010–2014 than in the time period of 1990–1994. This may be caused by the gradual drop in the marriage rate, the higher percentage of single people in the population and thus the lower selective effect of marriage on mortality (Fiala and Langhamrová 2016).

16.4 Decomposition of Life Expectancy Differences by Age

From a demographic standpoint, it is important to analyze not only the difference in overall life expectancy but also the contribution of individual age groups to this overall difference. For these purposes, the method which decomposes differences in life expectancy to the contribution of each age group is often used. This is why the decomposition of the overall difference of life expectancy by ten-year age intervals was calculated for each analyzed time period and each category of unmarried people. Of course, there cannot be any difference in the age group of 0–9, and the differences in the age group of 10–19 and 90–99 are insignificant. This is why these age groups are not shown in the following figures.

When comparing with married men and women, the biggest contributions to the difference in life expectancy at birth come mostly from men in the age groups of 50–59 and 60–69 and usually from women in the age of 60–69 and 70–79. However, the contributions differ, depending on marital status. During the first analyzed five-year time periods, the biggest contribution of men aged under 60 comes from single men, while the biggest contribution of men over 60 comes from divorced or widowed men. One of the main reasons may be the fact that young single men die more due to their irresponsibility, unhealthy lifestyle or some medical reason (which may also be why they did not get marry), while older single men are psychologically more stable than divorced or widowed men, some of whom may have a hard time dealing with the dissolution of their marriage or with the death of their long-time spouse. However, this was not the case during the past ten years, and in all age groups of men, single men contribute to the difference in life expectancy the most and widowed men the least, which corresponds to the overall difference in life expectancy at birth. The trend in women is more regular and, with some exceptions, single women always contribute the most and widows the least. See Figs. 16.5, 16.6, 16.7, 16.8, 16.9, 16.10, 16.11, 16.12, 16.13, and 16.14.

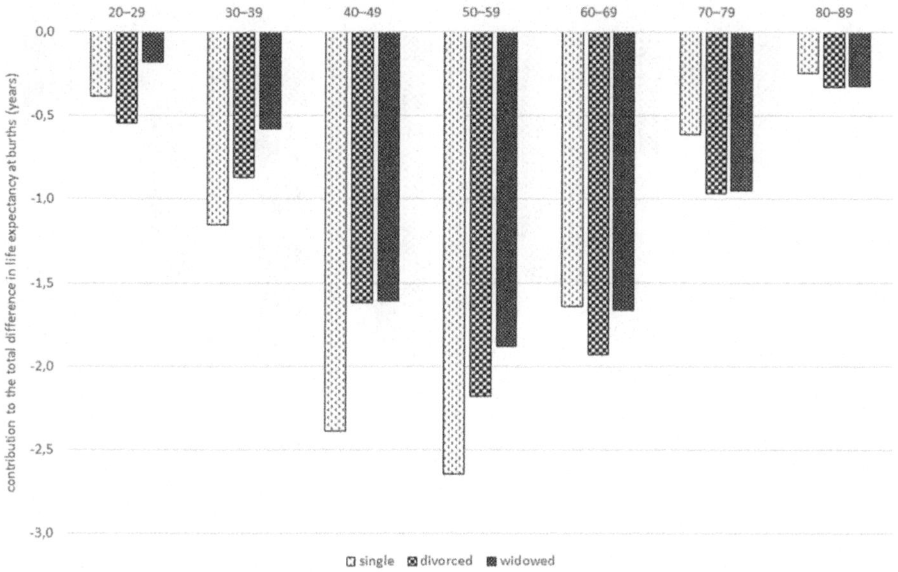

Source: data Czech Statistical Office, authors' calculation

Fig. 16.5 Decomposition by age in life expectancy at birth by marital status – 1990–1994 males (reference category – married)

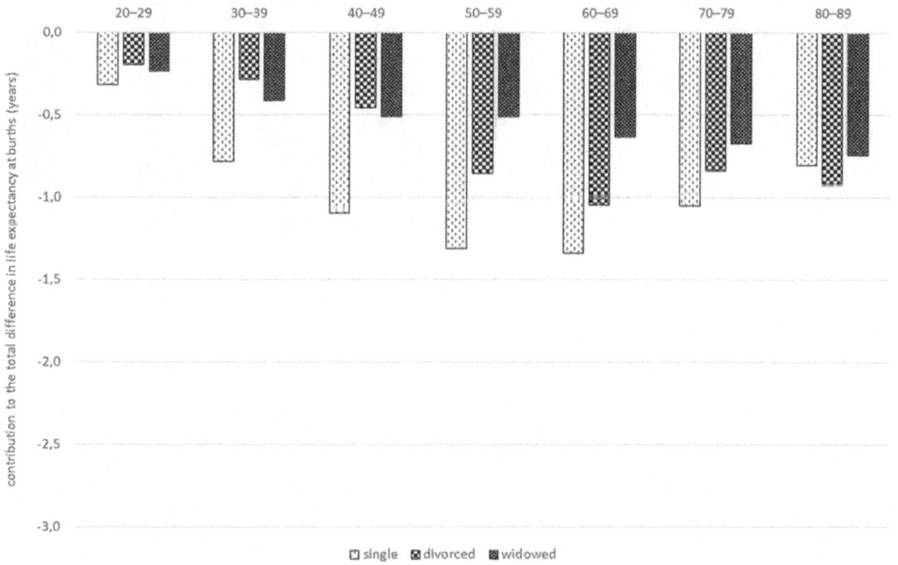

Source: data Czech Statistical Office, authors' calculation

Fig. 16.6 Decomposition by age in life expectancy at birth by marital status – 1990–1994 females (reference category – married)

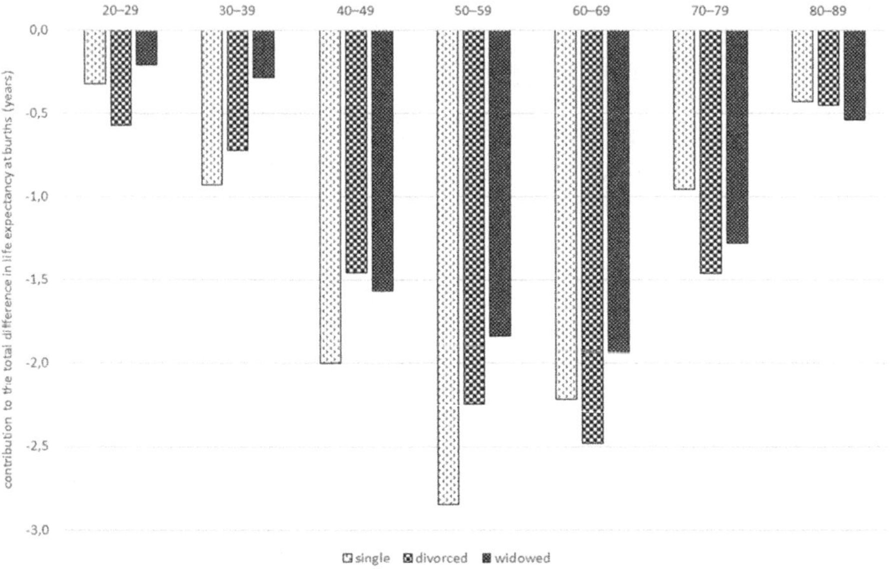

Source: data Czech Statistical Office, authors' calculation

Fig. 16.7 Decomposition by age in life expectancy at birth by marital status – 1995–1999 males (reference category – married)

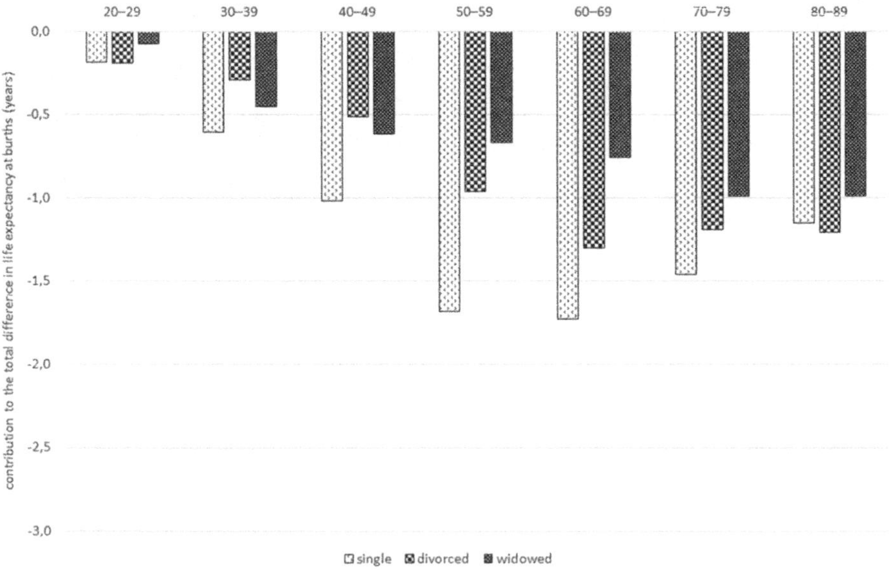

Source: data Czech Statistical Office, authors' calculation

Fig. 16.8 Decomposition by age in life expectancy at birth by marital status – 1995–1999 females (reference category – married)

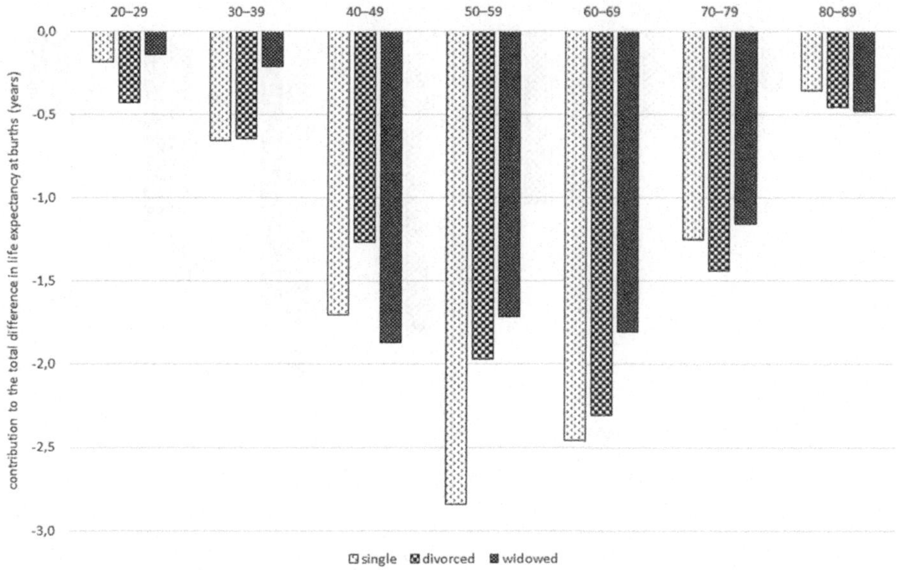

Source: data Czech Statistical Office, authors' calculation

Fig. 16.9 Decomposition by age in life expectancy at birth by marital status – 2000–2004 males (reference category – married)

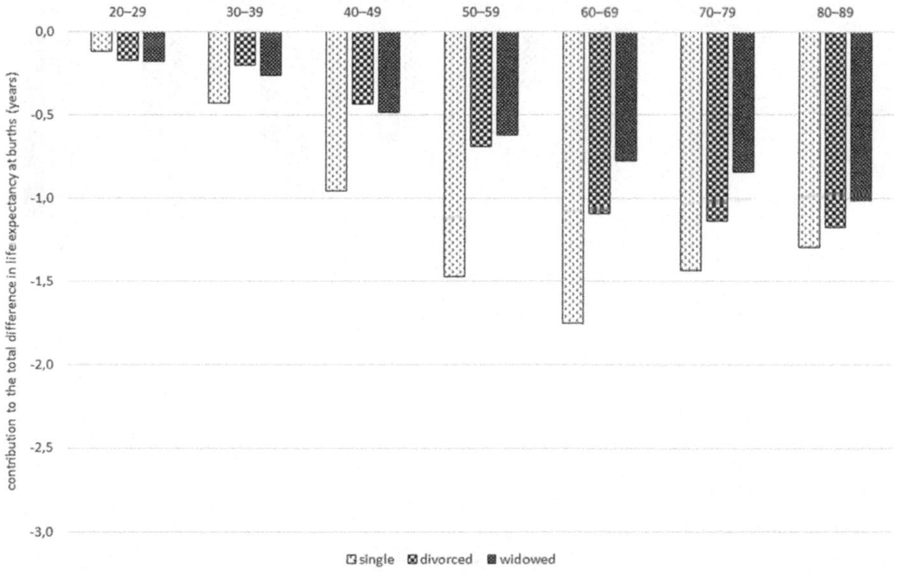

Source: data Czech Statistical Office, authors' calculation

Fig. 16.10 Decomposition by age in life expectancy at birth by marital status – 2000–2004 females (reference category – married)

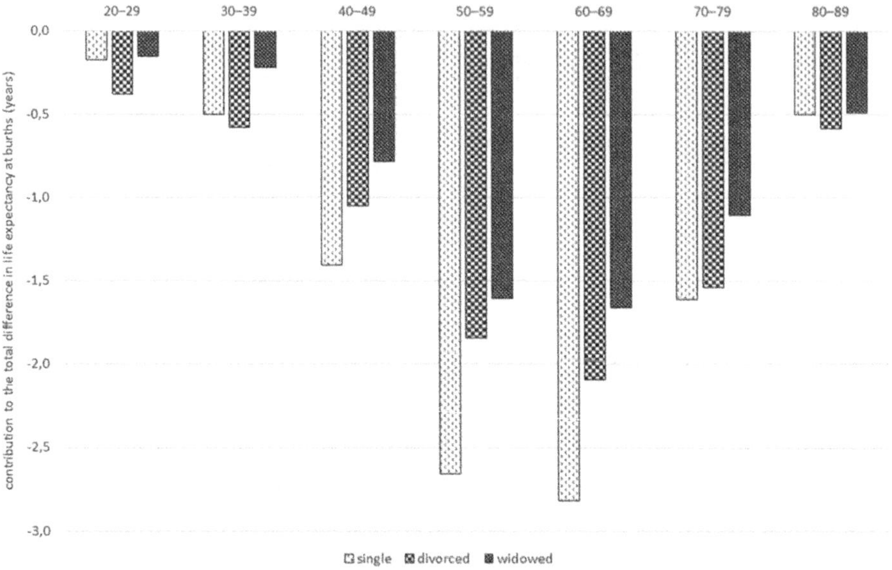

Source: data Czech Statistical Office, authors' calculation

Fig. 16.11 Decomposition by age in life expectancy at birth by marital status – 2005–2009 males (reference category – married)

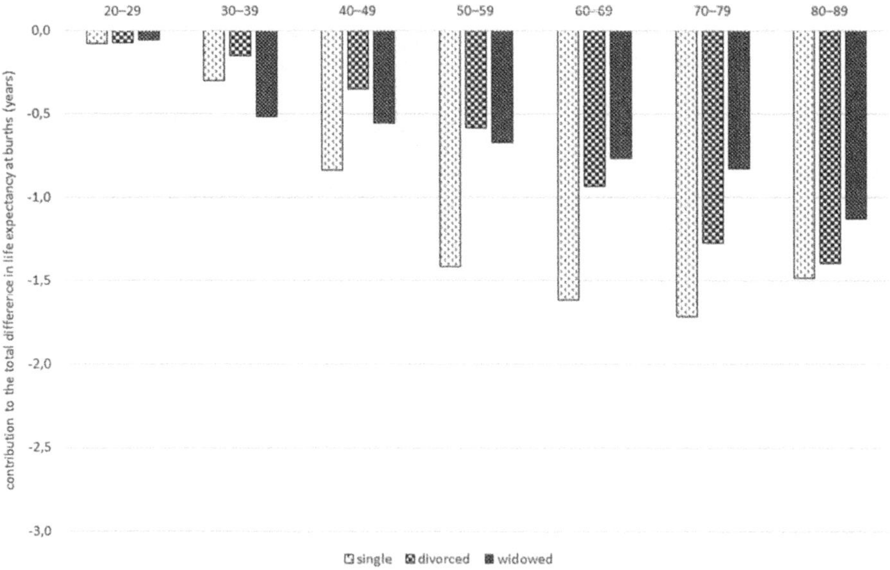

Source: data Czech Statistical Office, authors' calculation

Fig. 16.12 Decomposition by age in life expectancy at birth by marital status – 2005–2009 females (reference category – married)

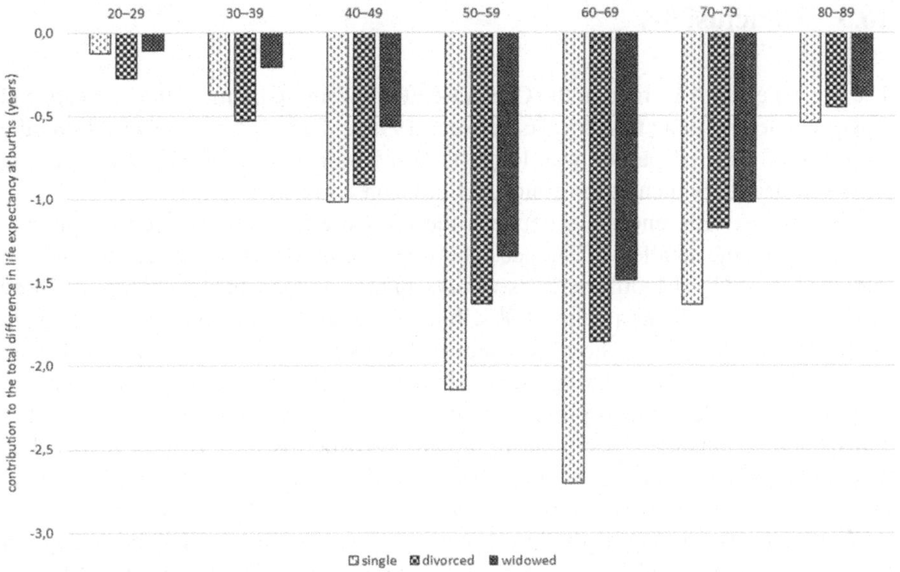

Source: data Czech Statistical Office, authors' calculation

Fig. 16.13 Decomposition by age in life expectancy at birth by marital status – 2010–2014 males (reference category – married)

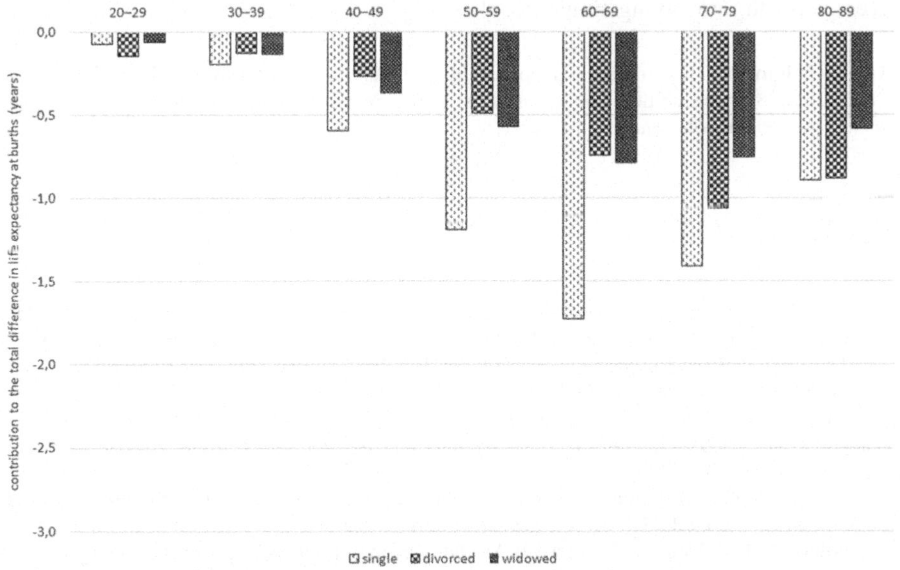

Source: data Czech Statistical Office, authors' calculation

Fig. 16.14 Decomposition by age in life expectancy at birth by marital status – 2010–2014 females (reference category – married)

16.5 Conclusions

The life expectancy of men in the Czech Republic went up by more than 8 years and that of women by more than 6 years between 1990 and 2014. After the year 1990, the mortality of married people was lower than the mortality of single, divorced and widowed people, which corresponds to European trends.

The biggest differences are between the life expectancy of married people and single people; the smallest difference is between the mortality of married people and widowed people. The difference is always bigger in men than in women. These differences were bigger in the 1990s, but this gradually changed after 2000. In 2010–2014 in particular, the differences in life expectancy by marital status were significantly smaller than during the previous five-year time period and smaller than in 1990–1994. This is also proven by the fact that the overall increase in the life expectancy of unmarried men during the analyzed period was slightly higher than that of married men and that the life expectancy of unmarried women increased more than the life expectancy of married women.

The main reason may be the lower marriage rate and thus a lower percentage of married people and a higher percentage of single people. This lessens the selective effect of marriage. While some physical or psychological handicap or an irresponsible lifestyle, which could also be the cause of the higher death rate of single people, used to often be the reason why people did not marry, nowadays there is probably a higher percentage of healthy and responsible people with an average or above-average death rate among single people.

Acknowledgment This article was supported by the Grant Agency of the Czech Republic No. GA ČR 15-13283S under the title *Projection of the Czech Republic Population According to Educational Level and Marital Status*.

References

Fiala, T., & Langhamrová, J. (2016). *Mortality differences by family status in the Czech Republic since 1993*. In: *STMDA*, Valetta, Malta, 1.-4.6.2016. https://onedrive.live.com/?authkey=%21AAQ6%5FVpgAZuZB4s&cid=CB6060F40BD0FF92&id=CB6060F40BD0FF92%21348&parId=CB6060F40BD0FF92%21106&o=OneUp

Hamplová, D. (2012). *Zdraví a rodinný stav: dvě strany jedné mince?* Str. 738–739.

Hamplová, D. (2009). *Life satisfaction, happiness and marital status in four central European countries* (pp. 131–132).

Parker-Pope, T. (2010). Is marriage good for your health? *New York Times*, 2010-04-14. http://www.nytimes.com/2010/04/18/magazine/18marriage-t.html

Pechholdová, M., & Šamanová, G. (2013). Mortality by marital status in a rapidly changing society: Evidence from the Czech Republic. *Demographic Research, 29*, 307–322. https://doi.org/10.4054/DemRes.2013.29.12. http://www.demographic-research.org/Volumes/Vol29/12/.

Rychtaříková, J. (1998). Úmrtnost v České republice podle rodinného stavu. *Demografie, 40*(2), 93–102.

Srb, V., & Boris, V. B. (1990). Úmrtnost obyvatelstva podle rodinného stavu 1950–1980. *Demografie, 31*(1), 37–41.

Chapter 17
Air Pollution and Health Risks: A Statistical Analysis Aiming at Improving Air Quality in an Alpine Italian Province

Giuliana Passamani and Matteo Tomaselli

17.1 Introduction

In recent years much more attention has been devoted to health risks caused by air pollution. The World Health Organization (WHO), using data collected by the Global Health Observatory (GHO), has estimated that air pollution caused 6.5 million deaths in 2012, with different estimated average values across the six WHO regions[1]: the highest value of 133.5 deaths (per 100,000 population) in the Western Pacific (Democratic People's Republic of Korea and China the worst country averages), and the lowest value of 20.3 deaths in the Americas. Europe shows an estimated average value of 64.2 deaths, with an estimated value of 35.2 deaths in Italy, while the Eastern European countries show very high estimated values. As WHO states: "The lower the levels of air pollution, the better the cardiovascular and respiratory health of the population will be, both long- and short-term".[2]

Among all the estimated deaths associated with air pollution, WHO underlines that 3.1 million premature deaths every year are estimated as a result of exposure to

[1]http://www.who.int/gho/phe/air_pollution_mortality/en/

[2]http://www.who.int/mediacentre/factsheets/fs313/en/, key fact 2.

G. Passamani (✉)
Department of Economics and Management, University of Trento, Trento, Italy
e-mail: giuliana.passamani@unitn.it

M. Tomaselli
Economics and Management, Doctoral School of Social Sciences, University of Trento, Trento, Italy
e-mail: matteo.tomaselli.1@unitn.it

© Springer International Publishing AG, part of Springer Nature 2018
C. H. Skiadas, C. Skiadas (eds.), *Demography and Health Issues*,
The Springer Series on Demographic Methods and Population Analysis 46,
https://doi.org/10.1007/978-3-319-76002-5_17

ambient air pollution, while the remaining are associated with household exposure to smoke[3]. The Organization points to key ambient air pollutants that pose health risks: particulate matter (PM), ozone (O_3), nitrogen dioxide (NO_2) and sulphur dioxide (SO_2). They are atmospheric aerosols and greenhouse gases which may also interact physically and chemically in the atmosphere, in such a way to make much more difficult forecasting their future variations in air pollution. The problem of ambient air pollution is widely recognized by the population, and it is particularly alarming when rainfalls are scarce for a prolonged period. The scientific community is active in monitoring ambient air pollution, both at the soil level through dedicated monitoring sites, and at the aerospace level through, for instance, the Copernicus Atmosphere Monitoring Service[4] promoted by the European Space Agency (ESA).

It has been shown in the specialized literature that air pollution undoubtedly effects human health, especially in large cities and in areas affected by heavy traffic roads, with undeniable negative consequences on the cardiovascular and respiratory systems (see Brunekreef and Holgat 2002; Kampa and Castana 2008). It is now widely accepted that air pollution is closely related to climate change, which may also effect human health through different pathways, thus increasing the overall negative balance of ambient pollution (Haines et al. 2006). One of the main aspects that characterises air pollution is its intrinsic temporal heterogeneity (mainly influenced by the meteorological conditions that determine long-term trends and cyclical behaviours, see Milionis and Davies 1994), and its spatial heterogeneity. For this reason, empirical analyses have recently adopted spatial regression models to assess the association between mortality and air pollution (see, for instance, Jerrett et al. 2005; Van der Wal and Janssen 2000; Burnett et al. 2001), thus accounting for spatial autocorrelation when more than one location in the geographic area under analysis is taken into consideration[5]. Other adopted approaches model the intertemporal dynamics through time-series regressions (Milionis and Davies 1994; Salcedo et al. 1999), hazard models (Hoek et al. 2002) or spline and other non-linear models (Dominici et al. 2002; Chelani and Devotta 2006).

When the emphasis of the analysis is on short-term health effects and on the observations of changes in repeated outcome variables, the commonly adopted technique is to use panel models (Yu et al. 2000; Janes et al. 2008). Recent developments have introduced heterogeneity in panel models, and, in fact, this is the approach that we adopt in this paper and that is described in Sect. 17.3.

Since it is not possible to review the whole literature here, we invite the interested reader to read O'Neill et al. (2003) and Dominici et al. (2003), and the compelling overview of air pollution consequences on health given by WHO (2013).

---

[3]http://www.who.int/airpollution/en/

[4]See https://atmosphere.copernicus.eu/

[5]By and large, not considering spatial autocorrelation does not substantially changes effect estimates. Moreover, spatial autocorrelation models can possibly underestimate standard errors. See Hoek et al. (2002) and Burnett et al. (2001)

This brief introduction has highlighted the importance of a comprehensive analysis of air quality and its determinants.

Our focus will be at local level, given the availability of information provided by the Provincial Environmental Protection Agency (APPA) of the Province of Trento, whose purpose is monitoring ambient quality. Even though we are not exploring, from a scientific point of view, their sources and characteristics, how they are formed and removed, we aim to understand the temporal evolution of the gaseous and aerosol pollutants, how they statistically interact among themselves and with atmospheric factors, such as temperature, wind and rain. We assume that a better comprehension of the dynamics of air pollutants and of the impact that meteorological variables have on them, possibly using stochastic models that can then be used for simulation, can surely help in deciding future local policy interventions aiming to reduce the pollution levels and to improve the quality of air.

Our data set is made up of daily time series observations on the main pollutants and meteorological variables registered at seven monitoring sites within the alpine province of Trento, which is located in the north-eastern part of Italy. It is mainly a mountainous area characterised by valleys, rivers and lakes of different dimensions. It is also intersected by two important trunk roads: the Brenner motorway, that crosses the province from north to south in the direction of Austria, and the Valsugana highway, that links Trento to the eastern part of Italy. The largest towns are located along the Brenner motorway and in the Valsugana valley. Though the air quality of the province may be considered overall good with respect to other provinces, it is indeed affected by important sources of pollution, above all in the valleys, where much of the population live. Therefore, pollution has a direct impact on the lives of the majority of the inhabitants of the area. Understanding pollution behaviour may thus be the first step towards the adoption of appropriate local policy measures, in order to limit pollution and its negative consequences on health.

The rest of the paper is organised as follows. First, we describe our data set and the air pollution levels for each monitoring site. Second, for each of them we compute the pollution factor, on which we then base our empirical analysis. The latter is divided into two parts: in the first, using an estimated panel data model, we remove the part explained by the weather variables from the pollution factors, while in the second part we study how the three main pollutants affect the unexplained part of the pollution factors. On this component, in fact, policy makers should focus.

17.2 Descriptive Analysis of Data and Possible Health Risks

The empirical analysis is based on daily data on air pollutants and meteorological variables collected and provided by the Trentino Environmental Protection Agency (APPA). Due to the availability of data, only two years, 2014 and 2015, and seven monitoring sites within the province of Trento are considered: Trento PSC (Trento 1 henceforth) and Rovereto, as urban and residential areas; Borgo Valsugana and Riva del Garda, as sub-urban sites, but with quite different climates, as the latter is mitigated by the winds coming from lake Garda, the largest Italian lake; Monte Gaza and Piana Rotaliana, as rural areas, and Trento VBZ (Trento 2 henceforth) which is an urban area afflicted by heavy traffic.

From a first descriptive analysis of the observed pollutants across the monitoring sites, we can detect the diverse characteristics of the distributions of the three pollutants that we consider: PM_{10}, NO_x, and O_3. The relative data are obtained from continuous measurements of each pollutant, the unit of measurement being μg/m^3. The first picture of Fig. 17.1 refers to vertical box-plot representations of the observed daily average values of PM_{10}, the particles with a diameter between 2.5 and 10 micrometres, which are produced by cars engines and other combustion processes. As expected, the calculated percentiles show that the distributions are asymmetric with quite a few large outliers. It's to be noted that, according to the European Environment Agency (EEA) air quality standards[6], values larger than 50 μg/m^3 put at risk people with respiratory disease. As can be seen from Table 17.1, the lowest sample average level is observed for Monte Gaza, the mountain area, and the highest is observed for Trento 2, the heavy traffic area. However, an average level as high as Trento 2 is also observed for Borgo Valsugana. The other monitoring sites show intermediate comparable average levels of PM_{10}. Therefore, it is straightforward to deduce a first raw relationship between the locations and the PM_{10} levels: the higher the traffic levels, the higher the PM_{10} levels.

The second picture of Fig. 17.1 refers to vertical box-plot representations of the observed daily maximum hourly average values of NO_x, nitrogen oxides, given by the combination of NO and NO_2, mainly originated by combustion processes. Again, the calculated percentiles show that the distributions are asymmetric with many very large outliers, except for Monte Gaza. According to EEA, hourly concentrations of NO_2 should not go above 200 μg/m^3 for more than 18 hours in any year and their annual average should not be greater than 40 μg/m^3. As we can observe, the most polluted area is Trento 2 where an increasing likelihood of respiratory symptoms and breathing discomfort in active children, the elderly, and people with lung disease such as asthma, and of possible respiratory effects in general population can be detected. As reported in Table 17.1, sample average levels of NO_x above 40 μg/m^3 are registered also for Trento 1, Rovereto, Borgo Valsugana and Piana Rotaliana.

The third picture of Fig. 17.1 refers to vertical box-plot representations of the observed daily maximum hourly average values of O_3, ozone, a pollutant that is originated by the action of daylight UV rays on the other pollutants, especially those produced during combustion processes. The box-plots show similar distributions for

[6]http://ec.europa.eu/environment/air/quality/standards.htm

the monitoring sites[7], with the only exception of Monte Gaza, a site characterized by somewhat higher levels of O_3. This is not surprising because the location of this site records high solar radiation levels throughout the year, which are the primary responsible for the generation of the ozone and hence for the unusual O_3 levels (for more details, see the Air Quality Reports, APPA 2014, 2015). The registered levels of ozone are such that, according to EEA, they do not seem to adversely effect human health.

Therefore, the pollutant for which most exceedances are registered is NO_x.

An analysis using the inverse distance weight spatial interpolations (without Monte Gaza) for the three pollutants, and depicting them in a spatial form where darker colours indicate relatively higher pollution levels, confirms the results emerged from the box-plot representations: Fig. 17.2 shows that, for what concern PM_{10} and NO_x, the rural and sub-urban areas are effectively less polluted than the traffic and urban areas (with the already recognized exception of Borgo Valsugana for the PM_{10} levels), while, for O_3 levels, the exposure to solar radiation is far more relevant than the distinction between urban or rural location, as the rural area Piana Rotaliana and the suburban area Riva del Garda are more polluted than the urban area Trento 1.

Finally, Fig. 17.3 shows the dynamics of the time series and their trend[8] for each monitoring site. Beyond the three air pollutants, we graph the dynamics of the daily average weather variables that we will consider for the analysis: temperature (°C), rain (mm), solar radiation (W/m^2), humidity (%), dew point (°C), wind run[9] (km), and atmospheric pressure (bar). With the understandable exception of rain that depends on local atmosphere phenomena especially in summer, all the variables exhibit comparable seasonal dynamics. Moreover, as expected, O_3 shows a behaviour that follows the dynamics of temperature and of solar radiation, in contrast with the behaviour of PM_{10} and NO_x.

With the available time series, we construct a slightly unbalanced panel data set including the daily average data for each monitoring site in which shorter periods of missing observations are filled through linear interpolation (longer periods of missing data are left blank). We also exclude the last five days of observations for 2015, since data are not available for all the monitoring sites. This data set represents the starting point of the following econometric empirical analysis.

[7] O_3 data are not available for Trento 2.

[8] The trend was obtained by applying the Hodrick and Prescott filter to each time series.

[9] Wind speed (km/h) has been excluded because it is strongly correlated with wind run.

17.3 An Unobserved Factor as Air Quality Indicator

Not having available an index measuring the short-term air quality situation as a whole at each monitoring site[10], we suggest a procedure for the estimation of a single unobserved common component that we consider an air pollution indicator for each site. Therefore, in order to compare air pollution levels across the different sites of the province of Trento, we look for a variable that summarizes the three pollutants in an indicator.[11]

To this purpose it is possible to adopt a methodology called Principal Component Factor Analysis (PCFA), which aims to extract meaningful linear combinations by decomposing the correlation matrix of a set of observed variables that may jointly explain a certain phenomenon, and provides the so-called common factors and the corresponding factor loadings. The common factors are thus latent variables which are described through their relationship with the variables of interest, while the factor loadings show the weight of each variable in explaining the factors. In details, for each site, given the observation y_{tj} on the j-th variable relative to time t, the common factors z_{tq}, for the same time t, contribute to explain it through the following relationship:

$$y_{tj} = z_{t1}\lambda_{1j} + z_{t2}\lambda_{2j} + \ldots + z_{tq}\lambda_{qj} + u_{tj} \tag{17.1}$$

where λ_{qj} is the factor loading, and u_{tj} is a unique component proper of the j-th variable.

The appropriate number q of unobserved factors, smaller than the number of observed variables, depends on their observed correlations, and can be chosen either on the basis of the eigenvalues obtained from the decomposition of the correlation matrix, or on the basis of the percentage of explained variance.

To avoid misleading results determined by "extreme" locations, two monitoring sites are excluded from the econometric empirical analysis: Monte Gaza and Trento 2, the first because it is located in a mountain area, and the second because it is devoted to the study of traffic pollution and of the specific pollutant CO which is not recorded at the other sites. For the remaining sites, the three considered air pollutants display well determined patterns (see Sect. 17.2) and high correlation coefficients: PM_{10} and NO_X are strongly and positively correlated for all the sites, as NO_X and O_3 are strongly but negatively correlated; PM_{10} and O_3 are also negatively correlated for each site, but the magnitude of the coefficient is lower (Table 17.2).

[10]We could have followed the procedure used by EEA which takes measurements of up to five key pollutants supported by modelled data and determines the index level that describes the current air quality situation at each monitoring station. The single index level would correspond to the poorest index level for any of five pollutants.

[11]Principal component factor analysis (see Passamani and Masotti 2016; Fontanella et al. 2007; Forni et al. 2000 for some applications) and principal component regression models (see Kumar and Goyal 2011 for an application) are techniques that are used to summarise the available information into one or more factors.

Given the small number of observed pollutants and their correlation structure, it is reasonable to expect that a single latent factor explains a high percentage of the observed variables variability, according to the following model:

$$y_t = \lambda z_t + u_t \tag{17.2}$$

where y_t represents the (3×1) vector of dependent variables, the three pollutants for each site, z_t the unobservable common factor, λ the (3×1) vector of factor loadings and u_t the (3×1) vector of disturbances. The results, in fact, give evidence of one factor z_t that we consider as an indicator of air pollution levels for each monitoring site as suggested by Passamani and Masotti (2016). By employing the PCFA discussed above, the indicator "summarises a complex situation in a single variable whose evolution can be compared in time and in space" (Passamani and Masotti 2016, p. 787)[12]. The dynamics of the pollution factor, or *PF*, for each site is shown in Fig. 17.4, where we can notice that it is characterised by a clear seasonal behaviour.

17.4 The Effect of Meteorological Variables on Air Quality

As weather is an important air pollution contributor in determining air quality, in the following we first aim to study the impact of the variables characterising weather, before focusing the attention on how to improve air quality.

A first aspect characterising our data is the seasonality, which affects both the pollution factors and the meteorological variables. Consequently, we could even detect a seasonal variation in the effects of air quality on health. The observation of seasonal patterns in Figs. 17.3 and 17.4 indicate that the winter season is characterised by higher volatility than the summer season. The heating systems and the higher usage of cars in cold days are probably the primary responsible for this phenomenon.

Another aspect that should be included into the analysis is the intrinsic intertemporal nature of pollution: today's pollutant levels directly affect tomorrow's levels and are determined by yesterday's levels. Therefore, a dynamic approach is essential to study the evolution of the pollution factor.

Finally, a last aspect that affects our data set and that has already emerged above is undoubtedly heterogeneity. The monitoring sites are remarkably different in terms of location, and this is responsible for the different levels observed throughout the period of analysis. This fact clearly emerges if we use a scatterplot for representing each pollution factor versus each meteorological variable, and show the different

[12]While Passamani and Masotti (2016) suggests a dynamic approach, for the purpose of this work we adopt a static principal component factor approach.

slopes for the partial relationships between them[13]. All these aspects are taken into consideration by the adopted panel estimation technique: the Dynamic Common Correlated Effects (DCCE).[14]

In the following of our analysis we adopt the DCCE panel time series estimation approach proposed by Pesaran (2004) which deals with all the aspects described in the previous paragraph. This estimator is implemented in Stata 13 by the command *xtdcce2* and it allows:

- the specification of a dynamic model;
- either homogeneous or heterogeneous slopes, thus fully considering the intrinsic heterogeneity characterising the monitoring sites;
- controlling for cross-sectional dependence, an aspect that we do not consider here.

Given the dependent variable z_{it} and the vector of explanatory variables x_{it}, where i indicates the cross-section unit and t the time unit, the stochastic model is:

$$\begin{aligned} z_{it} &= \rho_i z_{it-1} + \beta_i' x_{it} + \varepsilon_{it} \\ \varepsilon_{it} &= \gamma_i f_t + e_{it} \end{aligned} \tag{17.3}$$

where ρ_i is a heterogeneous coefficient measuring the effect of the lagged dependent variable, β_i is a vector of heterogeneous panel coefficients, f_t is an unobserved factor common to all the observed cross-section units and γ_i is a heterogeneous factor loading. Model (3) is estimated through:

$$\begin{aligned} z_{it} &= \rho_i z_{it-1} + \beta_i' x_{it} + \sum_{k=0}^{p} \delta_{i,k}' \bar{w}_{t-k} + \varepsilon_{it} \\ \bar{w}_t &= \left(\bar{z}_t, \bar{z}_{t-1}, \bar{x}_t\right) \end{aligned} \tag{17.4}$$

where the bar indicates the cross-section means and $p = \sqrt[3]{T}$, as suggested by Chudik and Pesaran (2015). The mean-group panel estimations are then computed as a simple mean of the heterogenous estimations:

$$\widehat{\pi}_{MG} = \frac{1}{N} \sum_{i=1}^{N} \widehat{\pi}_i \tag{17.5}$$

where $\widehat{\pi}_i = \left(\widehat{\rho}_i, \widehat{\beta}_i\right)$.

To study the general within-province relationship between air pollution and atmospheric variables including all data provided by the monitoring sites, we make use of the DCCE technique, where z_{it} corresponds to the value of the unobserved factor estimated at time t for each monitoring site i, and discussed in the previous section. In the vector of explanatory variables x_{it}, at time t for each monitoring site i, we include the meteorological variables that are commonly assumed to influence air pollution: temperature

[13]The graphs are available upon request.

[14]Stata package xtdcce2, see Ditzen(2016).

(*TOut*), wind run (*WRun*), rain (*R*), solar radiation (*SR*), humidity (*Hum*) and atmospheric pressure (*Press*)), the square of temperature, wind run and rain to capture the non-linear relationship emerged from analysing the aforementioned scatterplots, and three seasonal dummies to capture the seasonal impact of winter (*S1*), spring (*S2*) and autumn (*S3*). We checked the correlations between all these weather variables in order to avoid problems of multicollinearity in the estimation. The strongest correlation is between *Hum* and *Dew* and is equal to 0.77, whereas the other values are lower in absolute value. Therefore, by excluding *Dew*, it is plausible to exclude the problem of multicollinearity.

This approach estimates a coefficient for each monitoring site, then it provides the panel mean group estimates. Estimation results are shown in Table 17.3[15]. The first two columns are referred to the pooled-panel (homogeneous) model, while the third and the fourth columns are referred to the heterogeneous model described by Eq. (17.3).

Aggregate mean estimates of the heterogeneous model show significant values for each variable with the only exception of the seasonal dummies. Therefore, the level of the pollution factor depends positively on the previous-day level (while the second lag was not significant) and, as expected, it is negatively but not linearly affected by wind and rain, that directly reduce air pollution, while humidity and pressure have both a positive effect. This sign is, however, less easy to interpret. The temperature and the solar radiation are also negatively related to the pollution levels, since higher values may represent favourable conditions to avoid using cars and heating systems.

The pooled-panel model shows comparable coefficients, but the standard errors are somehow different (notably, *WRun* and the squared term $WRun^2$ are not significant). The largest difference is, however, in the R^2: the adjusted R^2 of the heterogeneous model is 0.86, while the adjusted R^2 of the pooled model is 0.15, a result that stresses the importance of considering heterogeneous slopes.

The next section aims to study the component of the pollution factor that is unexplained by the atmospheric variables, namely the residuals of the panel model in Table 17.3.

17.5 The Effect of the Pollutants on Air Quality

Atmospheric processes are quite complicated and they can lead to dispersion or concentration of air pollutants, thus affecting air quality. Even though we know that pollution at global level affects the evolution of weather and climate, at local level we cannot control the meteorological conditions and we can just measure their

[15]Estimations do not account for cross-sectional dependence, that emerges as a consequence of the common dynamics of the meteorological variables. When we attempted to deal with this it by implementing the correction allowed by the DCCE technique, residuals were still affected by cross-sectional dependence and, at the same time, results did not change much. As a consequence, the specification of the model should be improved in future analyses in order to cope with this problem. Nonetheless, it does not affect the analysis of the residuals (see the next section).

impact on air quality: this was the purpose of the previous section. In the following we aim to understand how we could improve air quality controlling for gases and particles in the atmosphere. Therefore, considering the estimated residuals $\widehat{\varepsilon}_{it}$, of the panel data analysis, as that part of pollution due mainly to human behaviour, the question is: "How can we reduce air pollution by reducing the pollutant levels?"

As can be seen in Fig. 17.5, the variability of the residuals differs from site to site, is not homoscedastic and it can be analysed in order to understand how it can be explained and controlled. To this purpose, for each site we regress the panel residuals obtained in the previous section, on the three main pollutants, as follows:

$$\widehat{\varepsilon}_t = \alpha' y_t + e_t \tag{17.6}$$

obtaining the results showed in Table 17.4.

As expected, the coefficients associated to the pollutants are positive and significant and they are much higher when the levels of the pollutants are lower, which means that reducing by a certain amount the single pollutant the effect on reducing the level of pollution is larger for the sites with lower levels of the same pollutant, keeping the other pollutants constant. These results could be used for simulating the effects on air pollution of adopting policies imposing any reduction in the limits of pollutant emissions.

17.6 Conclusions

Moving from the acknowledged fact that air pollution poses health risks and that being able to understand how to improve air quality is an important tool for informing public policy decisions, with our work we aim to suggest a statistical analytical procedure that can be used for a better understanding of the whole process. The procedure has been developed, first, to estimate a model able to describe the intertemporal relationship between air pollution and the available meteorological variables within the alpine province of Trento, and second, to examine the unexplained part of this relationship, which represents that part of the overall air pollution due to human behaviour and, therefore, could be controlled.

The province of Trento is characterised by heterogeneous landscapes, with a majority of rural areas and a relevant minority of urban and traffic areas. As expected, the panel data analysis shows that rain and the strength of wind are the main responsible of a (non-linear) decline in the air pollution levels, as well as the temperature. The impact of humidity and of solar radiation are, instead, less clear and probably reflect a seasonal effect.

For what concerns the component of air pollution unexplained by the atmospheric conditions, the empirical analysis shows the estimated effects on improving ambient air quality that can be obtained by reducing the levels of the pollutants.

Even though the positive consequences on health are very hard to be assessed, nevertheless, what we indicate is that air quality can be improved, because a part of it depends on population behavioural choices.

Appendix

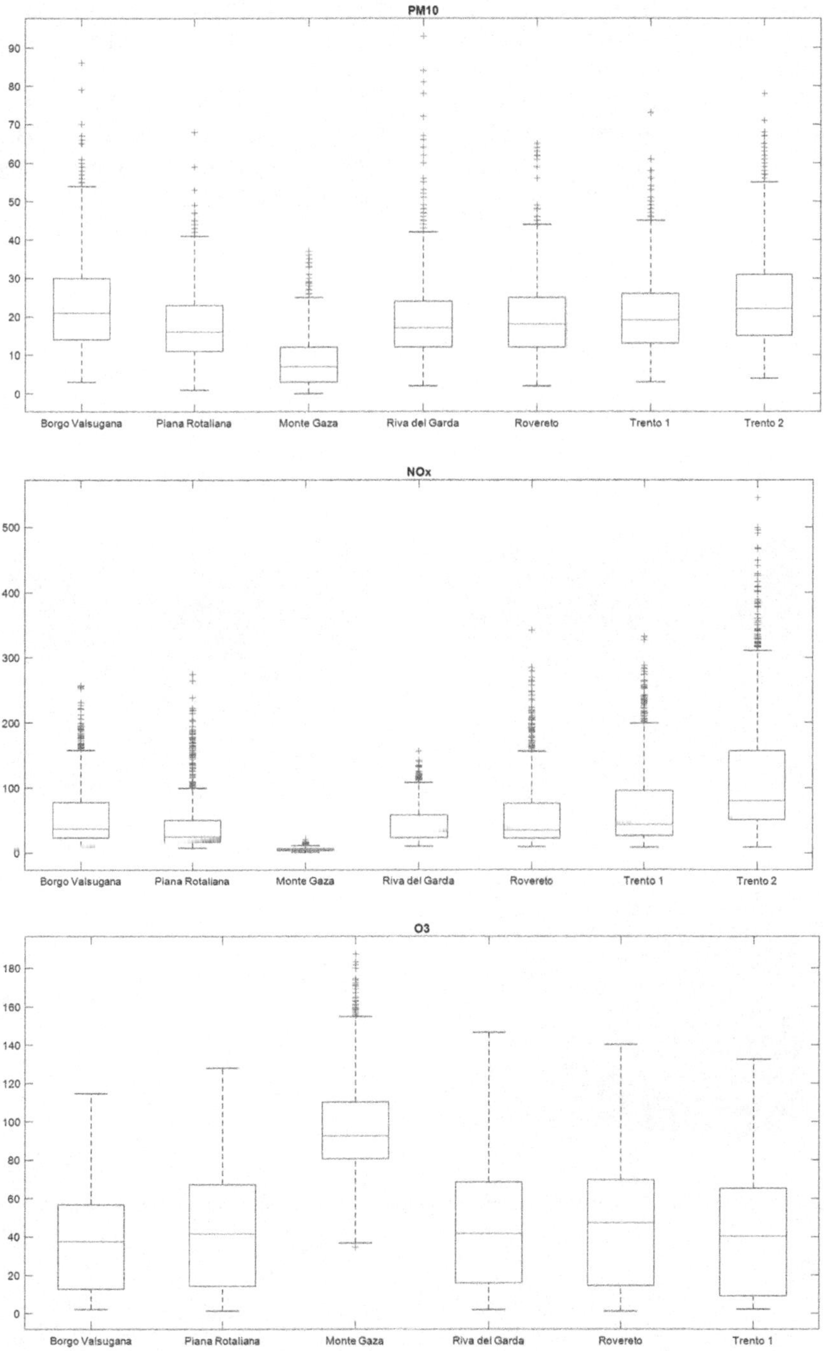

Fig. 17.1 Percentiles of the empirical distribution for each pollutant: boxplots with outliers

Table 17.1 Air pollutants: sample averages and standard deviations

	PM_{10}		NO_x		O_3	
	Mean	SD	Mean	SD	Mean	SD
Borgo	23.7643	12.8861	57.4694	48.7014	37.6219	25.7096
Piana Rotaliana	18.0970	9.42676	43.1551	43.7226	43.6120	30.7884
Monte Gaza	8.7599	7.2129	5.7444	2.6747	97.7400	24.5914
Riva del Garda	19.6321	11.6479	44.2184	27.6082	45.8782	32.6563
Rovereto	19.5082	10.1885	58.7943	54.7562	46.6496	33.2752
Trento 1	20.4828	10.1521	71.3097	63.4170	41.3936	31.9458
Trento 2	24.1767	12.7727	119.6250	96.8155	–	–

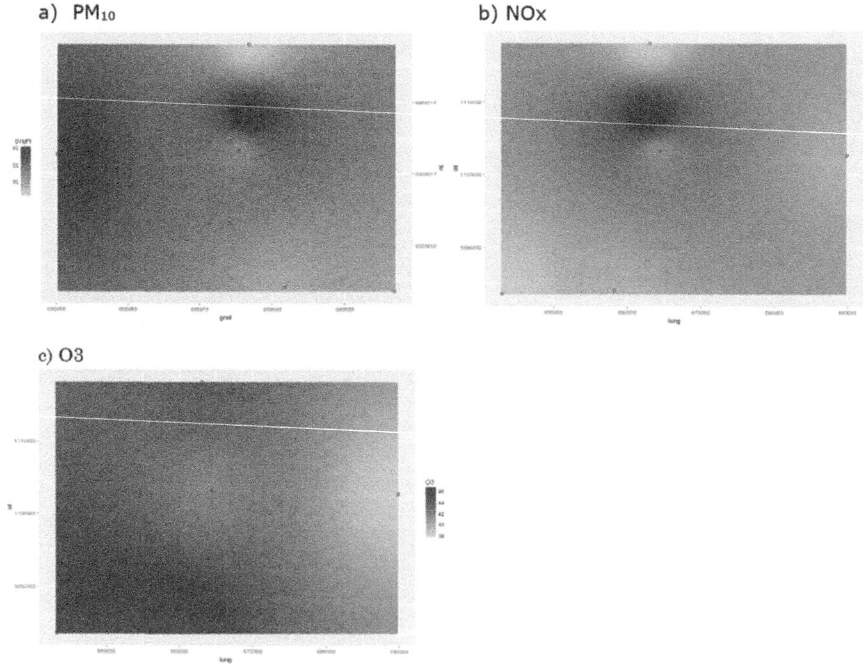

Fig. 17.2 Inverse distance weight interpolation for each pollutant, without Monte Gaza

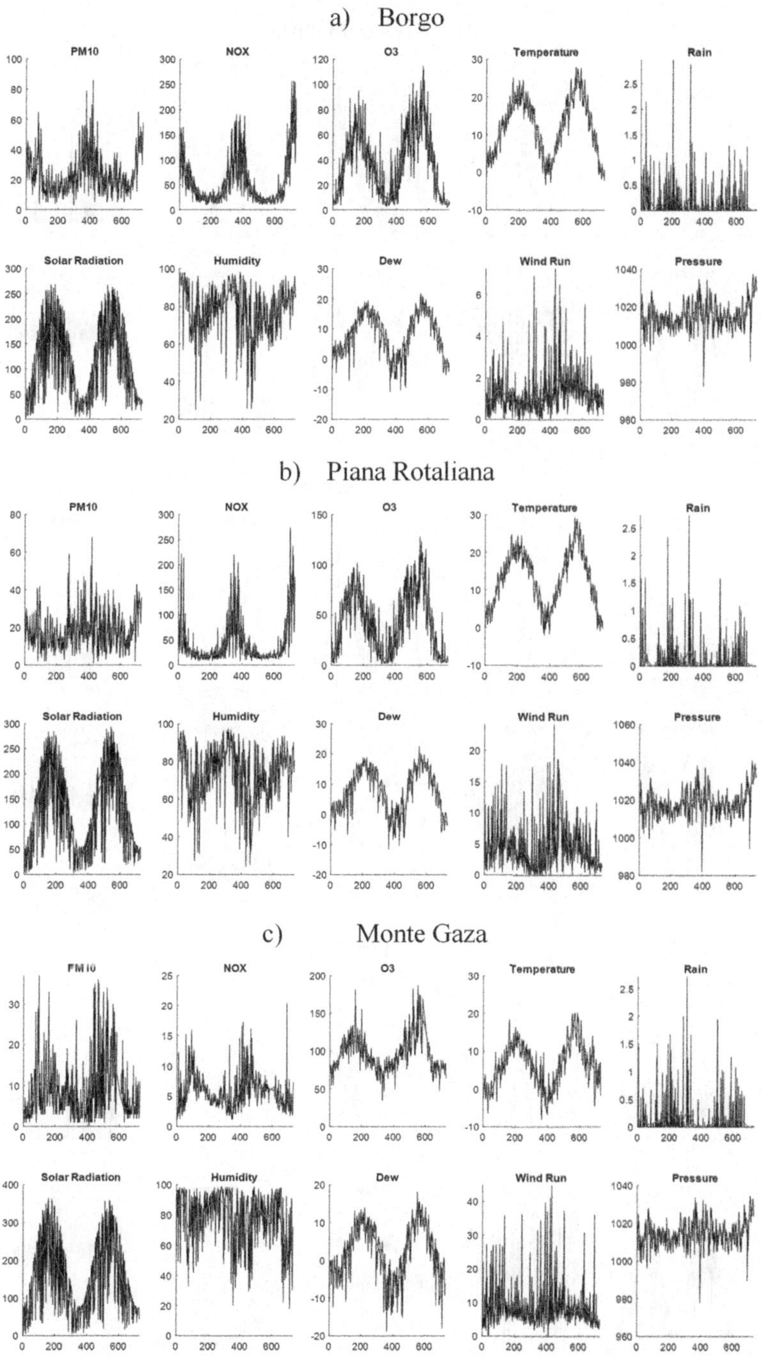

Fig. 17.3 Pollutants and meteorological variables: temporal dynamics and trend for each monitoring site

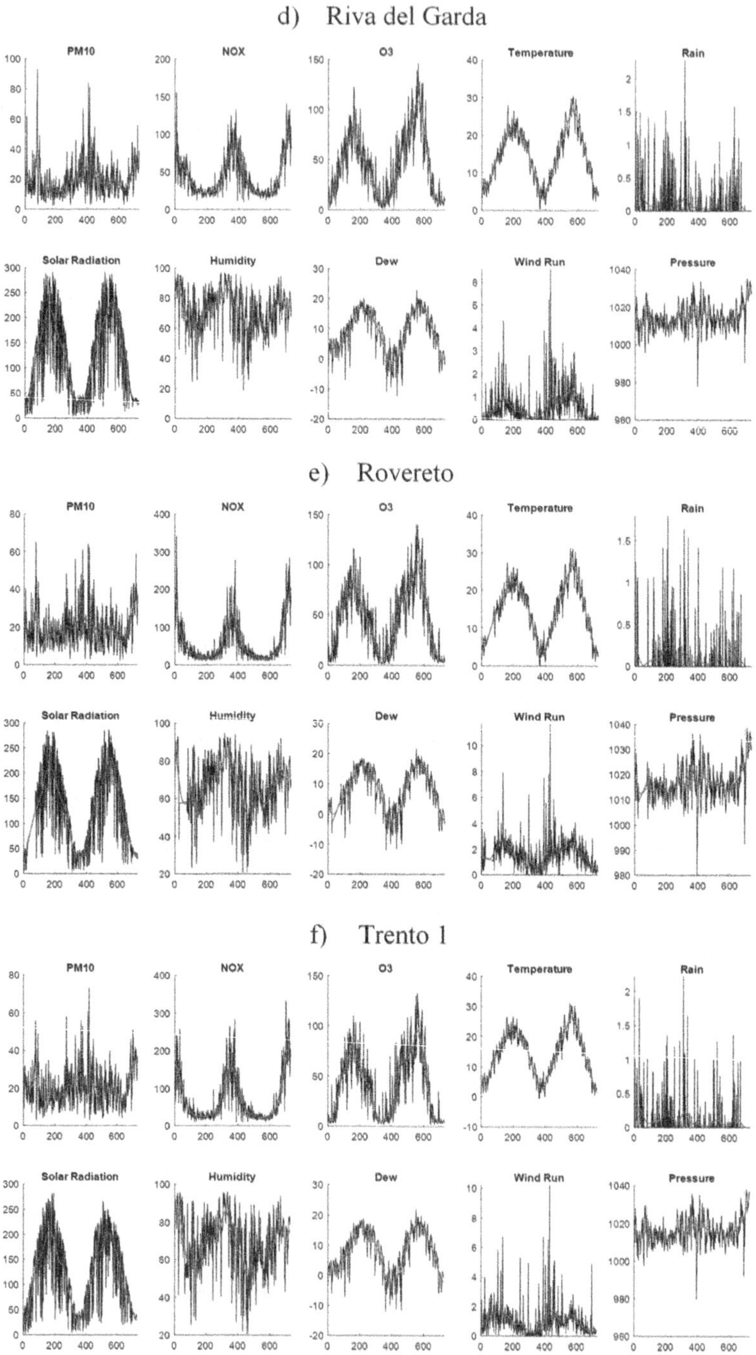

Fig. 17.3 (continued)

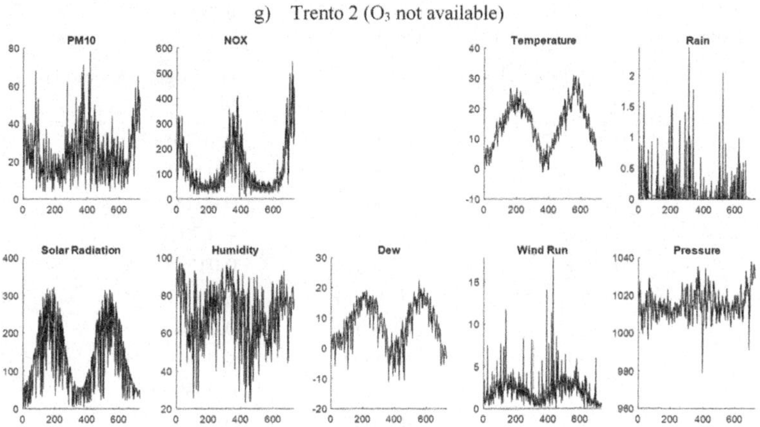

Fig. 17.3 (continued)

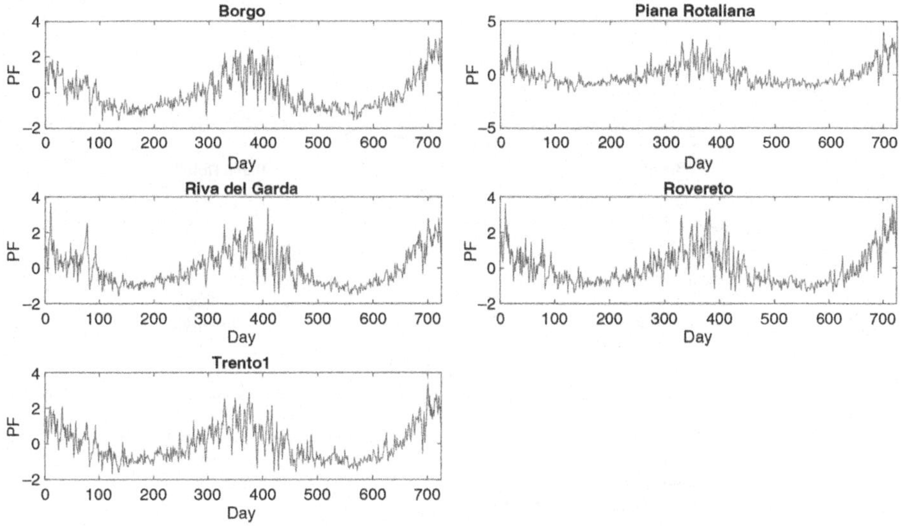

Fig. 17.4 Pollution factors (*PF*): dynamics for each monitoring site

Table 17.2 Air pollutants: correlations

	PM_{10}, NO_X	PM_{10}, O_3	O_3, NO_X
Borgo	0.6646	0.3962	0.6995
Piana	0.5100	0.1579	−0.6540
Riva	0.5478	0.2238	−0.7010
Rovereto	0.5488	0.2246	−0.7058
Trento 1	0.5116	0.2309	−0.7200

Table 17.3 Panel estimation (robust standard errors in parentheses; ***, ** and * indicate statistical significance at 1%, 5% and 10% level)

	Pooled model		Heterogeneous model	
Dep. Var.	PF		PF	
PF(−1)	0.4882***	(0.0178)	0.4670***	(0.0106)
TOut	−0.0742***	(0.0040)	−0.0803***	(0.0043)
$Tout^2$	0.0017***	(0.0002)	0.0018***	(0.0002)
WRun	−0.0984	(0.1414)	−0.2510***	(0.0470)
$WRun^2$	0.0038	(0.0092)	0.0134***	(0.0048)
R	−0.5013***	(0.1093)	−0.4055***	(0.1281)
R^2	0.1645***	(0.0446)	0.1564**	(0.0620)
SR	−0.0014***	(0.0002)	−0.0012***	(0.0003)
Hum	0.0085*	(0.0051)	0.0039***	(0.0009)
Press	0.0183***	(0.0030)	0.0134***	(0.0009)
S1	−0.0366	(0.0623)	−0.0333	(0.0552)
S2	−0.0141	(0.0180)	−0.0271	(0.0223)
S3	0.0427	(0.0454)	0.0453	(0.0373)
Cons.	/	/	−12.7663***	(1.0864)
N	3620		3620	
Adj. R^2	0.15		0.86	

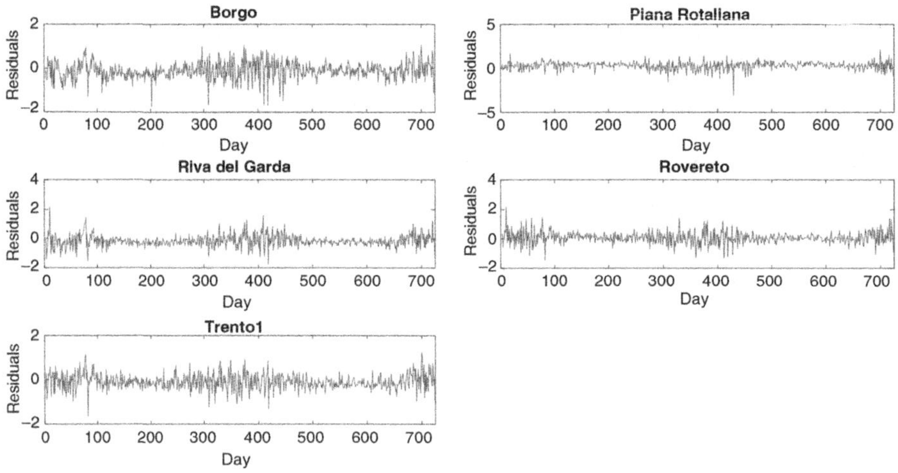

Fig. 17.5 Residuals from panel model for each monitoring site

Table 17.4 Analysis of the residuals (robust standard errors in parentheses; ***, ** and * indicate statistical significance at 1%, 5% and 10% level)

	Borgo	Piana Rotaliana	Riva del Garda	Rovereto	Trento 1
Dep. Var.	Residuals	Residuals	Residuals	Residuals	Residuals
PM_{10}	0.0091***	0.0122***	0.0162***	0.0160***	0.0150***
	(0.0015)	(0.0024)	(0.0015)	(0.0017)	(0.0015)
NO_X	0.0029***	0.0031***	0.0051***	0.0023***	0.0016***
	(0.0005)	(0.0007)	(0.0008)	(0.0005)	(0.0003)
O_3	0.0030***	0.0046***	0.0017***	0.0025***	0.0011**
	(0.0006)	(0.0007)	(0.0005)	(0.0006)	(0.0005)
Cons.	−0.6068***	−0.2535***	−0.7704***	−0.4909***	−0.5545***
	(0.0418)	(0.0480)	(0.0495)	(0.0464)	(0.0396)
N	724	724	724	724	724
Adj. R^2	0.2483	0.1869	0.4299	0.3247	0.3237

References

APPA Trento. (2014). *Air quality report 2014*. URL: http://www.appa.provincia.tn.it/binary/pat_appa_restyle/rapporti_annuali_aria/Rapporto_QA_2014.1475227470.pdf

APPA Trento. (2015). *Air quality report 2015*. URL: http://www.appa.provincia.tn.it/binary/pat_appa_restyle/rapporti_annuali_aria/Rapporto_QA_2015.1475227283.pdf

Brunekreef, B., & Holgate, S. T. (2002). Air pollution and health. *The Lancet, 360*(9341), 1233–1242.

Burnett, R., Ma, R., Jerrett, M., Goldberg, M. S., Cakmak, S., Pope, C. A., 3rd, & Krewski, D. (2001). The spatial association between community air pollution and mortality: A new method of analyzing correlated geographic cohort data. *Environmental Health Perspectives, 109*(Suppl 3), 375.

Chelani, A. B., & Devotta, S. (2006). Air quality forecasting using a hybrid autoregressive and nonlinear model. *Atmospheric Environment, 40*(10), 1774–1780.

Chudik, A., & Pesaran, M. H. (2015). Common correlated effects estimation of heterogeneous dynamic panel data models with weakly exogenous regressors. *Journal of Econometrics, 188*(2), 393–420.

Ditzen, J. (2016). *xtdcce2: Estimating dynamic common correlated effects in stata*. Heriot Watt University. URL: http://repec.org/usug2016/ditzen_uksug16.pdf

Dominici, F., Daniels, M., Zeger, S. L., & Samet, J. M. (2002). Air pollution and mortality: Estimating regional and national dose-response relationships. *Journal of the American Statistical Association, 97*(457), 100–111.

Dominici, F., Sheppard, L., & Clyde, M. (2003). Health effects of air pollution: A statistical review. *International Statistical Review, 71*(2), 243–276.

Fontanella, L., Ippoliti, L., & Valentini, P. (2007). Environmental pollution analysis by dynamic structural equation models. *Environmetrics, 18*, 265–283.

Forni, M., Hallin, M., Lippi, M., & Reichlin, L. (2000). The generalized dynamic-factor model: Identification and estimation. *The Review of Economics and Statistics, 82*, 540–554.

Haines, A., Kovats, R. S., Campbell-Lendrum, D., & Corvalan, C. (2006). Climate change and human health: Impacts, vulnerability and public health. *Public Health, 120*(7), 585–596.

Hoek, G., Brunekreef, B., Goldbohm, S., et al. (2002). Association between mortality and indicators of traffic-related air pollution in The Netherlands: A cohort study. *Lancet, 360*, 1203–1209.

Janes, H., Sheppard, L., & Shepherd, K. (2008). Statistical analysis of air pollution panel studies: An illustration. *Annals of Epidemiology, 18*(10), 792–802.

Jerrett, M., Burnett, R. T., Ma, R., Arden Pop, C., Krewski, D., Newbold, K. B., Thurston, G., Shi, Y., Finkelstein, N., Calle, E. E., & Thun, M. J. (2005). Spatial analysis of air pollution and mortality in Los Angeles. *Epidemiology, 16*, 727–736.

Kampa, M., & Castanas, E. (2008). Human health effects of air pollution. *Environmental Pollution, 151*(2), 362–367.

Kumar, A., & Goyal, P. (2011). Forecasting of air quality in Delhi using principal component regression technique. *Atmospheric Pollution Research, 2*(4), 436–444.

Milionis, A. E., & Davies, T. D. (1994). Regression and stochastic models for air pollution. Review, comments and suggestions. *Atmospheric Environment, 28*(17), 2801–2810.

O'Neill, M. S., Jerrett, M., Kawachi, I., Levy, J. I., Cohen, A. J., Gouveia, N., et al. (2003). Health, wealth, and air pollution: Advancing theory and methods. *Environmental Health Perspectives, 111*(16), 1861–1870.

Passamani, G., & Masotti, P. (2016). Local atmospheric pollution evolution through time series analysis. *Journal of Mathematics and Statistical Science, 2*(12), 781–788.

Pesaran, M. H. (2004). *General diagnostic tests for cross section dependence in panels* (CESifo Working Paper Series No. 1229).

Salcedo, R. L. R., Ferraz, M. A., Alves, C. A., & Martins, F. G. (1999). Time-series analysis of air pollution data. *Atmospheric Environment, 33*(15), 2361–2372.

Van der Wal, J. T., & Janssen, L. H. J. M. (2000). Analysis of spatial and temporal variations of PM 10 concentrations in the Netherlands using Kalman filtering. *Atmospheric Environment, 34*(22), 3675–3687.

WHO. (2013). *Review of evidence on health aspects of air pollution REVIHAAP Project*. URL: http://www.euro.who.int/__data/assets/pdf_file/0004/193108/REVIHAAP-Final-technical-report-final-version.pdf?ua=1

Yu, O., Sheppard, L., Lumley, T., Koenig, J. Q., & Shapiro, G. G. (2000). Effects of ambient air pollution on symptoms of asthma in Seattle-area children enrolled in the CAMP study. *Environmental Health Perspectives, 108*(12), 1209.

Chapter 18
AR Dynamic Evolving Neuro-Fuzzy Inference System for Mortality Data

Gabriella Piscopo

18.1 Introduction

In the last century the improvements in standards of living, the progress in medicine and the economic enhancements have driven human population to live better and longer. From an actuarial point of view, the decreasing trends in global mortality represent risk for insurers, which price their products on the basis of the historical mortality tables, and for governments, which have to plan health and pension policies. In this context, the so called longevity risk derives from improvements in mortality trend with systematic deviations of the number of the deaths from its expected values. In order to capture this trend and produce accurate mortality forecasts, stochastic models have been introduced. The most used is the Lee-Carter (LC) model (Lee and Carter 1992), whose main statistical tools are the least square estimation through the Singular Value Decomposition of the matrix of the log age specific mortality rate and the Box and Jenkins modelling and forecasting for time series. The LC is fitted to historic data and used to forecast long term mortality. However, strong structural changes have occurred in mortality patterns and several extensions have been proposed to overcome the limits of the model due to extrapolation based on the past data. Recently, Neural network (NN) and fuzzy inference system (FIS) have been introduced in the context of mortality data by Atsalaki et al. (2008). They implement an Adaptive Neuro-Fuzzy Inference System (ANFIS) model based on a first order Takagi Sugeno (TS) type FIS (Takagi and Sugeno 1985). They predict the yearly mortality in a one step ahead prediction scheme and use the method of trial and error to select the type of membership function that

G. Piscopo (✉)
Department of Economic and Statistical Sciences, University of Naples Federico II, Naples, Italy
e-mail: gabriella.piscopo@unina.it

© Springer International Publishing AG, part of Springer Nature 2018
C. H. Skiadas, C. Skiadas (eds.), *Demography and Health Issues*,
The Springer Series on Demographic Methods and Population Analysis 46,
https://doi.org/10.1007/978-3-319-76002-5_18

describe better the model. The least-squares and the backpropagation gradient descent methods are used for training the parameters of the FIS. They show that the ANFIS produces better results than the AR and ARIMA models for mortality projections. D'Amato et al. (2014) produce a comparative analysis between classical stochastic models and ANFIS implementing them on the Italian mortality dataset. Piscopo (2017) proposes an Integrated Dynamic Evolving Neuro-Fuzzy Inference System (DENFIS) for longevity predictions. DENFIS is introduced by Kasabov and Song (2002) for adaptive learning of dynamic time series predictions. It is an adaptive intelligent system where the learning process is updated thanks to a preliminary clusterization of the training data. The Evolving Clustering Method (ECM) is used to subdivide the input set and determine the position of each data in the input set. Kasabov and Song (2002) show that DENFIS effectively describes complex data and outperforms some existing methods. Wei et al. (2011) describe a fusion DENFIS model. In this paper we use an integrated AR-DENFIS model to produce mortality forecasts with an application to the Italian population and compare the results with the classical LC. The paper is organized as follows: in Sect. 18.2 we present the dynamic evolving neuro fuzzy procedure; in Section 18.3 we briefly describe the LC; in Sect. 18.4 we show a comparative application to Italian mortality dataset; final remarks are offered in Sect. 18.5.

18.2 The Dynamic Evolving Neuro Fuzzy System

The Dynamic Evolving Neuro Fuzzy System is an adaptive learning fuzzy system for dynamic time series prediction. It differs from the ANFIS because the fuzzy rules and parameters are dynamically updated as new informations come in the system; both use a TS architecture to implement learning and adaptation. Jang (1993) introduce the ANFIS: the procedure learn information from the data and Fuzzy Logic computes the membership function parameters that best allow the associated fuzzy inference system to track the given input/output data. A first order TS architecture is described in Fig. 18.1.

Let us assume that the FIS has two input x and y and one output z. A first order TS fuzzy model has the following rules:

Rule 1: if x is A_1 and y is B_1 then $f_1 = p_1x + q_1y + r_1$
Rule 2: if x is A_2 and y is B_2 then $f_2 = p_2x + q_2y + r_2$

The procedure follows the steps:
Let $O_{i,l}$ be the output of the node i in the layer l

1. Layer 1: Every node in this layer is an adaptive one with a node function

$$\begin{aligned} O_{1,i} &= \mu_{A_i}(x) \text{ for } i = 1, 2, \text{ or} \\ O_{1,i} &= \mu_{B_{i-2}}(x) \text{ for } i = 3, 4 \end{aligned} \tag{18.1}$$

where the typical membership functions depend on the premise parameters $a_i, b_i, c_{i,}$.

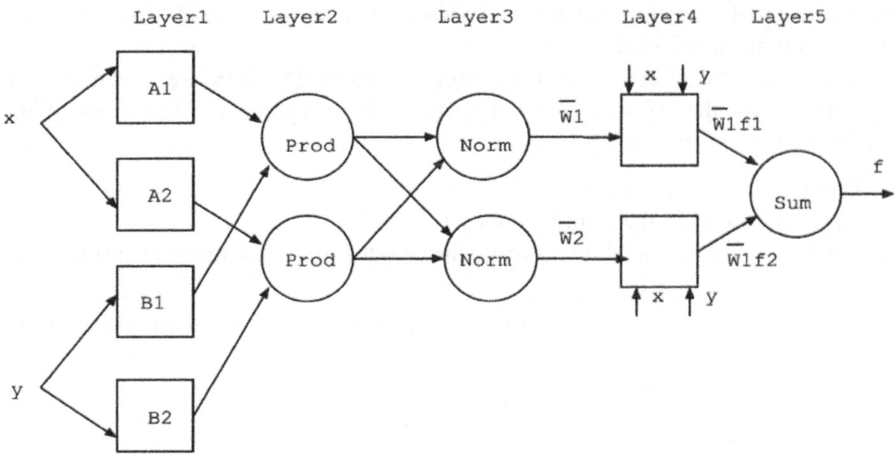

Fig. 18.1 Takagi- Sugeno Architecture

2. Layer 2: The output of each node is the product of all the incoming signals:

$$O_{2,i} = w_i = \mu_{A_i}(x) \cdot \mu_{B_i}(y), \quad i = 1, 2 \tag{18.3}$$

3. Layer 3: the outputs of this layer are the normalization of the incoming signals:

$$O_{3,i} = \bar{w}_i = \frac{w_i}{w_1 + w_2}, \quad i = 1, 2 \tag{18.4}$$

4. Layer 4: each node in this layer is an adaptive node with a node function

$$O_{4,1} = \bar{w}_i f_i - \bar{w}_i (p_x + q_i y + r_i) \tag{18.5}$$

$p_i, q_i, r_i,$ are the consequent parameters.

5. Layer 5: the ith output of this layer is computed as the summation of the all incoming signals $\sum_i \bar{w}_i f_i$

In the hybrid learning algorithm the consequent parameters are identified by the least square estimation while the premise parameters are updated by gradient descent.

The DENFIS uses TS model where the fuzzy rules are created dynamically and the learning process is driven by the ECM procedure. The ECM is introduced to create a partition of the input space. Once a threshold value Dthr is set, a first cluster of inputs from the training data is extracted and its radius is set equal to zero. Another sample is extracted: if the distance between its centre and that of the existing cluster is less than the value of the parameter Dthr then the vector extracted is incorporated in the first cluster and the centre is updated and the radius increased; otherwise another cluster is created. A cluster will not be modified anymore when its radius becomes equal to Dthr. We refer to (Kasabov and Song 2002) for a detailed description of the ECM algorithm.

Once the clusters are created, the fuzzy rules of DENFIS are generated and updated within the partitioned input space using a TS model. The steps of the DENFIS are the following:

1. Define the training data set
2. Apply the ECM to the training data set
3. For each cluster create the fuzzy rule through the triangular membership function

$$\mu(x) = mf(x, a, b, c) = \max(\min((\mathrm{x} - \mathrm{a})/(\mathrm{b} - \mathrm{a}), (\mathrm{c} - \mathrm{x})/\mathrm{c} - \mathrm{b})), 0) \quad (18.6)$$

where x is the input vector, b is the cluster centre, $a = b - d \times Dthr$, $c = b + d \times Dthr$, d is a parameter of the width of the triangular function.

4. The consequent parameters of the TS procedure are calculated through a weighted least square estimation. In particular, the weighs are represented by $1 - d_j$ where d_j is the distance between the j-th sample and the corresponding cluster centre.
5. The fuzzy rules and the parameters are updated when a new cluster is created or the existing clusters are modified. When the ECM stops, the output of the system is generated according to the TS procedure.

18.3 The Lee Carter Model

In order to model the mortality separately for each i population without considering dependence between groups, the widely used Lee Carter Model (LC) describes the mortality rates at age x and time t as follows:

$$m_{xt,i} = \exp\left(\alpha_{x,i} + \beta_{x,i} k_{t,i} + u_{xt,i}\right) \quad (18.7)$$

where $m_{xt,\ i}$ is the sum of an age specific parameter independent of time $\alpha_{x,\ i}$ and a component given by the product of a time-varying parameter $k_{t,\ i}$, reflecting the general level of mortality and the parameter $\beta_{x,\ i}$, representing how rapidly or slowly mortality at each age varies when the general level of mortality changes. The model is fitted to historical data through the Singular Value Decomposition of the matrix of the observed mortality rates. The estimated time varying parameter is modelled as a stochastic process; standard Box and Jenkins methodology are used to identify an appropriate ARIMA model according which $k_{t,\ i}$ are projected.

18.4 An Application to Mortality Dataset

In this work we apply AR-DENFIS to mortality forecasts and compare the results with the LC.

In order to define the number of inputs of the DENFIS in the mortality dataset, we firstly apply an AR scheme; then we compare the results of mortality forecasts obtained by the LC and AR-DENFIS. The data used are taken from the Human Mortality Database (2008). We work on the mortality rates m_t for the Italian males aged 50, collected from t = 1940 up to t = 2012. The data, considered by single calendar year, are split into training dataset from 1940 up to 1993 and test dataset from 1994 up to 2012. The AR is fitted to the whole time serie and the order equal to 2 is chosen minimizing the Akaike Information Criterion; consequently, in our DENFIS we introduce two input variable x_1 and x_2 (mortality one and two years before) and one output y (mortality one step ahead).

Firstly, we implement the DENFIS on the training dataset, setting the value of Dthr equal to 0.1, the maximum number of iteration equal to 10, the parameter d equal to 2, the step size of the gradient descent equal to 0.01. Once the DENFIS is created, the mortality rate is projected on the testing period and the results are compared with the realized mortality.

In the second step of our application, we implement the LC. We fit the model on the male population aged between 0 and 100, considering years between 1940 and 1993; the parameter kt is derived and shown in Fig. 18.2; a random walk model is fitted on the serie of kt and is projected from 1994 up 2012 through a Monte Carlo simulation with n = 1000 paths. Finally the value of projected mortality rates for male aged 50 are derived using Eq. (18.7).

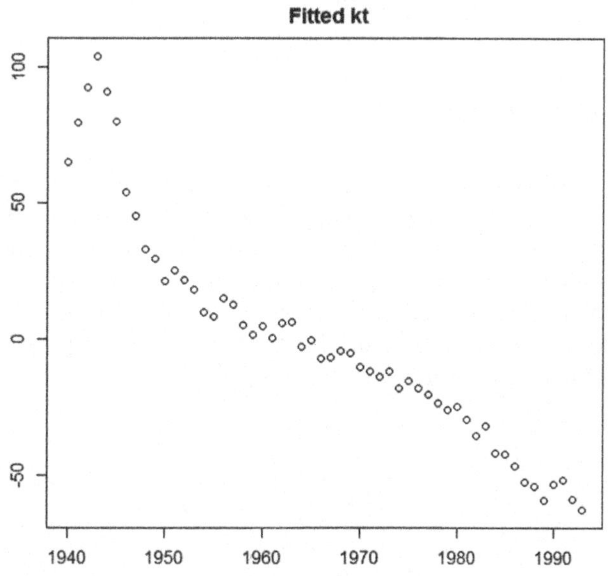

Fig. 18.2 The fitted parameter kt of the LC

Table 18.1 The mortality rates realized vs projected through LC and DENFIS

T	Realized	DENFIS	LC
1994	0.00461	0.004458675	0.005083814
1995	0.00413	0.004593811	0.005004209
1996	0.00409	0.004354364	0.004934666
1997	0.00388	0.004143083	0.004868312
1998	0.00390	0.004003856	0.004802357
1999	0.00371	0.003933489	0.004728343
2000	0.00359	0.003829500	0.004659374
2001	0.00359	0.003684567	0.004591524
2002	0.00316	0.003637632	0.004525431
2003	0.00334	0.003384584	0.004462271
2004	0.00312	0.002780000	0.004403274
2005	0.00305	0.002780000	0.004347287
2006	0.00297	0.002780000	0.004286747
2007	0.00304	0.002780000	0.004222623
2008	0.00294	0.002780000	0.004164231
2009	0.00292	0.002780000	0.004100000
2010	0.00278	0.002780000	0.004049956
2011	0.00288	0.002780000	0.003990748
2012	0.00286	0.002780000	0.003937622

Table 18.2 RMSE in the LC and DENFIS

	LC	**DENFIS**
MSE	1.219046e-06	5.726724e-08

The MSE of the LC and DENFIS are compared. The results are shown in Tables 18.1 and 18.2.

18.5 Final Remarks

In this paper we have applied an integrated AR-DENFIS procedure to forecasts mortality and have compared the results with the standard LC. The backtesting procedure highlights the improvements in mortality forecasts moving from LC to DENFIS: the mean square error decreases and the projected mortality trend appears more similar to the realized trend. In particular, the DENFIS catches the improvements in mortality realized in the last years better than the LC. This feature makes it attractive to handle with the longevity risk.

References

Atsalakis, G., Nezis, D., Matalliotakis, G., Ucenic, C. I., & Skiadas, C. (2008). *Forecasting mortality rate using a neural network with fuzzy inference system* (No 0806. Working Papers). University of Crete. Department of Economics. http://EconPapers.repec.org/RePEc:crt:wpaper:080

D'Amato V., Piscopo G., & Russolillo M. (2014). Adaptive Neuro-Fuzzy Inference System vs Stochastic Models for mortality data. In *Smart innovation, systems and technologies* (Vol. 26, pp. 251–258). Berlin: Springer.

Human Mortality Database. (2008). University of California, Berkeley (USA), and Max Planck Institute for Demographic Research (Germany). www.mortality.org

Jang, J. S. R. (1993). ANFIS: Adaptive-Network-based Fuzzy Inference Systems. *IEEE Transaction on Systems, Man and Cybernetics, 23*, 665–685.

Kasabov, N. K., & Song, Q. (2002). DENFIS: Dynamic evolving neuro-fuzzy inference system and its application for time series-prediction. *IEEE Transaction on Fuzzy System, 10*(2), 144–154.

Lee, R. D., & Carter, L. R. (1992). Modelling and forecasting U.S. mortality. *Journal of American Statistical Association, 87*, 659–671.

Piscopo, G. (2017). Dynamic evolving neuro fuzzy inference system for mortality prediction. *International Journal of Engineering Research and Application, 7*, 26–29.

Takagi, T., & Sugeno, M. (1985). Fuzzy identification of systems and its application to modelling and control. *IEEE Transactions on Systems, Man and Cybernetics, 15(1)*, 116–132.

Wei, L. Y., Cheng, C. H., & Wu, H. H. (2011). Fusion ANFIS Model based on AR for forecasting EPS of leading industries. *International Journal of Innovative Computing, Information and Control, 7(9)*, 5445–5458.

Chapter 19
Empirical Power Study of the Jackson Exponentiality Test

Frederico Caeiro and Ayana Mateus

19.1 Introduction

Let X be a continuous random variable with distribution function (df)

$$F(x) = P(X \leq x) = 1 \exp(-\lambda x), \quad x > 0. \tag{19.1}$$

Then X has exponential distribution with parameter $\lambda > 0$ and we will use the notation Exp (λ) to refer to this distribution. Note that if $X \sim \text{Exp}(\lambda)$, then $\lambda X \sim \text{Exp}$ (1). The exponential distribution is the adequate model for the time between two consecutive events in a Poisson process with intensity λ. This is a very simple mathematical model with a lot of useful statistical properties. Many of those properties are summarized in Ahsanullah and Hamedani (2010); Balakrishnan and Basu (1995); Johnson et al. (1994), among others.

The problem of testing exponentiality against other alternatives has received in the last decades a lot of attention from different researchers (see Alizadeh Noughabi and Arghami 2011; Brilhante 2004; Doksum 1984; Henze and Meintanis 2005; Kozubowski et al. 2009; Stephens 1986 and references therein). Possible alternative models, which extend the exponential distribution, are the gamma distribution, the Weibull distribution, the generalized Pareto distribution and the Tsallis or q-exponential distribution.

In this paper we revisit the Jackson statistic used to test exponentiality against a general alternative. In Sect. 19.2 we introduce the Jackson statistic test and we

F. Caeiro (✉) · A. Mateus
Faculdade de Ciências e Tecnologia & Centro de Matemática e Aplicações (CMA), Universidade Nova de Lisboa 2829-516, Caparica, Portugal
e-mail: fac@fct.unl.pt; amf@fct.unl.pt

© Springer International Publishing AG, part of Springer Nature 2018
C. H. Skiadas, C. Skiadas (eds.), *Demography and Health Issues*,
The Springer Series on Demographic Methods and Population Analysis 46,
https://doi.org/10.1007/978-3-319-76002-5_19

review several exact and asymptotic properties. For statistical power comparison, Lilliefors exponentiality test is also considered in this work. In Sect. 19.3 we present and discuss the empirical power of the Jackson test, computed for different alternative distributions.

19.2 Testing Exponentiality

Suppose X_1, X_2, ... X_n are independent and identically distributed random variables with common unknown continuous distribution. We wish to test the null hypothesis

$$\mathrm{H}_0 : X \sim \mathrm{Exp}(\lambda)$$

for some unspecified parameter $\lambda > 0$, against H_1: the distribution of X is not exponential. In what follows we will focus on the Jackson exponentiality test. For the statistical comparison we will also consider Lilliefors exponentiality test.

19.2.1 Jackson Exponentiality Test

Jackson test was introduced in Jackson (1967) and discussed in Caeiro et al. (2016). The test is based on the statistic

$$J_n = \frac{\sum_{i=1}^{n} m_i X_{(i)}}{\sum_{i=1}^{n} X_i}, \tag{19.2}$$

with $X_{(i)}$ the i-th ascending order statistic and

$$m_i = \lambda E\left(X_{(i)}\right) = \sum_{j=1}^{i} (n - j + 1)^{-1}, i = 1, \ldots, n.$$

Since this statistic test can be expressed as a function of the scaled random variables λX_i, the null distribution of J_n does not depend on the value of the parameter λ. With some algebra, Eq. (19.2) could be expressed in terms of the standardized spacings $S_i = (n - i + 1)(X_{(i)} - X_{(i-1)})$, $i = 1, \ldots, n$ with $X_0 \equiv 0$, that is,

$$J_n = \frac{\sum_{i=1}^{n} c_i S_i}{\sum_{i=1}^{n} S_i},$$

with $c_i = 1 + m_{i-1}$, $i = 1, \ldots, n$ ($m_0 \equiv 0$). The statistic test, J_n, can take values between $c_1 = 1$ and $c_n \sim \gamma + \ln n$, where γ denotes the Euler-Mascheroni constant. Without prior knowledge about the alternative distribution, the critical region for Jackson test is two-tailed. The exact null df was presented in Jackson (1967) and is given by

$$P(J_n \leq x) = \sum_{k=1}^{n} \frac{(x - c_k)^{n-1} I_{(0,\infty[}(x - c_k)}{\prod_{j=1, j \neq k}^{n} (c_j - c_k)}, \quad 1 < x < c_n, \tag{19.3}$$

where I_A denotes the indicator function on the set A($I_A(x) = 1$ if $x \in A$ and $I_A(x) = 0$ otherwise). This df was implemented in R programming language (R Core Team, 2015) and the computer code is available in Caeiro et al. (2016). Unless we use a arbitrary precision package to compute the df in Eq. (19.3), we can obtain inaccurate values for $n > 100$, due to floating-point inaccuracy in R software. In Table 19.1 we provide several quantiles of probability p from the df in (19.3). Table 19.1 extends Table 1 from Caeiro et al. (2016).

The limit distribution of $\sqrt{n}(J_n - 2)$ is the standard normal distribution (Jackson 1967). Since the rate of converge of $\sqrt{n}(J_n - 2)$ to the limit distribution is slow, Caeiro et al. (2016) studied a more a accurate approximation for the df, for nite sample sizes. The approximation, based on Edgeworth expansion (Abramowitz and Stegun 1972), is

$$P(J_n \leq x) \approx \Phi(z) - \phi(z)\left\{\gamma_1 \frac{z^2 - 1}{6} + (\gamma_2 - 3)\frac{z^3 - 3z}{24} + \gamma_1^2 \frac{z^5 - 10z^3 + 15z}{72}\right\}$$

where $z = (x - \mu)/\sigma$, ϕ and Φ are the density function and the df of the standard normal distribution and $\sigma^2 = \mu_2 = \mu_2' - \mu^2, \gamma_1 = \mu_3/\sigma^3$ and $\gamma_2 = \mu_4/\sigma^4$ with $\mu_3 = \mu_3' - 3\mu\mu_2' + 2\mu^2$ and $\mu_4 = \mu_4' - 4\mu\mu_3' + 2\mu^2$ and

$$\mu = \mu_1' = \frac{\sum_{i=1}^n c_i}{n}, \quad \mu_2' = \frac{\sum_{i=1}^n c_i^2 + \left(\sum_{i=1}^n c_i\right)^2}{n(n+1)},$$

$$\mu_3' = \frac{2\sum_{i=1}^n c_i^3 + 3\left(\sum_{i=1}^n c_i\right)\sum_{i=1}^n c_i^2 + \left(\sum_{i=1}^n c_i\right)^3}{n(n+1)(n+2)},$$

$$\mu_4' = \frac{6\sum_{i=1}^n c_i^4 + 8\left(\sum_{i=1}^n c_i\right)\sum_{i=1}^n c_i^3 + 3\left(\sum_{i=1}^n c_i^2\right)^2 + 6\left(\sum_{i=1}^n c_i\right)^2\sum_{i=1}^n c_i^2 + \left(\sum_{i=1}^n c_i\right)^4}{n(n+1)(n+2)(n+3)}.$$

Table 19.1 Exact quantiles from the null distribution of the Jackson statistic

p													
n	0.005	0.01	0.025	0.05	0.1	0.25	0.5	0.75	0.9	0.95	0.975	0.99	0.995
3	1.037	1.053	1.083	1.118	1.167	1.264	1.377	1.511	1.629	1.689	1.731	1.769	1.788
4	1.092	1.116	1.158	1.199	1.251	1.346	1.468	1.600	1.727	1.801	1.859	1.918	1.952
5	1.146	1.173	1.218	1.260	1.312	1.410	1.531	1.665	1.793	1.871	1.936	2.007	2.051
6	1.192	1.220	1.266	1.308	1.361	1.458	1.579	1.712	1.840	1.920	1.988	2.066	2.115
7	1.231	1.260	1.306	1.349	1.401	1.497	1.617	1.748	1.876	1.956	2.025	2.106	2.159
8	1.264	1.294	1.340	1.382	1.435	1.530	1.647	1.777	1.904	1.983	2.053	2.135	2.190
9	1.294	1.323	1.369	1.411	1.463	1.557	1.673	1.801	1.926	2.004	2.074	2.156	2.212
10	1.320	1.349	1.395	1.437	1.488	1.581	1.694	1.820	1.943	2.021	2.090	2.172	2.229
11	1.343	1.372	1.417	1.459	1.509	1.601	1.713	1.837	1.958	2.035	2.103	2.185	2.241
12	1.364	1.393	1.438	1.479	1.529	1.619	1.729	1.851	1.970	2.046	2.114	2.195	2.251
13	1.382	1.411	1.456	1.497	1.546	1.635	1.743	1.863	1.981	2.055	2.122	2.202	2.258
14	1.400	1.428	1.473	1.513	1.561	1.649	1.756	1.874	1.989	2.063	2.129	2.208	2.263
15	1.415	1.444	1.488	1.527	1.575	1.662	1.767	1.883	1.997	2.069	2.135	2.213	2.268
16	1.430	1.458	1.501	1.541	1.588	1.674	1.778	1.892	2.004	2.075	2.139	2.217	2.271
17	1.443	1.471	1.514	1.553	1.600	1.684	1.787	1.899	2.010	2.080	2.143	2.219	2.273
18	1.456	1.484	1.526	1.564	1.611	1.694	1.795	1.906	2.015	2.084	2.146	2.222	2.274
19	1.468	1.495	1.537	1.575	1.621	1.703	1.803	1.912	2.019	2.087	2.149	2.223	2.276
20	1.478	1.506	1.547	1.585	1.630	1.711	1.810	1.918	2.023	2.090	2.151	2.225	2.276
21	1.489	1.516	1.557	1.594	1.639	1.719	1.816	1.923	2.027	2.093	2.153	2.225	2.276
22	1.498	1.525	1.566	1.603	1.647	1.726	1.822	1.927	2.030	2.095	2.155	2.226	2.276
23	1.507	1.534	1.574	1.611	1.655	1.733	1.828	1.932	2.033	2.097	2.156	2.226	2.276
24	1.516	1.542	1.582	1.619	1.662	1.740	1.833	1.935	2.035	2.099	2.157	2.226	2.276
25	1.524	1.550	1.590	1.626	1.669	1.746	1.838	1.939	2.038	2.101	2.158	2.226	2.275
30	1.559	1.584	1.622	1.657	1.698	1.771	1.858	1.954	2.047	2.106	2.160	2.224	2.270
35	1.587	1.612	1.648	1.681	1.721	1.790	1.874	1.964	2.053	2.109	2.159	2.221	2.264

40	1.611	1.634	1.669	1.701	1.739	1.806	1.886	1.972	2.056	2.110	2.158	2.216	2.258
45	1.630	1.653	1.687	1.718	1.754	1.819	1.896	1.979	2.059	2.110	2.156	2.212	2.251
50	1.647	1.669	1.702	1.732	1.767	1.830	1.904	1.983	2.061	2.110	2.154	2.207	2.245
55	1.662	1.683	1.716	1.744	1.779	1.839	1.911	1.987	2.062	2.109	2.151	2.203	2.239
60	1.675	1.696	1.727	1.755	1.789	1.847	1.916	1.991	2.063	2.108	2.149	2.198	2.233
65	1.687	1.707	1.738	1.765	1.797	1.854	1.921	1.994	2.063	2.107	2.147	2.194	2.228
70	1.697	1.717	1.747	1.773	1.805	1.860	1.926	1.996	2.063	2.106	2.144	2.190	2.223
75	1.706	1.726	1.755	1.781	1.812	1.866	1.930	1.998	2.064	2.105	2.142	2.187	2.218
80	1.715	1.734	1.763	1.788	1.818	1.871	1.933	2.000	2.064	2.104	2.140	2.183	2.214
85	1.723	1.741	1.770	1.794	1.824	1.876	1.936	2.001	2.063	2.102	2.138	2.180	2.210
90	1.730	1.748	1.776	1.800	1.829	1.880	1.939	2.003	2.063	2.101	2.136	2.177	2.206
95	1.737	1.755	1.782	1.806	1.834	1.884	1.942	2.004	2.063	2.100	2.134	2.174	2.202
100	1.743	1.761	1.787	1.811	1.839	1.887	1.944	2.005	2.063	2.099	2.132	2.171	2.198

19.2.2 Lilliefors Exponentiality Test

To be able to compare the power of the Jackson exponentiality test, we also considered the Lilliefors test (Gibbons and Chakraborti, 2011; Lilliefors, 1969), which is a Kolmogorov-Smirnov type test. The test statistic is

$$D_n = \sup_x \mid F_n(x) - F_0(x) \mid , \tag{19.4}$$

with $F_0(x) = 1 - \exp(-x/\bar{x}), x > 0$ the exponential df in (19.1) and λ estimated by $1/\bar{x}$, where $\bar{x}$ denotes the sample mean and $F_n(x)$ is the empirical distribution function. The test statistic in Eq. (19.4) is equivalent to

$$D_n = \max\{D_n^+, D_n^-\},$$

with

$$D_n^+ = \max_{1 \le i \le n} \left(\frac{i}{n} - Y_i \right), D_n^- = \max_{1 \le i \le n} \left(Y_i - \frac{i-1}{n} \right)$$

and $Y_i = 1 - \exp(-X_{(i)}/\bar{X})$. The test rejects the null hypothesis of exponentiality, at the significance level α, if D_n is greater than a critical value with $P(D_n >$ *crit. value*$) = \alpha$. Since the parameter λ of the exponential distribution is estimated, the critical values for the Kolmogorov-Smirnov test are no longer valid. Lilliefors (1969) made a Monte Carlo simulation study, based on 5000 runs, to compute critical values for the test statistic D_n in (19.4). Since those critical values were computed from a small number of runs and values for even sample sizes were interpolated, we also conducted a monte carlo simulation study, based on 100,000 runs, to compute critical values for the statistic D_n in (19.4) with a smaller standard error. In Table 19.2 we present the simulated critical values for D_n for n= 3(19.1)20 and n = 25(19.5)100 at the significance levels α = 0.20, 0.10, 0.05, 0.025, 0.02, 0.01, 0.005. The values presented in Table 19.2 were computed in R language, with the computer code:

```
# Function to compute critical values for Lilliefors
Exponentiality test ksexp.crit <- function(n, runs=10^5,
alpha=0.05){

lambda <- 1

sim.ks <- replicate(runs, {x <- rexp(1000, rate=lambda)[1,n];

ks.test(x,"pexp",rate=1/mean(x))$statistic})

return(quantile(sim.ks, probs=1-alpha))

}
```

Table 19.2 Critical values for D_n at the significance level α and sample size n

α	0.20	0.10	0.05	0.025	0.02	0.01	0.005
3	0.451	0.511	0.551	0.578	0.585	0.601	0.612
4	0.401	0.445	0.485	0.522	0.532	0.559	0.582
5	0.361	0.405	0.442	0.474	0.484	0.512	0.537
6	0.332	0.373	0.408	0.440	0.449	0.475	0.500
7	0.310	0.348	0.381	0.412	0.421	0.447	0.470
8	0.292	0.327	0.359	0.387	0.396	0.421	0.444
9	0.276	0.311	0.341	0.367	0.376	0.401	0.423
10	0.263	0.296	0.324	0.350	0.358	0.381	0.403
11	0.251	0.283	0.311	0.336	0.343	0.365	0.386
12	0.242	0.272	0.299	0.323	0.330	0.351	0.371
13	0.233	0.262	0.288	0.311	0.318	0.339	0.359
14	0.224	0.253	0.278	0.301	0.308	0.328	0.347
15	0.217	0.245	0.270	0.292	0.298	0.317	0.337
16	0.211	0.237	0.261	0.283	0.289	0.310	0.329
17	0.205	0.230	0.254	0.274	0.280	0.300	0.319
18	0.199	0.224	0.247	0.267	0.273	0.292	0.309
19	0.194	0.219	0.240	0.261	0.267	0.285	0.302
20	0.189	0.213	0.234	0.254	0.260	0.277	0.295
25	0.170	0.192	0.211	0.228	0.233	0.249	0.263
30	0.156	0.175	0.193	0.209	0.214	0.228	0.243
35	0.145	0.163	0.179	0.195	0.199	0.213	0.225
40	0.136	0.153	0.169	0.182	0.187	0.199	0.212
45	0.128	0.145	0.159	0.172	0.176	0.188	0.200
50	0.122	0.137	0.151	0.164	0.168	0.179	0.190
60	0.111	0.126	0.139	0.150	0.154	0.164	0.174
70	0.103	0.116	0.128	0.139	0.143	0.153	0.162
80	0.097	0.109	0.120	0.130	0.133	0.142	0.151
90	0.091	0.103	0.113	0.123	0.126	0.134	0.142
100	0.087	0.098	0.108	0.117	0.120	0.127	0.135

Remark: To be able to reproduce the critical values, the command set.seed (19.1) must be used before ksexp.crit.

19.3 Power Comparison and Conclusions

19.3.1 Methodology

We present in this section the simulated Power values of the Jackson and Lilliefors tests. Results are based on a Monte Carlo simulation study with 100,000 samples of size $n = 5$, 10, 20, 50 and 100. The level of significance considered was $\alpha = 0.05$. We considered the two following alternatives to the exponential distribution: the gamma and Weibull distributions with density function given respectively by,

$$f(x) = \frac{\lambda^\theta x^{\theta-1}}{\Gamma(\theta)} \exp(-\lambda x), \quad x > 0 \quad (\theta > 0, \lambda > 0) \tag{19.5}$$

and

$$f(x) = \lambda\theta(\lambda x)^{\theta-1} \exp\left\{-(\lambda x)^\theta\right\}, \quad x > 0 \quad (\theta > 0, \lambda > 0). \tag{19.6}$$

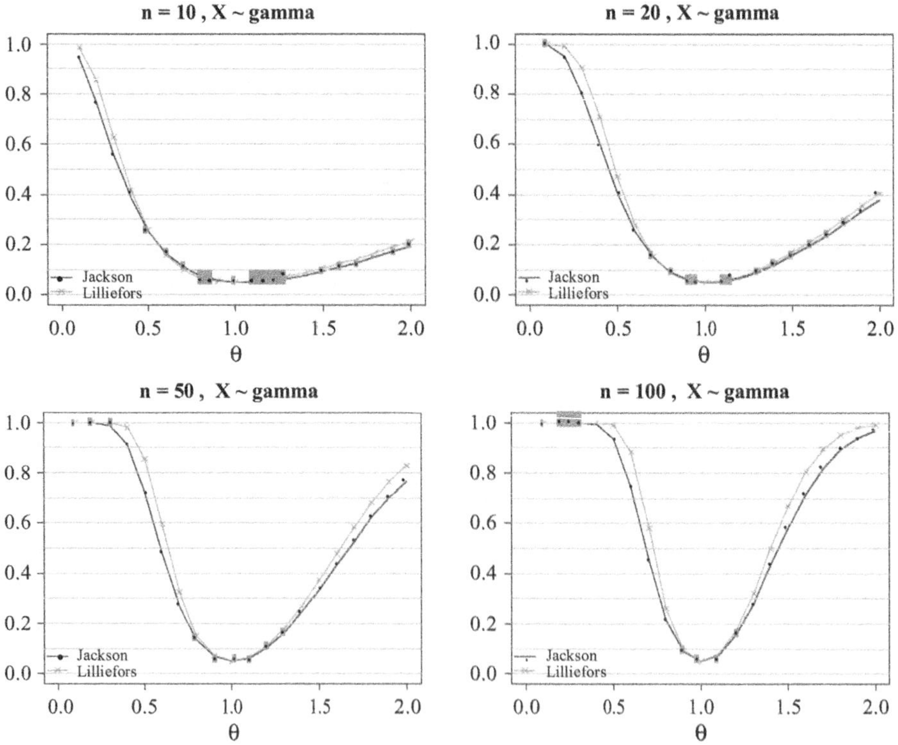

Fig. 19.1 Simulated Power curve for the statistic tests J_n and D_n and $\alpha = 0.05$, for the gamma model

When $\theta = 1$ those models reduce to the exponential distribution with parameter λ. Thus testing the exponential hypothesis is equivalent to test the null hypothesis $H_0 : \theta = 1$. For the power study, we considered $\lambda = 1$ and $\theta = 0.1(0.1)2$.

Although we considered the models in (19.5) and (19.6) we assume to have no knowledge of the alternative distribution. Therefor the critical region for Jackson test is two-tailed and for Lilliefors test is one-tailed. The critical values used in the simulation study are the ones available in Tables 19.1 and 19.2.

19.3.2 Results and Conclusions

In Figs. 19.1 and 19.2 and in Tables 19.3 and 19.4 we present the simulated power values at a significance level $\alpha = 0.05$. Results for $n = 5$ are only available in the tables. Results of this simulation study indicated that both exponentiality tests exhibit a similar statistical power, almost identical when the alternative hypothesis was nearly exponential (θ close to 1). The studied tests have a reasonable power, for

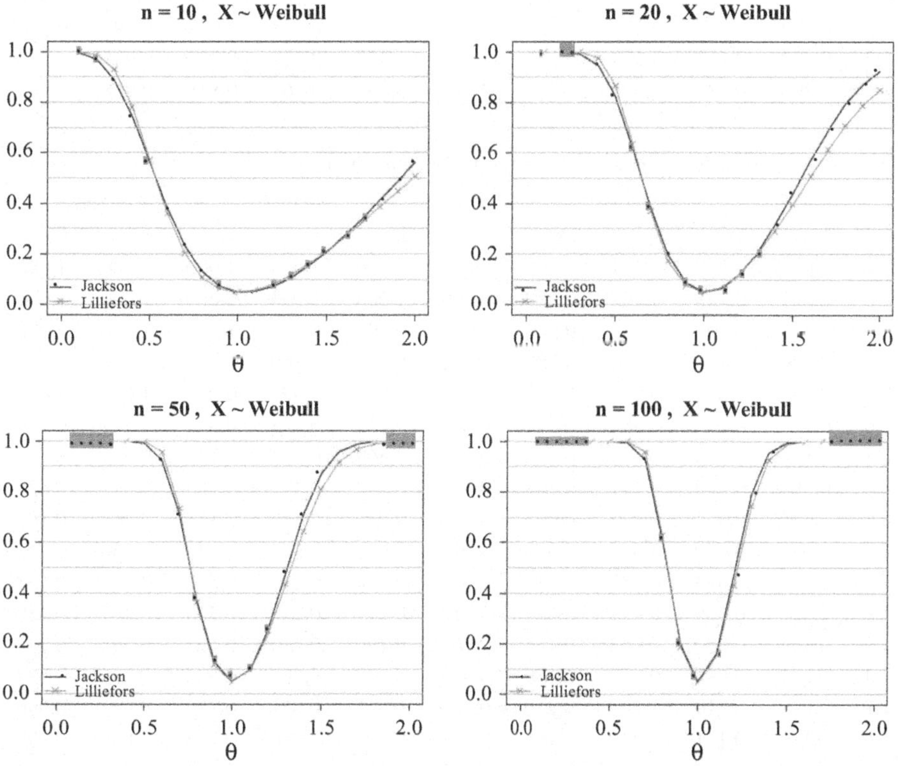

Fig. 19.2 Simulated Power curve for the statistic tests J_n and D_n and = 0:05, for the Weibull model

Table 19.3 Simulated power of the tests for the gamma alternative

	n = 5		n = 10		n = 20		n = 50		n = 100	
θ	J_n	D_n	J_n	D_n	J_n	D_n	J_n	D_n	J_n	D_n
0.1	0.736	0.770	0.943	0.985	0.998	1.000	1.000	1.000	1.000	1.000
0.2	0.518	0.499	0.762	0.853	0.949	0.991	1.000	1.000	1.000	1.000
0.3	0.357	0.316	0.556	0.627	0.800	0.906	0.987	0.999	1.000	1.000
0.4	0.247	0.202	0.383	0.414	0.597	0.707	0.909	0.980	0.995	1.000
0.5	0.173	0.134	0.254	0.257	0.405	0.471	0.722	0.855	0.935	0.990
0.6	0.122	0.093	0.166	0.159	0.254	0.280	0.480	0.595	0.744	0.883
0.7	0.090	0.068	0.108	0.098	0.151	0.155	0.272	0.327	0.453	0.581
0.8	0.067	0.055	0.076	0.067	0.091	0.088	0.138	0.151	0.214	0.260
0.9	0.058	0.052	0.058	0.054	0.061	0.058	0.071	0.071	0.088	0.093
1.0	0.049	0.050	0.051	0.052	0.049	0.051	0.050	0.050	0.050	0.050
1.1	0.047	0.051	0.051	0.054	0.053	0.056	0.062	0.067	0.078	0.082
1.2	0.049	0.057	0.055	0.061	0.068	0.072	0.102	0.110	0.158	0.176
1.3	0.050	0.062	0.065	0.076	0.091	0.100	0.163	0.181	0.283	0.322
1.4	0.055	0.069	0.077	0.088	0.121	0.132	0.245	0.269	0.433	0.499
1.5	0.062	0.078	0.095	0.107	0.158	0.171	0.336	0.374	0.584	0.670
1.6	0.066	0.084	0.110	0.125	0.197	0.211	0.433	0.478	0.715	0.804
1.7	0.075	0.095	0.129	0.144	0.238	0.255	0.527	0.584	0.819	0.895
1.8	0.080	0.102	0.152	0.168	0.286	0.306	0.622	0.682	0.894	0.950
1.9	0.090	0.113	0.174	0.191	0.333	0.357	0.701	0.765	0.940	0.979
2	0.097	0.121	0.194	0.212	0.381	0.405	0.767	0.828	0.968	0.992

Table 19.4 Simulated power of the tests for the Weibull alternative

	n = 5		n = 10		n = 20		n = 50		n = 100	
θ	J_n	D_n	J_n	D_n	J_n	D_n	J_n	D_n	J_n	D_n
0.1	0.899	0.938	0.997	1.000	1.000	1.000	1.000	1.000	1.000	1.000
0.2	0.768	0.785	0.968	0.989	0.999	1.000	1.000	1.000	1.000	1.000
0.3	0.618	0.600	0.885	0.928	0.992	0.999	1.000	1.000	1.000	1.000
0.4	0.470	0.423	0.743	0.782	0.946	0.976	1.000	1.000	1.000	1.000
0.5	0.336	0.279	0.563	0.571	0.824	0.865	0.992	0.998	1.000	1.000
0.6	0.227	0.176	0.382	0.361	0.618	0.637	0.924	0.956	0.997	0.999
0.7	0.148	0.108	0.233	0.203	0.385	0.369	0.706	0.733	0.929	0.956
0.8	0.094	0.070	0.131	0.108	0.197	0.172	0.377	0.365	0.613	0.628
0.9	0.063	0.054	0.073	0.062	0.087	0.075	0.130	0.115	0.200	0.187
1.0	0.049	0.050	0.050	0.050	0.050	0.051	0.051	0.049	0.050	0.048
1.1	0.047	0.054	0.053	0.059	0.065	0.070	0.099	0.098	0.159	0.151
1.2	0.053	0.065	0.074	0.082	0.118	0.119	0.253	0.235	0.467	0.430
1.3	0.064	0.080	0.107	0.116	0.201	0.196	0.480	0.435	0.794	0.744
1.4	0.081	0.098	0.152	0.159	0.313	0.290	0.708	0.644	0.955	0.927
1.5	0.099	0.119	0.208	0.210	0.440	0.397	0.872	0.810	0.995	0.986
1.6	0.119	0.141	0.270	0.265	0.571	0.508	0.956	0.915	1.000	0.998
1.7	0.143	0.167	0.339	0.324	0.691	0.614	0.989	0.967	1.000	1.000
1.8	0.169	0.195	0.414	0.386	0.792	0.708	0.998	0.989	1.000	1.000
1.9	0.197	0.223	0.490	0.448	0.870	0.788	1.000	0.997	1.000	1.000
2.0	0.226	0.251	0.565	0.507	0.923	0.850	1.000	0.999	1.000	1.000

sample sizes $n \geq 50$. Lilliefors test is usually more powerful for the gamma alternative and θ not close to 1. For the Weibull alternative and $\theta > 1$, Jackson test is more powerful.

Acknowledgements This research was partially supported by National Funds through FCT (Fundação para a Ciência e a Tecnologia), through the project UID/MAT/00297/2013 (Centro de Matemática e Aplicações).

References

Abramowitz, M., & Stegun, I. A. (1972). *Handbook of mathematical functions, Applied mathematics series* (Vol. 55, 10th ed.). Washington, DC: National Bureau of Standards, US Government Printing Office.

Ahsanullah, M., & Hamedani, G. G. (2010). *Exponential distribution*. New York: Nova Science Publishers.

Alizadeh Noughabi, H., & Arghami, N. R. (2011). Testing exponentiality based on characterizations of the exponential distribution. *Journal of Statistical Computation and Simulation, 81*(11), 1641–1651. https://doi.org/10.1080/00949655.2010.498373.

Balakrishnan, N., & Basu, A. P. (1995). *Exponential distribution: Theory, methods and applications*. Boca Raton: CRC Press.

Brilhante, M. F. (2004). Exponentiality versus generalized Pareto - a resistant and robust test. *REVSTAT – Statistical Journal, 2*(1), 2–13.

Caeiro, F., Marques, F. J., Mateus, A., & Atal, S. (2016). A note on the Jackson exponentiality test. *AIP Conference Proceedings, 1790*, 080005. https://doi.org/10.1063/1.4968686.

Doksum, K. A., & Yandell, B. S. (1984). Tests for exponentiality. In P. R. Krishnaiah & P. K. Sen (Eds.), *Handbook of statistics 4: Nonparametric methods* (Vol. 4, pp. 579–611). Amsterdam: North-Holland.

Gibbons, J. D., & Chakraborti, S. (2011). *Nonparametric statistical inference*. Boca Raton: CRC Press.

Henze, N., & Meintanis, S. G. (2005). Recent and classical tests for exponentiality: A partial review with comparisons. *Metrica, 61*, 29–45.

Jackson, O. A. Y. (1967). An analysis of departures from the exponential distribution. *Journal of the Royal Statistical Society, B*(29), 540–549.

Johnson, N. L., Kotz, S., & Balakrishnan, N. (1994). *Continuous univariate distributions* (Vol. 1, 2nd ed.). New York: Wiley.

Kozubowski, T. J., Panorska, A. K., Qeadan, F., Gershunov, A., & Rominger, D. (2009). Testing exponentiality versus Pareto distribution via likelihood ratio. *Communications in Statistics – Simulation and Computation, 38*(1), 118–139.

Lilliefors, H. W. (1969). On the Kolmogorov-Smirnov test for the exponential distribution with mean unknown. *Journal of the American Statistical Association, 64*(325), 387–389.

Stephens, M. A. (1986). Tests for the exponential distribution. In R. B. D'Agostino & M. A. Stephens (Eds.), *Goodness-of-fit techniques* (pp. 421–459). New York: Marcel Dekker Inc.

R Core Team (2015). *A language and environment for statistical computing*. Vienna: R Foundation for Statistical Computing. URLhttp://www.R-project.org/

Chapter 20
An Intervention Analysis Regarding the Impact of the Introduction of Budget Airline Routes to Maltese Tourism Demographics

Maristelle Darmanin and David Suda

20.1 Introduction

Intervention analysis looks for dynamic changes in a time series following an intervention. The seminal paper related to intervention analysis is that by Box and Tiao (1975). This intervention, in actual practice, could take the form of an event, procedure, law or policy intended to change a particular trend. Transportation and tourism time series are time series which are expected to be impacted by external events that are known to have occurred at a particular point in time. By understanding the extent of the impact of an intervention on a time series, policy makers would be able to quantify the extent of the impact and adjust policy to cater for inferred change. Intervention analysis has often been used to study the effects of policy, procedure or other events on transportation and tourism. In (Vaziri et al. 1990), the impact of fare and service changes on transportation in Kentucky during the period 1975-1985 is studied. In (Park et al. 2016), the impact on passenger ridership of the opening of a new railway line in Soeul is investigated. A study from a tourism perspective is found in (Min et al. 2011), where the impact of SARS in 2003 on Japanese tourism to Taiwan is assessed.

The relatively small size of the Maltese islands means that changes in policies and interventions may prove to have a significant effect on the economy. Tourism is an important pillar of the Maltese economy, and the impact of the introduction of low cost carriers, which have been introduced in 2006, to Maltese tourism has never

M. Darmanin
National Statistics Office, Valletta, Malta
e-mail: maristelle.darmanin@gov.mt

D. Suda (✉)
University of Malta, Msida, Malta
e-mail: david.suda@um.edu.mt

© Springer International Publishing AG, part of Springer Nature 2018
C. H. Skiadas, C. Skiadas (eds.), *Demography and Health Issues*,
The Springer Series on Demographic Methods and Population Analysis 46,
https://doi.org/10.1007/978-3-319-76002-5_20

before been studied. In this paper we look at how the introduction of these new routes has impacted on the volume and pro le of tourists visiting Malta during the above mentioned period. The analysis is based on variables derived from the Tourstat survey (https://nso.gov.mt/en/nso/Sources and Methods/Unit C3/Popula tion and Tourism Statistics/Pages/Inbound-Tourism.aspx) carried out by the National Statistics Office in Malta. This is a tourism survey carried out monthly using a two-stage sampling technique consisting of clustering and systematic sampling stages. The survey is carried out at departure terminals at randomly picked time-intervals, and tourists visiting Malta are selected systematically and interviewed as they are entering the departures lounge towards the end of their stay. The results from this survey are then projected for the whole tourist population. For the analysis, we consider the period 2003-2012 on a monthly basis. We shall be looking at two interventions – the introduction of low cost routes to Pisa and London in October 2006, and a considerable addition of new routes (namely Bologna, Marseille and other European airports in Spain, Denmark and Poland) in March 2010. Due to numerous time series data sets at our disposal, from here onwards we shall only present those series where intervention eventually proved to be significant.

When carrying out intervention analysis, the following assumptions will be taken into consideration. First of all, apart from the noise of the series, the only exogenous impact shall be presumed to be that of the event or the intervention itself. Secondly, the temporal delimitations of the intervention are presumed to be known, such as the time of onset, the durations and the time of termination of the input event. Lastly, it is ensured that a sufficient number of observations in the series should be available before and after the onset of the event for the researcher to separately model the pre-intervention time series and the post-intervention time series.

20.2 Building the Intervention Model

Building an intervention model typically follows these steps. A model is constructed for change, which describes what is expected to occur given knowledge of the known intervention (or interventions). Data analysis is then worked out appropriately based on that model. A pre-intervention model is first obtained, based on the data prior to the first intervention. A SARIMA (seasonal autoregressive moving average) model is typically used at this stage, but not exclusively. This is then followed by an analysis on the whole data set including the intervention. This is usually chosen after the selected model is used to generate forecasted values for the period after the intervention, and the differences between the actual values after the intervention and the forecasted values are visually analysed. The typical intervention model is given by

$$Y_t = f(\theta, \mathbf{I}, t) + N_t \tag{20.1}$$

where Y is the original or appropriately transformed series, f represents the dynamic model for the intervention effects and is a function of the parameter set θ, the intervention variables **I** and the time t, and N represents the underlying time series with no intervention, which may either be completely random or modeled by some time series model of endogenous variables. Diagnostic checks are then carried out on the fitted model, and if serious deficiencies are uncovered, the model needs to be modified. The diagnostic checking which occurs at this stage is the testing of the significance of model parameters, where one also includes post-intervention data, and analysis of residuals. In this paper we shall assume that N is modeled by SARIMA. A SARIMA (p,d,q) $(P,D,Q)_s$ with no constant term is given by the equation

$$(1-B)(1-B^s)\phi(B)\Phi(B^s)N_t = \theta(B)\Theta(B^s)Z_t \tag{20.2}$$

where B is the backward operator, Z is a white noise process and:

1. $\phi(z) = 1 - \phi_1 z - \ldots - \phi_p z^p$
2. $\Phi(z) = 1 - \Phi_1 z - \ldots - \Phi_P z^P$
3. $\theta(z) = 1 + \theta_1 z - \ldots - \theta_q z^q$
4. $\Theta(z) = 1 + \Theta_1 z - \ldots - \Theta_Q z^Q$

If we include the constant term, we replace N_t in (20.2) with $\tilde{N}_t \equiv N_t - \mu$ for non-zero constant term μ. We now look into possible ways of modeling intervention.

20.2.1 Dynamic Models for Intervention

A model for intervention can contain both single and multiple interventions. For a single intervention, the dynamic model in (20.1) is given by

$$f(\theta, I, t) = \chi_t = \frac{\omega(B)}{\delta(B)} I_t \tag{20.3}$$

where

1. $\omega(z) = 1 - \omega_1 z - \ldots - \omega_r z^r$
2. $\delta(z) = 1 - \delta_1 z - \ldots - \delta_s z^s$
3. $\omega(z)$ and $\delta(z)$ have roots outside the unit circle
4. χ_t represents the dynamic transfer from a single intervention I
5. $\theta = (\omega_1 \ldots, \omega_r, \delta_1 \ldots, \delta_s)$

Furthermore, we call the term $\frac{\omega(z)}{\delta(z)}$ in (20.3) the transfer function, as it relates the exogenous input I_t with the observed process Yat time$t$. The generalisation of (20.3) for multiple interventions is given by

$$f(\theta, \mathbf{I}, t) = \sum_{j=1}^{k} \chi_{tj} = \sum_{j=1}^{k} \frac{\omega_j(B)}{\delta_j(B)} I_t^{(j)} \tag{20.4}$$

where

1. $\omega_j(z) = 1 - \omega_{1j}z - \ldots - \omega_{r_j j}z^{r_j}$
2. $\delta_j(z) = 1 - \delta_{1j}z - \ldots - \delta_{s_j j}z^{s_j}$
3. for all j, $\omega_j(z)$ and $\delta_j(z)$ have roots outside the unit circle
4. $\mathbf{I} = (I^{(1)}, \ldots, I^{(j)})$
5. χ_{tj} represents the dynamic transfer from the jth intervention $I^{(j)}$
6. $\theta = (\omega_{11}, \ldots, \omega_{r_k k}, \delta_{11}, \ldots, \delta_{s_k k})$

The two most common types of intervention variables I_t^j are the step intervention and the pulse intervention. The step intervention $S^{(T,j)}$ represents an intervention at time T that remains in effect thereafter, hence causing a permanent change in state. In this case:

$$S_t^{(T,j)} = \begin{cases} 0, t < T \\ 1, t \geq T \end{cases} \tag{20.5}$$

The pulse intervention $P^{(T,j)}$, on the other hand, represents an intervention at time Twhose change in state is only temporary. In this case

$$P_t^{(T,j)} = \begin{cases} 0, t \neq T \\ 1, t = T \end{cases} \tag{20.6}$$

Sometimes, however, the intervention effect may also be seasonal. This is likely to cause model misspecification if not catered for. Specifically devised for our purpose, we shall also consider a periodic pulse intervention to model one of our time series. Denoting it by $P^{(d,t,j)}$, we de ne this as follows

$$P_t^{(d,T,j)} = \begin{cases} 1, t = T + j + bd \\ 0, t \neq T + j + bd \end{cases} \tag{20.7}$$

where $a \in \{0, 1, d - 1\}$ and $b \in \mathbb{Z}^+$. To cater for multiple periodic pulse intervention effects, one can consider these within the context of a multiple intervention model of the type (4).

We next discuss the polynomial terms in (20.3) and (20.4). The ω_j-polynomials are responsible for the delay in the effect of the intervention variable, while the δ_j-polynomials are responsible for the type of change in the mean after the effect of the intervention. For example, if $\omega_j(z) = \widetilde{\omega}$, then the effect of the intervention of the mean is immediate, while if $\omega_j(z) = \widetilde{\omega}z^k$ for $k > 0$, then the effect of the intervention is delayed by$k$. On the other hand, $\delta_j(z) = 1$ suggests an abrupt change in mean after the effect of the intervention, $\delta_j(z) = 1 - \widetilde{\delta}z$ where $\widetilde{\delta} \in (0, 1)$ suggests a gradual change in mean after the effect of the intervention, while $\delta_j(z) = 1 - z$ suggests a

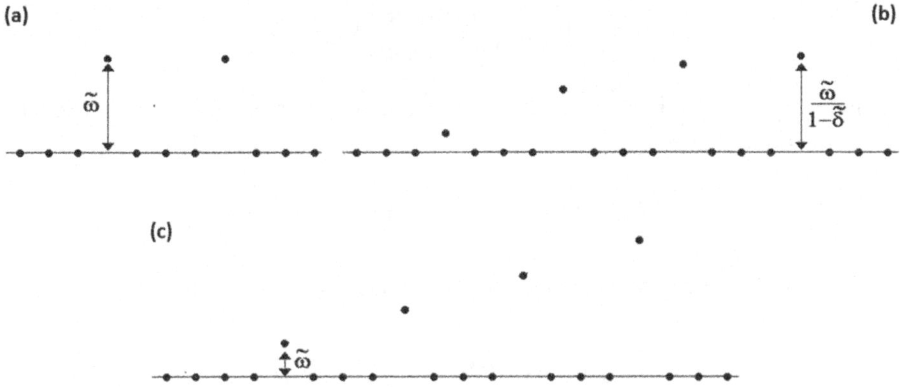

Fig. 20.1 The response to a periodic pulse intervention with $d = 4$ for the following transfer functions: (**a**)$\omega(z) = \widetilde{\omega}, \delta(z) = 1$, (**b**) $\omega(z) = \widetilde{\omega}, \delta(z) = 1 - z^4$ and (**c**) $\omega(z) = \widetilde{\omega}, \delta(z) = 1 - \widetilde{\delta} z^4$

linear increase/decrease without bound. For illustrations of the different effects to the mean level for different combinations of ω_j -polynomials and δ_j -polynomials applied to interventions of the type (5) and (6), see (Box 1975), Sect. 2. For interventions of the type (7), we shall only apply $\omega_j(z) = \widetilde{\omega}_j$, due to the fact that the intervention effect for a particular month will only be expected to occur in that month. On the other hand, in the denominator, we shall assume either that $\delta_j(z) = 1$, $\delta_j(z) = 1 - \widetilde{\delta}_j z^d$ or $\delta_j(z) = 1 - z^d$. In the latter, we allow for gradual change along the seasonal streaks of the intervention. The forms for $\omega_j(z)$ and $\delta_j(z)$ mentioned in this paragraph are the only ones we shall consider moving forward (Fig. 20.1).

Preliminary analysis for deciding which intervention model is most appropriate is not unique. One approach for selecting an adequate intervention model is through plots of the differences between the actual values after intervention and the forecasted values. We opt to use moving average plots which have smoothed out the noise and seasonal effects, hence bringing to the fore the underlying patterns of the data. This will be elaborated on in Sect. 3. Ultimately, these are just graphical indications, and the resulting model may not correspond to what one expects from preliminary analysis.

20.2.2 Inference for the Intervention Model

We now discuss estimation for the intervention model in (20.1). Given a time series of length $N + d + sD$, the likelihood may be obtained in terms of an N-dimensional vector $\mathbf{W}$ whose t^{th} element is given by

$$W_t = (1 - B)^d (1 - B^s)^D (Y_t - f(\theta, \mathbf{I}, t))$$

where

$$W_t = \left\{ \frac{\theta(B)\Theta(B^s)}{\phi(B)\Phi(B^s)} \right\} Z_t$$

is stationary. Let β be the vector SARIMA and intervention parameters in 1. Then the likelihood function is

$$L(\beta, \sigma_z^2 | \mathbf{W}) = (2\pi\sigma_z^2)^{-\frac{N}{2}} |\mathbf{M}|^{\frac{1}{2}} \exp\left\{ -\frac{S(\beta)}{2\sigma_z^2} \right\}$$

where $\sigma_z^2 \mathrm{M}^{-1}$ is the covariance matrix of $\mathbf{W}$ and

$$S(\beta) = \mathbf{W}'\mathbf{M}\mathbf{W} = \sum_{t=0}^{N} E[Z_t | \mathbf{W}, \beta]$$

Least squares estimation may be applied as a good alternative when MLE becomes infeasible to implement because of the model's strong non-linearity. Furthermore, two alternative approaches to estimation are suggested by (Box 1975). The first approach uses the same parameters obtained at pre-intervention stage and just estimates the intervention parameters. In this case we would be looking at a quasi-likelihood or quasi-least squares problem. This appears to be less ideal but may sometimes lead to more manageable optimisation, however this was never necessary in our case. The second approach, on the other hand, will apply maximum likelihood estimation or least squares estimation (typically non-linear least squares estimation) to the whole model. When the intervention is abrupt or gradual, i.e. $\delta(z) = 1, \delta(z) = 1 - \widetilde{\delta} z \, \mathrm{or} \, \delta(z) = 1 - \widetilde{\delta} z^d$, maximum likelihood may be used by applying a number of available software packages. When $\delta(z) = 1 - z$ or $\delta_j(z) = 1 - z^d$, estimating (20.1) becomes a restricted least squares problem. For the purpose of restricted least squares estimation, (20.1) may be rewritten as

$$(1 - B)^d (1 - B^s)^D \left\{ \frac{\phi(B)\Phi(B^s)}{\theta(B)\Theta(B^s)} \right\} (Y_t - f(\theta, \mathbf{I}, t)) = Z_t \qquad (20.8)$$

Methods for transforming (20.8) into regression form can be found in (Cryer and Chan 2010), Chap. 11, and the parameters are then estimated via the usual non-linear least squares techniques.

20.2.3 Goodness of Fit Measures and Residual Diagnostics

The following goodness of fit measures are used to select the best intervention model. In the following, we denote by $\widehat{Y}_t$ the one-step ahead predictor of Y_t.

1. Mean absolute error (MAE) : $MAE = \frac{1}{T} \sum_{t=1}^{T} | Y_t - \widehat{Y}_t |$;

2. Mean absolute percentage error (*MAPE*): $MAPE = \frac{100}{T}\sum_{t=1}^{T} \mid \frac{Y_t - \widehat{Y}_t}{Y_t} \mid$;
3. Maximum absolute error (*MaxAE*): $MaxAE = \max_t \mid Y_t - \widehat{Y}_t \mid$;
4. MaxAPE (*MaxAPE*): $MaxAPE = 100\max_t \mid \frac{Y_t - \widehat{Y}_t}{Y_t} \mid$;
5. Normalised BIC(*NBIC*) : $NBIC = p \ln T - 2 \ln L$, where L is the model likelihood and p is the number of parameters to be estimated. When the likelihood is not known, we can approximate this by $NBIC = \ln(MSE) + p \ln(T)$, where $MSE = \frac{1}{T}\sum_{t=1}^{T}\left(Y_t - \widehat{Y}_t\right)^2$ For independent identically distributed normal disturbances, the two are equivalent.

Furthermore, one can also apply the Ljung-Box test or other tests for serial correlation on the error terms to ensure that the white noise hypothesis is satisfied.

20.3 Results

The limitation with intervention analysis is that it is based on the assumption that the model specification is correct and no other exogenous occurrences have influenced the data. Furthermore, the size of the pre-intervention and post-intervention data set may also hinder a proper specification of the model. A more detailed discussion of the limitations of intervention analysis can be found in e.g. (Yaffee and McGee 2000). We shall therefore perform preliminary analysis on the data to identify some characteristics of the data after the noise and seasonality have been smoothed, to avoid having gross misspecifications in the model and erroneous identification of the intervention.

20.3.1 Preliminary Analysis Using Moving Averages

We shall plot prior moving averages of order 12 over the French tourism series, package tourism series and Italian tourism series – three series that we have identified to be influenced by the mentioned interventions. We opt for prior moving averages rather than centred ones, as these are better for identifying the exact occurrence of the intervention effect. From Fig. 20.2, we can see from the moving average that the French tourism model appears to show a linear and unbounded increase in tourism following the addition of new routes, including Marseille, in March 2010. The package tourism moving averages, after the March 2010 intervention, shows a gradual increase which quickly reaches a plateau. The Italian tourism

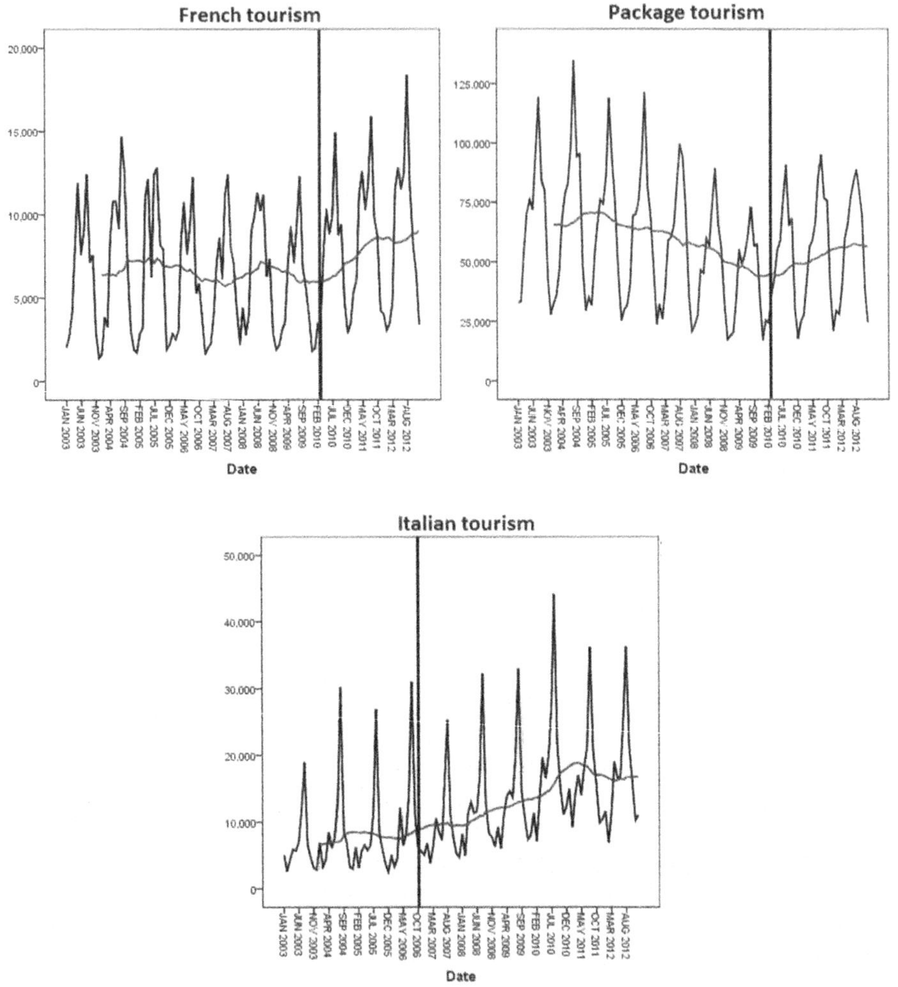

Fig. 20.2 Original series (black solid line) and prior moving average of order 12 (grey solid line) for the following tourism series: French (top left), package (top right) and Italian (bottom). Black vertical line denotes the time of the intervention

model, on the other hand, also appears to show an increase which reaches a plateau after a few years.

Despite the characteristics evident in Fig. 20.2, the modeling aspect may lead us to different models altogether. Sometimes, what appears to be the ideal model ends up not being estimable. Furthermore, there are instances where it may be di cult to capture all features, and we may be forced to opt for some features rather than others. Nonetheless, in this paper we present intervention models where the white noise hypothesis via the Ljung-Box test is not rejected at the 0.05 level of significance and, furthermore, we shall ensure that the SARIMA part of the model is causal and invertible after first order and seasonal differencing.

20.3.2 Model Fitting and Diagnostics

In this section we discuss models and their diagnostics for the aforementioned series where this was estimable. We select the model with the best good-ness of t criteria which satisfies the required model assumptions. Due to the permanent nature of our interventions, we have not considered the pulse interventions in (20.5), but the step interventions in (20.4) failed, we applied the periodic pulse interventions in (20.6) for each month. When implementing an intervention model of the type (4), we have attempted estimation for $\omega(z) = \widetilde{\omega} z^k$ for various lags k and $\delta(z)$ for all the aforementioned forms. We take $k = 0, 1, 2, 3$ when $\delta(z) = 1$ and $k = 0, 1$ otherwise. For some cases, the parameters for the models could not be estimated due to numerical instability. For an intervention model of the type (6), we have considered $\omega(z) = \widetilde{\omega}$ in conjunction with $\delta(z) = 1, \delta(z) = 1 - \widetilde{\delta} z^d$ and $\delta(z) = 1 - z^d$. We have also allowed for multiple interventions, however none of the time series considered found more than one intervention to be significant. The time series where intervention was deemed to have a significant impact were monthly French tourist numbers, monthly package tourist numbers and monthly Italian tourist numbers. For the French tourism series and package tourism series, the step intervention model was sufficient and the significant intervention was the one occurring in March 2010. This was expected for the French tourism time series, as this corresponded to the intervention where the Marseille route was introduced. On the other hand, for the Italian tourist time series, the periodic pulse intervention model was found to be more appropriate and the significant intervention was the one occurring in October 2006. This means that the introduction of the Pisa route in October 2006 left an impact on Italian tourism volumes, but the introduction of the Bologna route in March 2010 does not appear to have had a significant impact. The fitted models and the results are the following.

We first look at the step intervention model for French tourism time series. With reference to the model in (20.1), N is represented by a *SARIMA* $(0, 0, 0)(1, 1, 0)_{12}$. On the other hand, we take $\omega(z) = \omega z$ and $\delta(z) = 1 - z$. The two coefficients that need estimating $\boldsymbol{\Phi}$, and $\widetilde{\omega}$, we obtained through non-linear least squares estimation after transforming (20.7) into regression form. The parameters, standard errors and corresponding 95% confidence intervals are found in Table 20.1.

The goodness of fit statistics for this model are $MAE = 1120.74$, $MAPE = 14.9$, $MaxAE = 4903.4$, $MaxAPE = 92.92$, $NBIC = 14.46$ and $R^2 = 0.86$. The Ljung-Box statistic for the 18th lag is 18.898 and the p-value is 0.4. Fitting a similar model but with $\omega(z) = \widetilde{\omega}$ was unsuccessful. Models with $\omega(z) = \widetilde{\omega} z^k$ for $k = 0, 1, \ldots 3$ and $\delta(z) = 1$ were also successfully fitted, but the Ljung-Box test was rejected at 0.05 level of significance in all cases, with p-values extremely close to zero.

Table 20.1 Parameter estimates for the French tourism intervention model

Estimate	Standard Error	95% Lower Bound	95% Upper Bound
−0.45	0.09	−0.62	−0.27
656.79	132.33	394.04	919.53

Table 20.2 Goodness of t tests and Ljung-Box statistic for the package tourist intervention model at $k = 0, 1, 2, 3$

k	R^2	MAE	MAPE	MaxAE	MaxAPE	NBIC	Ljung-Box	
0	0.93	5166.58	9.63	18642.62	40.4	17.81	16.44	(p = 0:42)
1	0.94	5128.23	9.53	18462.64	40.68	17.81	18.29	(p = 0:31)
2	0.94	5075.65	9.44	18741.43	40.4	17.79	17.31	(p = 0:37)
3	0.94	5111.37	9.51	18542.7	40.87	17.79	18.62	(p = 0:29)

Table 20.3 Parameter estimates for the package tourism intervention model at $k = 2$

Parameter	Estimate	Standard Error	p-value
ϕ	0.57	0.08	0
Φ	−0.46	0.09	0
$\tilde{\omega}$	4686.06	2028.95	0.02

Table 20.4 Parameter estimates for the Italian tourism intervention model

Parameter	Estimate	Standard Error	p-value
μ	10734.55	1173.76	0
ϕ	0.52	0.09	0
Θ	−0.52	0.11	0
$\tilde{\omega}_7$	8335.69	2253.92	0
$\tilde{\omega}_8$	12271.77	3510.25	0
$\tilde{\delta}_8$	0.51	0.18	0.01
$\tilde{\omega}_9$	4743.29	2241.27	0.04

The next series we shall look into is the package tourism time series, again applying the step intervention model. With reference to the model in (20.1), N is represented by a *SARIMA* $(1, 0, 0)(1, 1, 0)_{12}$. On the other hand, we take $\omega(z) = \tilde{\omega}z^k$ for $k = 0, 1, 2, 3$ and $\delta(z) = 1$. Other types of intervention models were also attempted but the model fitting was unsuccessful. There are three coefficients that needed estimating: ϕ, $\boldsymbol{\Phi}$ and $\tilde{\omega}$. These are obtained via maximum likelihood estimation. To select the optimal k, we look at the goodness of t statistics for various $k = 0, 1, 2$ in Table 20.4 when maximum likelihood estimation is applied.

In Table 20.2, the superior goodness of t statistics are marked in bold. Since the intervention model at $k = 2$ had the best *MAE* and *MAPE*, and the joint best R^2, *MaxAPE* and *NBIC* with other models having different k, we opt for this model. The parameters, standard errors and p-values for the intervention model at k=2 are found in Table 20.3.

We finally look at the Italian tourism time series. The first attempt was to t intervention models with $\omega(z) = \tilde{\omega}z^k$ and all possible $\delta(z)$. While the models were estimable when $\delta(z) = 1$ and $\delta(z) = 1 - Z$, these led to residuals with significant short term correlation. An analysis of raw monthly pre-intervention and post-intervention means led us to suspect that seasonality in the intervention effect was the issue. The post-intervention increase in the raw mean for the month of July was 8402.58 (the highest) in comparison to the pre-intervention raw mean, while the increase for February was 3283. We therefore implement the periodic pulse intervention model, and we shall assign a periodic pulse to each month of the year. Hence we have a model of the type (1), where the dynamic model is of the multiple type in (20.3). We consider combinations of the cases where $\omega_j(z) = \widetilde{\omega}_j$, and $\delta_j(z)$ is either equal 1, $1 - \widetilde{\delta}_j z^{12}$ or $1 - z^{12}$. Hence, we look at an intervention model of the form

$$f(\theta, \mathbf{I}, t) = \sum_{j=1}^{12} \frac{\widetilde{\omega}_j}{\delta_j(z)} P_t^{(12,T,j)}$$

where T corresponds to October 2006, the 46th data point. With reference to the model in 1, N is represented by a $SARIMA(1;0;0)\,(0;0;1)_{12}$ with constant term. On the other hand, the best model is obtained when $\omega(z) = \widetilde{\omega}$ and $\delta(z) = 1$ for July and September, while $\delta(z) = 1 - \widetilde{\delta}_z{}^{12}$ for August. We use maximum likelihood estimation to estimate μ, ϕ, Θ_1,Θ_2 , the $\widetilde{\omega}_j'$s and δ_8 The periodic pulse interventions for July, August and September were found to be significant. The significant parameters, standard errors, and p-values are found in Table 20.4. The goodness of t statistics for this model are $MAE = 2572.57$, $MAPE = 29.77$, $MaxAE = 18175.44$, $MaxAPE = 165.56$, $NBIC = 16.92$ and $R^2 = 0.77$. The Ljung-Box statistic for the 18 th lag is 13.17 and the p-value is 0.66.

Based solely on the obtained model fits, we deduce the following. French tourism has increased linearly after removing the SARIMA dynamics of the model, at an estimated rate of 656.79 every month. The response to the intervention appears to have occurred with a delay of one month, as k=1 for the dynamic model explaining intervention. On the other hand, after removal of the SARIMA dynamics, package tourism appears to have increased by an estimated 4686.06 in the post-intervention months. Indeed, package tourism appeared to have been on the decline for quite a few years prior to the 2010 intervention. The response to the interventions appears to have happened with a two month lag (k=2). What we may be seeing here is the response of the tourism industry to the introduction of a significant number of low cost routes in March 2010, by offering more worthwhile deals to the potential Maltese tourism market. It is also likely that package deals have now been making use of inexpensive routes created by the competition to lower their prices. Finally, for the Italian tourism market, the periodic pulse intervention was found to be significant for the months of July, August, and September. We have a sudden estimated increase of 8115.29, on removal of the SARIMA effect, in the post-intervention July months. For September, the sudden estimated increase is of 4571.45. On the other hand, for August, the post-intervention effect is increasing asymptotically to 25044.43. A plot of the original series, fitted values of one-step predictors and lower/upper 95% confidence levels can be seen in Fig. 20.3.

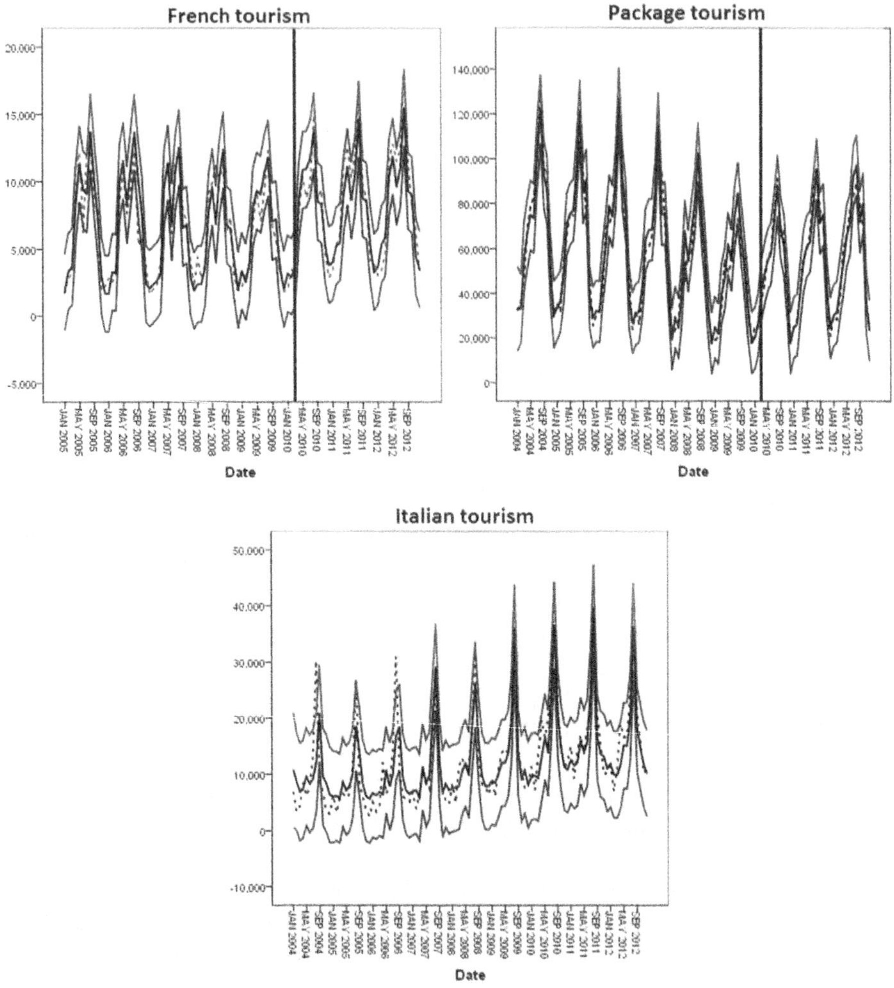

Fig. 20.3 Original series (black dashed line), fitted series (black solid line), lower and upper 95% confidence levels (lower and upper grey solid lines) for the following tourism series: French (top left), package (top right) and Italian (bottom). Black vertical line denotes the time of the intervention

20.4 Conclusion

Intervention analysis is a useful way of assessing the impact of policy on time series. In this paper, we have presented three cases where the introduction of new routes was found to have a significant impact, either on the intended tourism market or on other areas. Intervention was found to be significant for French and Italian tourism, where an increase in tourists from this country is detected, and package tourism, where the tourism industry appears to have responded to the introduction of low cost airlines. Furthermore, we see that the intervention did not affect Italian tourism equally for all months – only the effects for the months of July, August and September were found to be significant. Interestingly, intervention was not found to have led to a significant increase in British tourists in 2006, or a significant increase in tourists from other EU countries in 2010, despite the addition of new routes from Spain, Denmark and Poland.

Intervention analysis is not without its pitfalls. The amount of data available pre-intervention and post-intervention may affect both model selection and estimation. A complex transfer function may also complicate the estimation problem. Indeed, sometimes we may need to settle for simpler and less informative models. Furthermore, we need to be careful not to falsely attribute changes in the dynamics of a time series to intervention effects. These are all issues we have encountered when performing the analysis. A careful exploratory analysis of the data and being well informed about the context that one is dealing with may help avoid these mistakes. Nonetheless, intervention analysis is an effective and important tool for detecting effect of a sudden change, whether intended or unintended, and is also capable of influencing future policy and decision-making.

References

Box, G. E. P., & Tiao, G. C. (1975). Intervention analysis with applications to economic and environmental problems. *Journal of the American Statistical Association, 70*(349), 70–79.

Cryer, J. D., & Chan, K. S. (2010). *Time series analysis: With applications in R* (2nd ed.). New York: Springer.

https://nso.gov.mt/en/nso/Sources and Methods/Unit C3/Population and Tourism Statistics/Pages/Inbound-Tourism.aspx

Min, J. C. H., Lim, C., & Kung, H. H. (2011). Intervention analysis of SARS on Japanese tourism demand for Taiwan. *Quality and Quantity, 45*(1), 91–102.

Park, M. S., Eom, J. K., Heo, T. Y., & Song, J. (2016). Intervention analysis of the impact of opening a new railway line on passenger ridership in Soeul. *KSCE Journal on Civil Engineering, 20*(6), 2524–2534,

Vaziri, M., Hutchinson, J., & Kermanshah, M. (1990). Short-term demand for specialized transportation. *Journal of Transportation Engineering, 116*(1), 105–121.

Yaffee, R. A., & McGee, M. (2000). *An introduction to time series analysis and forecasting: With applications of SAS and SPSS.* New York: Academic Press.

Chapter 21
Investigating Southern Europeans' Perceptions of Their Employment Status

Aggeliki Yfanti, Catherine Michalopoulou, Aggelos Mimis, and Stelios Zachariou

21.1 Introduction

In all large-scale sample surveys, demographic and socio-economic variables are included as background variables which "in addition to providing general contextual/collateral information, they are used as independent variables, as socio-economic covariates of attitudes, behavior, or test scores, etc. and in all sorts of statistical models, in particular, as exogenous factors in causal analysis" (Braun and Mohler 2003: 101). Furthermore, background variables have been and will continue to be used in order to assess the quality of the realized sample by carrying out detailed comparisons of their distributions to the more recent available respective census data (Braun and Mohler 2003), since "it is only sound practice to test a theoretical result empirically" (Stephan and McCarthy 1958: 134). In the case of the employment status, i.e. one of the occupational background variables, because of its great overtime variability, the census data available for such comparisons is most of the time outdated. Recognition of this fact "leads us to consider alternatives, especially the possibility of comparing the results obtained by one sample survey on such . . . [a variable] with the results obtained by other sample surveys" (Stephan and McCarthy 1958: 156). In this respect, the more appropriate "other [such] sample survey" that provides updated information is the Labour Force Survey (LFS) and, in this instance, the European Union Labour Force Survey (EU-LFS). However, the measurement of the employment status as a background variable included in all

A. Yfanti (✉) · C. Michalopoulou · A. Mimis
Panteion University of Social and Political Sciences, Athens, Greece
e-mail: aggelikiyfanti@panteion.gr; kmichal@panteion.gr; mimis@panteion.gr

S. Zachariou
Hellenic Statistical Authority, Piraeus, Greece
e-mail: s.zachariou@statistics.gr

© Springer International Publishing AG, part of Springer Nature 2018
C. H. Skiadas, C. Skiadas (eds.), *Demography and Health Issues*,
The Springer Series on Demographic Methods and Population Analysis 46,
https://doi.org/10.1007/978-3-319-76002-5_21

large-scale sample survey and the census is defined on the basis of how people perceive it, whereas the EU-LFS measurement of the employment status is based on a synthesized economic construct computed using a number of variables according to the ILO conventional definitions that classify the population of working age (15 years or more) into three mutually exclusive and exhaustive categories: employed, unemployed and inactive. These two measurements are not comparable and their results will differ since a composite economic construct would normally deviate from people's perceptions.

In the literature, the debate on the definition or concept especially of unemployment is of long standing (see for a review Yfanti et al. 2017). As Gauckler and Körner (2011: 186) pointed out, "measuring the ILO employment status in household surveys and censuses is challenging in several respects…The ILO defines employment in the broadest term, whereby one hour per work counts as being employed. A small job of one hour per week is enough. Such a definition will sometimes be in conflict with the respondent's everyday life perception." Eurostat (2009: 58), presenting an extensive analysis on whether the ILO definitions capture all unemployment and meet current and potential user needs, concluded that "there is no need for a revision of the ILO labour force concept when it is looked at from an economic perspective or when it is considered for international comparability… However, there is a point to make concerning the ILO definition of unemployment. It intends to capture only a restricted part of the whole labour reserve, i.e. the one showing a strong attachment to the labour market. It is not meant to measure the entire labour reserve. Jones and Riddell (1999), based on their results that indicated a substantial heterogeneity within the non-employed and a distribution of degrees of labour force attachment to be separated into distinct groups that displayed different behaviour, proposed that additional information appears necessary to identify activities such as "wait unemployment." Furthermore, Brandolini et al. (2004), discussing the heterogeneity of the labour market groups and the difficulty of a single definition of unemployment, pointed out the existence of large differences not only among countries, but also among socio-demographic groups within the same country.

All these "grey areas" of labour force attachment make the analysis difficult as the ILO conventional definitions do not reflect individuals' situation in the labour market as they perceive it. It is in this respect that Eurostat decided in 2006 to include the self-perceived employment status as a supplementary indicator to the ILO concepts intended to capture all these complexities. In 2011, de la Fuente (2011) briefly discussed the coverage problems of self-perceived unemployment and the three new Eurostat indicators that were introduced as supplementary to the unemployment rate based on the results of EU-LFS for 2010. Gauckler and Körner (2011) investigated the comparability of the employment status measurement in the German LFS and Census of 2011. The purpose of this paper is, by obtaining a demographic and social "profile" of agreement and disagreement between Southern Europeans' declared self-perceptions of their employment status and the ILO conventional definitions, to investigate whether or not conflicting and coinciding perceptions differ overtime within-nations and cross-nationally.

21.2 Method

21.2.1 Prerequisites for Comparability

The EU-LFS is a set of independent national multipurpose large-scale sample surveys conducted by the respective statistical offices of the member countries, providing quarterly and annual results on labour participation and those outside the labour force. The survey population is defined centrally as all persons aged 15 years or more living in private households, excluding persons in compulsory military or community service and those residing in collective dwellings. Therefore, the survey population overtime within-nations and cross-national comparability is ensured (Kish 1994).

The self-perceived employment status included in the EU-LFS is an optional variable for the participating countries, provided only in the annual datasets. It is available for most countries with the exception of Germany, UK and Norway. Although this variable was first introduced in 2006, Eurostat (2008) changed the reference period in 2008 and consequently there is an issue of comparability. In this respect, it was decided to base the analysis on the 2008–2014 datasets for the following Southern European countries: Greece, Italy, Portugal and Spain.

Also, the Eurostat (2008) instruction that, "this question shouldn't in any case precede the questions on the labour status according to the ILO definition or the questions on the registration at the public employment office" has to be considered for comparability. Because this is a perception question, i.e. sensitive to its placement in the questionnaire (Stephan and McCarthy 1958), the questionnaires of the four countries under investigation complied with this instruction allowing for overtime within-nations and cross-national comparability. Furthermore, it was decided to report the results for the age group 15–74 so as to allow for comparability with the ILO conventional definition of unemployment (Fig. 21.1; see also de la Fuente 2011).

21.2.2 The ILO Conventional Definitions of the Employment Status

Figure 21.1 presents the detailed EU-LFS measurement of the employment status based on a number of variables according to the ILO conventional definitions.

The variable WSTATOR measures the labour status during the reference week for all respondents aged 15 years or more according to the conventional definitions that were adopted by the ILO as agreed at the 13th and 14th International Conference of Labour Statisticians (Hussmanns et al. 1990). This variable takes the value one (1) when respondents did any work for pay or profit for one hour or more, including family work during the reference week. The second value (2) refers to respondents who despite of having a job or business did not work during the reference week

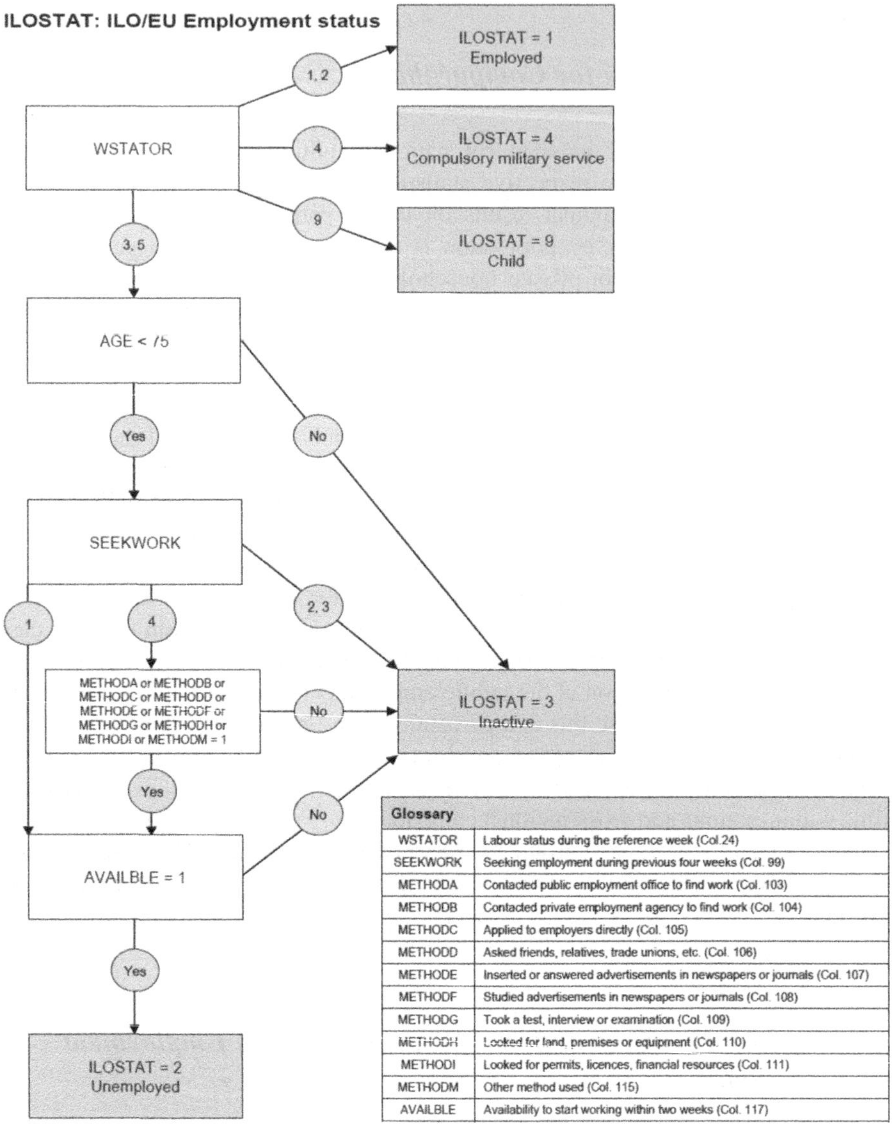

Glossary	
WSTATOR	Labour status during the reference week (Col.24)
SEEKWORK	Seeking employment during previous four weeks (Col. 99)
METHODA	Contacted public employment office to find work (Col. 103)
METHODB	Contacted private employment agency to find work (Col. 104)
METHODC	Applied to employers directly (Col. 105)
METHODD	Asked friends, relatives, trade unions, etc. (Col. 106)
METHODE	Inserted or answered advertisements in newspapers or journals (Col. 107)
METHODF	Studied advertisements in newspapers or journals (Col. 108)
METHODG	Took a test, interview or examination (Col. 109)
METHODH	Looked for land, premises or equipment (Col. 110)
METHODI	Looked for permits, licences, financial resources (Col. 111)
METHODM	Other method used (Col. 115)
AVAILBLE	Availability to start working within two weeks (Col. 117)

Fig. 21.1 The ILO conventional definitions of the employment status used in the EU-LFS. Reproduced from "EU Labour Force Survey database user guide," by Eurostat, 2016: 55

because they were temporarily absent. The third value (3) is assigned to respondents who were not working because of lay-off. The fourth value (4) indicates the respondent who was a conscript on compulsory military service or community service. Value five (5) designates respondents who did not work nor had a job or business during the reference week. As shown in Fig. 21.1, the definition of the

Table 21.1 The EU-LFS self-perceived employment status definition (all respondents aged 15 years or more)

Carries out a job or profession, including unpaid work for a family business or holding, including an apprenticeship or paid traineeship, etc.	1
Unemployed	2
Pupil, student, further training, unpaid work experience	3
In retirement or early retirement or has given up business	4
Permanently disabled	5
In compulsory military service	6
Fulfilling domestic tasks	7
Other inactive person	8
Not applicable (child less than 15 years)	9
No answer	^

unemployed applies only to respondents aged 15–74 years. Also, a number of variables is used that define whether respondents were seeking employment, the methods for doing so and their availability to start work immediately within two weeks (see for a detailed description, Eurostat 2016).

21.2.3 The EU-LFS Self-Perceived Employment Status Definition

In Table 21.1, the question measuring the self-perceived employment status is presented as is the case in all large-scale sample surveys and the census which differs from the ILO multivariate definition.

As shown, this is a perception question that gives the respondents the chance to identify they own employment status. The implementation rules for this variable (MAINSTAT) as defined by Eurostat (2008) specify that the main activity status represents self-perception regarding the respondents' activity status. For instance, students with small jobs will in general present themselves as students. The eighth response category (value 8) includes also respondents who cannot say whether they were "carrying out a job or profession" and those who do not fit into other categories or were on an extended leave from work (Eurostat 2008: 109). The instruction for the deliverance of this question according to the Eurostat good practices rules is that the interviewers have to read out the question and all the response categories.

21.2.4 Statistical Analyses

In order to ensure measurement overtime within-nations and cross-national comparability, all measures-variables have to be standardized (Kish 1994). In this respect, the variable measuring self-perceived employment status is first recoded into the three categories of the employed, unemployed and inactive according to the ILO conventional definitions. Then, the recoded variable is cross-tabulated with the ILO variable that is computed as presented in Fig. 21.1. The diagonal defines the "agreement" group, i.e. people's perceptions coinciding with the ILO conventional definitions. The off diagonal cases define the "disagreement" group, i.e., people's perceptions in conflict with the ILO conventional definitions. Then a demographic and social "profile" of both groups is obtained based on their demographic and social characteristics: gender (male, female), age (15–24, 25–34, 35–44, 45–54, 55–64 and 65–74), marital status (single, married, and other, i.e. widowed, divorced or legally separated) and highest level of educational attainment (primary, secondary and tertiary). Note that, initially, extensive checks were carried out for each category and based on these results it was decided to combine coinciding and conflicting perceptions into the before mentioned two groups.

21.3 Results

In Table 21.2, Southern Europeans' overall perceptions of their employment status as they compare to the ILO conventional definitions are presented.

As shown, more than 90% of Southern Europeans perceptions coincide overall with the ILO conventional definitions: 96.1–97.6% (Greece); 92.3–93.7% (Italy); 90.0–95.0% (Portugal); 97.1–97.8% (Spain). However, the number of people with

Table 21.2 Southern Europeans' overall perceptions of their employment status as they agree or disagree to the ILO conventional definitions (15–74; *N* in 000s)

Country	2008	2009	2010	2011	2012	2013	2014
Greece							
Agree %	97.6	97.3	97.3	96.7	96.2	96.1	96.1
Disagree %	2.4	2.7	2.7	3.3	3.8	3.9	3.9
N	8,328	8,303	8,305	8,308	8,313	8,184	8,135
Italy							
Agree %	93.9	93.7	93.4	93.2	93.1	92.5	92.3
Disagree %	6.1	6.3	6.6	6.8	6.9	7.5	7.7
N	45,337	45,563	45,685	45,800	45,866	45,556	45,626
Portugal							
Agree %	95.0	94.7	94.8	91.7	90.6	90.0	90.9
Disagree %	5.0	5.3	5.2	8.3	9.4	10.0	9.1
N	8,140	8,141	8,123	8,116	8,060	7,907	7,860
Spain							
Agree %	97.8	97.6	97.6	97.1	97.6	97.5	97.7
Disagree %	2.2	2.4	2.4	2.9	2.4	2.5	2.3
N	34,650	34,809	34,673	34,683	34,494	34,602	34,477

Table 21.3 Southern Europeans' (aged 15–74) perceptions coinciding with the ILO conventional definitions of the employed, unemployed and inactive (%)

Country	2008	2009	2010	2011	2012	2013	2014
Greece							
Employed	99.4	99.3	99.2	99.0	98.9	99.1	99.2
Unemployed	81.5	82.7	85.7	85.4	87.1	87.5	86.6
Inactive	97.3	96.9	97.4	97.4	96.9	96.8	97.0
Italy							
Employed	99.8	99.8	99.7	99.8	99.8	99.8	99.8
Unemployed	40.8	43.2	43.7	42.6	49.0	49.4	49.8
Inactive	96.9	97.2	97.4	97.7	97.4	97.7	97.7
Portugal							
Employed	99.9	100.0	99.9	99.7	99.7	99.7	99.8
Unemployed	67.0	70.6	74.1	66.0	67.3	65.4	62.5
Inactive	92.1	91.8	91.8	88.0	86.5	86.6	88.3
Spain							
Employed	99.3	99.2	99.2	98.9	98.9	98.8	99.0
Unemployed	87.6	90.6	91.8	91.3	93.8	93.6	93.8
Inactive	97.5	97.7	97.6	97.5	97.7	97.7	97.8

conflicting perceptions amounts to a considerable total ranging from 4,143,000 to 5,543,000: 202,000–319,000 (Greece); 2,759,000–3,499,000 (Italy); 407,000–791,000 (Portugal); 775,000–934,000 (Spain).

In Table 21.3, Southern Europeans' perceptions of their employment status coinciding with the ILO conventional definitions of the employed, unemployed and inactive are presented.

As shown, more than 98.8% of Southern Europeans agree with the ILO conventional definition in perceiving themselves as employed: 98.9–99.4% (Greece); 99.7–99.8% (Italy); 99.7–100.0% (Portugal); 98.8–99.3% (Spain). Also, more than 88% agree in perceiving themselves as inactive: 96.9–97.4% (Greece); 96.9–97.7% (Italy); 88.0–92.1% (Portugal); 97.5–97.8% (Spain). However, they do disagree with the ILO conventional definition in perceiving themselves as unemployed: 81.5–87.5% (Greece); 40.8–49.8% (Italy); 66.0–74.1% (Portugal); 87.6–93.8% (Spain). Italians disagree more remarked in perceiving themselves as unemployed than the Portuguese people, Greeks and Spaniards.

These findings indicate that a thorough investigation of the demographic and social characteristics of the "agreement" and "disagreement" groups is necessary in order to assess whether or not their distributions differ. In Tables 21.4, 21.5, 21.6 and 21.7, the demographic and social "profile" of Southern Europeans' coinciding and conflicting perceptions with the ILO conventional definitions is presented for Greece, Italy, Portugal and Spain, respectively.

The investigation of the "agreement" and "disagreement" groups for 2008–2014 (Tables 21.4, 21.5, 21.6, 21.7) shows that they do differ in terms of their demographic and social "profile": Greeks with conflicting perceptions are mainly women

Table 21.4 The demographic and social "profile" of coinciding and conflicting perceptions with the ILO conventional definitions: Greece (%)

Variable	2008	2009	2010	2011	2012	2013	2014
Gender							
Agree							
Male	49.6	49.6	49.6	49.6	49.7	49.2	49.3
Female	50.4	50.4	50.4	50.4	50.3	50.8	50.7
Disagree							
Male	41.6	42.9	43.2	46.9	45.9	43.9	43.8
Female	58.4	57.1	56.8	53.1	54.1	56.1	56.2
Age*							
Agree							
15–24	13.6	13.2	13.1	13.0	12.8	13.5	13.4
25–34	19.3	18.8	18.5	18.2	17.7	17.6	17.1
35–44	20.2	20.4	20.6	20.7	20.6	20.1	20.1
45–54	18.1	18.4	18.5	18.7	19.0	18.9	19.2
55–64	15.6	16.0	16.2	16.3	16.4	16.3	16.4
65–74	13.3	13.2	13.1	13.2	13.4	13.7	13.8
Disagree							
15–24	22.1	22.3	19.4	16.9	15.5	16.3	14.3
25–34	25.0	28.1	26.6	25.4	23.1	23.4	24.2
35–44	19.1	17.9	19.4	21.3	23.1	23.4	22.6
45–54	14.7	14.3	16.7	17.6	19.0	18.8	18.8
55–64	11.3	10.7	11.3	12.5	13.6	13.4	15.0
65–74	7.8	6.7	6.8	6.3	5.7	4.7	5.1
Marital status							
Agree							
Single	31.5	30.8	30.7	31.3	31.8	32.9	33.2
Married	60.9	61.3	61.2	60.5	59.8	58.7	58.5
Other	7.6	7.9	8.1	8.3	8.3	8.4	8.3
Disagree							
Single	43.1	45.5	41.0	39.3	38.0	39.4	38.1
Married	51.0	48.2	51.4	53.7	56.6	54.4	54.9
Other	5.9	6.3	7.7	7.0	5.4	6.3	7.0
Education							
Agree							
Primary	28.8	28.4	27.6	26.0	24.6	23.6	22.4
Secondary	52.9	53.1	52.9	53.2	54.0	54.1	54.4
Tertiary	18.3	18.4	19.5	20.8	21.3	22.3	23.1
Disagree							
Primary	27.2	24.1	25.7	26.6	22.4	21.0	21.0
Secondary	55.9	57.6	58.6	57.2	59.9	59.6	59.7
Tertiary	16.8	18.3	15.8	16.2	17.7	19.4	19.4

*All the results are at significant at $p < 0.001$.

Table 21.5 The demographic and social "profile" of coinciding and conflicting perceptions with the ILO conventional definitions: Italy (%)

Variable	2008	2009	2010	2011	2012	2013	2014
Gender							
Agree							
Male	49.7	49.5	49.4	49.3	49.4	49.2	49.2
Female	50.3	50.5	50.6	50.7	50.6	50.8	50.8
Disagree							
Male	46.4	48.2	49.5	50.3	49.4	50.2	50.5
Female	53.6	51.8	50.5	49.7	50.6	49.8	49.5
Age*							
Agree							
15–24	12.8	12.8	12.8	12.7	12.7	12.7	12.7
25–34	17.0	16.4	16.0	15.5	15.3	14.5	14.3
35–44	21.2	21.2	21.1	21.0	20.7	20.2	19.9
45–54	18.3	18.7	19.2	19.6	20.0	20.4	20.8
55–64	16.3	16.5	16.7	16.9	16.8	17.0	17.0
65–74	14.4	14.4	14.3	14.3	14.6	15.1	15.3
Disagree							
15–24	21.7	21.0	20.5	20.2	19.5	18.3	17.3
25–34	28.6	29.6	28.1	27.6	25.4	25.4	24.9
35–44	24.2	24.3	24.7	23.9	24.4	24.2	23.9
45–54	15.4	16.0	17.0	17.6	19.1	20.0	20.9
55–64	8.4	7.9	8.7	9.4	10.5	11.0	11.8
65–74	1.7	1.2	1.1	1.2	1.1	1.1	1.1
Marital status*							
Agree							
Single	31.0	31.2	31.3	31.6	32.3	32.5	32.9
Married	59.4	59.1	58.8	58.4	57.3	56.6	57.0
Other	9.6	9.7	9.8	10.0	10.4	10.8	10.1
Disagree							
Single	48.5	49.2	49.0	49.7	48.2	48.9	48.4
Married	45.1	44.8	44.3	43.5	44.1	43.0	44.1
Other	6.5	6.1	6.7	6.9	7.7	8.1	7.5
Education*							
Agree							
Primary	18.9	17.9	16.9	15.8	14.9	14.2	13.0
Secondary	69.3	70.2	71.0	71.8	72.0	72.1	72.8
Tertiary	11.7	11.9	12.2	12.4	13.1	13.7	14.2
Disagree							
Primary	13.1	11.8	11.6	11.1	10.6	9.8	8.9
Secondary	76.8	78.7	78.4	79.3	79.2	80.0	80.6
Tertiary	10.2	9.6	10.1	9.6	10.2	10.2	10.4

*All the results are at significant at $p < 0.001$.

Table 21.6 The demographic and social "profile" of coinciding and conflicting perceptions with the ILO conventional definitions: Portugal (%)

Variable	2008	2009	2010	2011	2012	2013	2014
Gender							
Agree							
Male	49.9	49.3	49.3	49.1	49.1	48.1	47.9
Female	50.6	50.7	50.7	50.9	50.9	51.9	52.1
Disagree							
Male	40.0	42.7	42.1	47.3	48.4	48.2	48.3
Female	60.0	57.3	57.9	52.7	51.6	51.8	51.7
Age*							
Agree							
15–24	15.2	14.9	14.5	14.2	14.1	14.2	14.1
25–34	20.3	20.0	19.7	19.4	18.6	16.8	16.2
35–44	19.7	19.9	20.0	20.6	21.0	20.9	20.9
45–54	18.0	18.2	18.5	18.7	19.0	19.4	19.4
55–64	15.1	15.3	15.4	15.3	15.4	16.1	16.4
65–74	11.7	11.6	11.9	11.9	12.0	12.7	13.1
Disagree							
15–24	11.0	10.0	10.2	12.6	13.0	13.1	13.2
25–34	15.0	15.0	14.0	13.7	13.3	12.8	12.2
35–44	13.7	14.6	14.9	13.1	14.0	14.8	14.0
45–54	15.9	15.7	16.8	17.7	17.2	17.4	18.2
55–64	21.3	21.3	21.3	22.6	23.1	23.5	23.8
65–74	23.0	23.4	22.7	20.2	19.4	18.3	18.5
Marital status							
Agree							
Single	27.3	27.4	27.4	32.7	33.8	34.1	33.6
Married	65.0	64.6	64.5	57.0	55.5	55.1	55.7
Other	7.7	8.0	8.1	10.3	10.7	10.8	10.7
Disagree							
Single	21.4	20.1	19.4	28.4	30.5	31.5	32.0
Married	69.0	69.3	69.7	59.8	57.7	56.6	56.0
Other	9.6	10.6	10.9	11.8	11.8	11.9	12.0
Education*							
Agree							
Primary	52.0	49.6	47.7	42.9	40.7	39.0	36.7
Secondary	36.0	38.0	39.2	42.0	42.8	43.9	44.4
Tertiary	11.9	12.4	13.2	15.1	16.7	17.2	18.9
Disagree							
Primary	71.5	70.4	70.9	63.2	59.8	56.6	53.8
Secondary	22.9	24.9	23.9	29.3	32.4	35.1	36.6
Tertiary	5.7	4.6	5.2	7.6	7.7	8.2	9.6

*All the results are at significant at $p < 0.001$.

Table 21.7 The demographic and social "profile" of coinciding and conflicting perceptions with the ILO conventional definitions: Spain (%)

Variable	2008	2009	2010	2011	2012	2013	2014
Gender							
Agree							
Male	50.2	50.1	50.0	49.9	49.7	49.9	49.8
Female	49.8	49.9	50.0	50.1	50.3	50.1	50.2
Disagree							
Male	43.2	45.3	45.2	45.8	46.2	45.5	44.2
Female	56.8	54.7	54.8	54.2	53.8	54.5	55.8
Age*							
Agree							
15–24	13.0	12.8	12.4	12.1	11.9	11.7	11.5
25–34	22.0	21.5	20.9	20.0	19.2	18.3	17.4
35–44	21.6	21.8	22.1	22.3	22.5	22.7	22.7
45–54	17.9	18.3	18.7	19.2	19.6	20.1	20.4
55–64	14.5	14.5	14.7	14.9	15.3	15.2	15.5
65–74	11.0	11.2	11.2	11.4	11.6	11.9	12.4
Disagree							
15–24	22.7	17.9	20.0	18.7	18.7	19.2	19.6
25–34	25.7	25.7	23.5	25.2	21.9	20.6	19.3
35–44	21.4	23.3	22.5	22.6	22.5	22.8	20.8
45–54	15.7	17.5	18.3	17.0	18.5	18.8	20.5
55–64	12.8	13.7	13.6	14.6	16.5	16.5	17.2
65–74	1.7	2.0	2.1	1.9	1.8	2.2	2.6
Marital status*							
Agree							
Single	33.7	33.9	33.9	34.0	34.4	35.7	36.1
Married	57.9	57.6	57.4	57.2	56.5	54.1	53.7
Other	8.4	8.5	8.7	8.8	9.0	10.1	10.3
Disagree							
Single	46.5	41.6	43.1	43.1	43.6	45.1	46.0
Married	47.5	49.3	49.3	48.8	49.9	47.6	44.4
Other	6.1	9.1	7.6	8.0	6.5	7.3	9.6
Education*							
Agree							
Primary	25.2	24.7	23.8	22.3	20.7	19.7	16.4
Secondary	49.0	49.1	49.9	49.9	50.8	50.9	53.1
Tertiary	25.8	26.2	26.3	27.8	28.5	29.3	30.5
Disagree							
Primary	20.0	23.6	21.6	21.6	20.2	18.3	15.3
Secondary	57.9	54.7	57.4	56.1	56.3	57.4	60.3
Tertiary	22.1	21.7	21.0	22.3	23.5	24.3	24.5

*All the results are at significant at $p < 0.001$.

(53.1–58.4%), aged 25–34 years (23.1–28.1%), married (48.2–56.6%) with secondary education (55.9–59.9%); Italians with conflicting perceptions are mainly men and women aged 25–34 years (25.4–29.6%), single (48.2–49.7%) with secondary education (76.8–80.6%); Portuguese people with conflicting perceptions are mainly women (51.6–60.0%), aged 65–74 (20.2–23.4%) in 2008–2010 and 55–64 (22.6–23.8%) in 2011–2014, married (56.0–69.7%) with primary education (53.8–71.5%); Spaniards with conflicting perceptions are mainly women (54.2–56.8%) aged 25–34 (23.5–25.7%) in 2008–2011 and 35–44 (20.8–22.8%) in 2012–2014, married (44.4–49.9%) with secondary education (54.7–60.3%).

21.4 Conclusions

The surprisingly high percentages of Southern Europeans' perceptions of their employment status in agreement with the ILO conventional definitions indicate that this question should precede and not follow the questions on the labour status according to the ILO conventional definitions or the questions on the registration at the public employment office as is the Eurostat instruction to participating countries. It is common practice in social sample survey research to place perception questions before concepts are made quite clear or as Oppenheim (1992) pointed out: "We try, as much as possible, to avoid putting ideas into respondents' minds". This result is in line with Gauckler and Körner (2011) who proposed that the self-perceived employment status question should be asked first in their belief that this might provide radically different results. These findings have to be taken into account, since as Schwarz (1987) argued, cognitive issues raised from the questionnaire may have important implications on questionnaire design and survey operations.

The demographic and social "profile" of conflicting perceptions in Greece and Spain is quite similar (young married women with secondary education). In the cases of Italy and Portugal, it differs as it is young single men and women with secondary education and older married women with primary education, respectively. However, within each country the pattern is in the main systematic overtime. These results imply that there is some kind of "bias" introduced by the ILO conventional definitions of the employed, unemployed and inactive and further research is required as Gauckler and Körner (2011) carried out on the "main status effect".

References

Brandolini, A., Cipollone, P., & Viviano, E. (2004). *Does the ILO definition capture all unemployment? (Temi di discussione del Servizio Studi 529).* Roma: Banca d'Italia.

Braun, M., & Mohler, P. P. (2003). Background variables. In J. A. Harkness, F. J. R. Van de Vijver, & P. P. Mohler (Eds.), *Cross-cultural survey methods.* Hoboken, New Jersey: Wiley.

de la Fuente, A. (2011). *New measures of labour market attachment: 3 new Eurostat indicators to supplement the unemployment rate (Statistics in Focus 57),* Eurostat, European Commission.

Eurostat. (2008). *Labour Force Survey revised explanatory notes* (to be applied from 2008Q1 onwards), European Commission.
Eurostat. (2009). *Task Force on the quality of the Labour Force Survey: Final report*. European Commission.
Eurostat. (2016). *EU Labour Force Survey database user guide*. European Commission.
Gauckler, B., & Körner, T. (2011). Measuring the employment status in the Labour Force Survey and the German census 2011: Insights from recent research at Destatis. *Methoden –Daten–Analysen, 5*(2), 181–205.
Hussmanns, R., Mehran, F., & Verma, V. (1990). *Surveys of economically active population, employment, unemployment and underemployment: An ILO manual on concepts and methods*. Geneva: International Labour Office.
Jones, S. R. G., & Riddell, W. C. (1999). The measurement of unemployment: An empirical approach. *Econometrica, 67*(1), 147–162.
Kish, L. (1994). Multipopulation survey designs: Five types with seven shared aspects. *International Statistical Review, 62*(2), 167–186.
Oppenheim, A. N. (1992). *Questionnaire design, interviewing and attitude measurement* (new edition). London: Continuum.
Schwarz, N. (1987). *Cognitive issues of Labour Force Surveys in a multinational context: Issues and findings*. Paper prepared for the OECD Working Party on Employment and Unemployment Statistics, Paris, April, 14–16.
Stephan, F. F., & McCarthy, P. J. (1958). *Sampling opinions: An analysis of survey procedure*. Westport: Greenwood Press.
Yfanti, A., Michalopoulou, C., & Zahariou, S. (2017). *The decision of how to measure unemployment is a political and not a statistical question: Evidence from the European Labour Force Survey: 2008–2014*. Manuscript in preparation.

Part VI
Health Sciences, Demography, Risk and Insurance

Chapter 22
Risk Factors of Severe Cognitive Impairment in the Czech Republic

Kornélia Svačinová Cséfalvaiová and Jitka Langhamrová

22.1 Introduction

Due to an expected increase of demented persons, another objective of the PhD thesis is to find risk factors for the occurrence of dementia. In the event that is known as risk factors associated with dementia, and medicine can find a way to delay disease or prevented. The aim is to evaluate the applied statistics and draw conclusions regarding the demographic and medical issues associated with dementia. It is as important as the mathematical (theoretical) statistics. Application statistics troubleshooting from another department is equally important for statistics, demography and biomedicine. In the Czech Republic lacks an effective national measures in the field of dementia and mental disorders – National Action Plan for Alzheimer's disease was accepted until the beginning of 2016.

In general, particular disease, e.g., diabetes, cardiovascular disease or poor physical and mental condition, also increase the risk of occurrence. The situation is complicated by the fact that the individual may suffer at the same time at more than one simultaneously disease: diabetes, hypertension or heart disease. Equally important is appreciated that not all AIDS patients with a given disease visit the practitioner and are introduced into the statistics. Therefore, a number of diseases which are characterized by, but not limited too course of the patient, e.g., Elevated blood pressure, it can be seen only very roughly. One approach to solving this problem is to try to model development morbidity from chronic disease on the basis of knowledge of the risk factors.

K. Svačinová Cséfalvaiová (✉) · J. Langhamrová
Department of Demography, Faculty of Informatics and Statistics, University of Economics, Prague, Czech Republic
e-mail: k.csefalvaiova@seznam.cz; langhamj@vse.cz

© Springer International Publishing AG, part of Springer Nature 2018
C. H. Skiadas, C. Skiadas (eds.), *Demography and Health Issues*,
The Springer Series on Demographic Methods and Population Analysis 46,
https://doi.org/10.1007/978-3-319-76002-5_22

The source of data used is the SHARE database (The Survey of Health, Aging and Retirement in Europe), which by its multidisciplinary nature provides a comprehensive picture of the aging process in Europe. The results in the dissertation are of significance with respect to the issue of dementia useful material for future analysis and professionals.

22.2 Data – The Survey of Health, Ageing and Retirement in Europe (SHARE)

The aim of SHARE (The Survey of Health, Aging and Retirement in Europe) is creating a longitudinal data set across Europe consisting of persons older than 50 years and their families.

Among the main topics of multidisciplinary research include demography, family, education, physical and mental health, cognitive function, medical care and risks, quality of life, employment and income, housing, income and consumption of households, social support, etc. Data set SHARE provides full advice socio-demographic variables, variables relating to lifestyle and physical and mental health, which help to elucidate acting factors. The investigation so far to the 5 waves in different European countries, including CR. It was on a panel database of microdata from the area of the economic situation, health, social and family bonds. It provides real-tracking data on a sample of 123,000 individuals (more than 293,000 interviews) 27 European countries and Israel older than 50 years. Czech Republic was involved in the project in a second wave of investigations in 2006. The variables characterizing the state of physical and mental health and variables from which it was possible to calculate a variable cognitive function, found only in the second, fourth and fifth wave investigation, were therefore used in the dissertation data exclusively from these waves. One drawback SHARE investigation that do not include people in social devices. Estimates of the incidence of dementia seniorskej population differ. In institutionalized senioroch it is always higher than in senioroch living alone (Nikolai et al. 2013). As shown Jagger et al. (2000). The prevalence of dementia is significantly increased in social and health devices as in households. Since demented persons require intensive care, it is in a certain phase of the disease necessary to have these persons transferred to social facilities (Hallauer 2002). The most frequent group of respondents were consisted of age less than 60 years (37.62%), followed by annual 60–69 (35.16%), annual 70–79 (19.23%), annual 80–89 (7.64%) and the smallest proportion represented persons older than 90 years (0.35%). The relative proportions of the age categories are shown in Fig. 22.1.

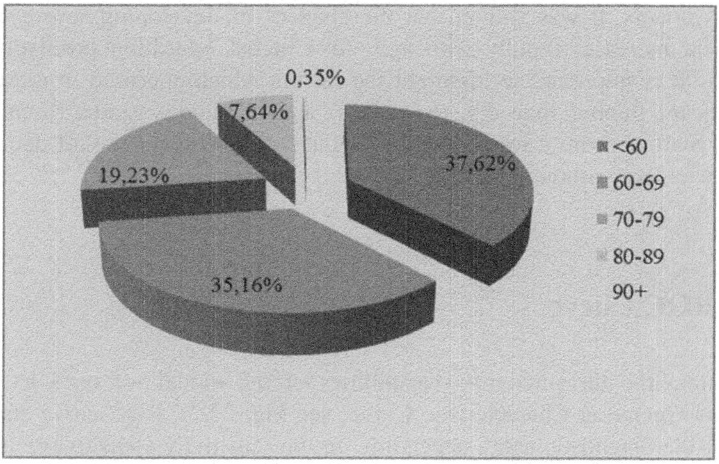

Fig. 22.1 Age structure of the respondents
Source: data SHARE (2015), own construction

22.3 Determinants of Occurrence of Dementia

In the literature there exist several risk factors of dementia. From these results it can be assumed that higher education and active lifestyle reduce the chance of developing dementia. Furthermore, some diseases such as diabetes and cardiovascular diseases or poor physical and mental health should generally increase the chances of developing dementia. The aim of this part is the analysis and identification of factors that affect the risk of severe cognitive impairment in the Czech Republic. Researchers question is whether there are any assumptions or risk factors, which when exposed to a certain person more frequently, thereby increasing their chances of developing a cognitive disorder? Admission variables related to socio-demographic characteristics, physical and mental health and lifestyle were drawn from the SHARE, which were described in Sect. 22.2.

Multi-dimensional analysis can exclude relationships that exist between the explanatory variables. To determine associations between basic demographic characteristics and other variables, and severe cognitive impairment model was constructed logistic regression. Alltogether we constructed four models of logistic regression.

After the analysis of risk factors for severe cognitive impairment and by looking for associations between socio-demographic variables, variables of physical and mental health, social characteristics and development of severe cognitive impairment the fourth model was created that includes variables, which were in the previous models confirmed as significant.

In all models, it was shown that the chances of developing severe cognitive impairment increases rapidly with age. Also higher education positively affects cognition. It is important to highlight the factors which appeared in most models as significant (higher than e.g., education) and the family status (living with a partner). Starting from a model there is about 6 times higher risk of dementia for persons who live without a partner.

22.4 ROC Curve

To illustrate the discriminating capabilities of the model we used ROC curve (Received Operation Characteristic Curve; see Fig. 22.2). ROC curve enables the ability of the diagnostic assay depending on the sensitivity (sensitivity) and specificity (accuracy) and minimize the consequences of erroneous diagnostic decisions. In a square of a unit we receive content: diagonal (and area under the diagonal size of about 0.5), when the model has no ability to classify and units are classified into groups randomly; a curve under the diagonal (defining the area of greater than 0.5) for certain models with better or worse discrimination capability; ROC curve confluent with the left upright and the upper horizontal side of the square in a situation where model classifies perfectly and the quality is best expressed by the entire unit area of a square (Hebák et al. 2015). The closer the ROC curve in the upper left corner, the higher the overall accuracy of the test (Zweig and Campbell 1993). In case the model no discriminatory property and units are randomly assigned to the given categories, the ROC curve has a diagonal shape (dashed line).

Value of McFadden's pseudo R-square is in this case, it was 0.41, and the value of Kendal tau is equal to 0.14. Statistics AUC value is 0.938 (see Fig. 22.3). By these criteria, the best is the final model (see Fig. 22.3).

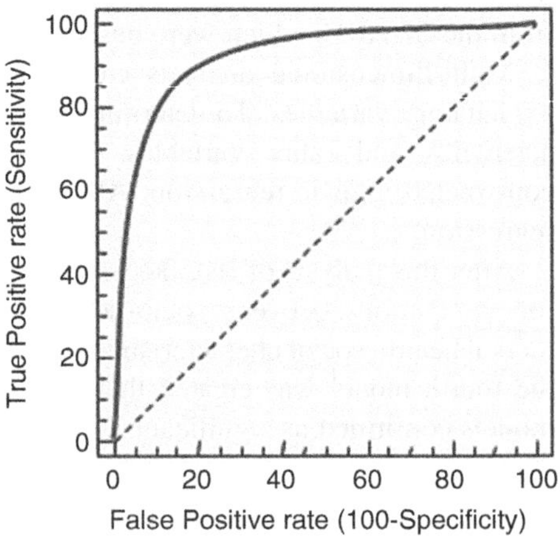

Fig. 22.2 ROC Curve
Source: MedCalc (2016)

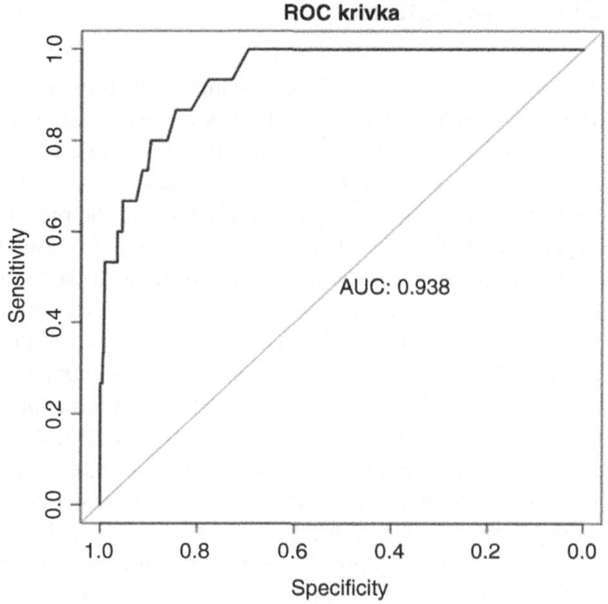

Fig. 22.3 ROC Curve
Source: own calculation

22.5 Risk Factors of Dementia in the Literature

Due to the complexity of dementia syndrome, and factors that increase the risk of disease, has heretofore been unambiguously identified relatively few risk factors. Risk factors, such as e.g., Age, family history and inheritance can not be changed, but recent investigations indicate that there are other risk factors that can be influenced. Some factors are still debatable and others have been repeatedly confirmed in the existing studies. Jorm (1994) is under research and Short form of the Informant Questionnaire on Cognitive Decline in the Elderly (IQCODE): Development and cross-validation discloses Down syndrome as a possible risk factors for Alzheimer's disease. During the 60s and 70s of the twentieth century the aluminum appeared to be a possible risk factor causing Alzheimer's disease. This suspicion led to concerns about the everyday use of aluminum through Pot film beverage cans antiperspirants. Since then, studies have not confirmed the statistical significance of aluminum in the incidence of dementia and Alzheimer's disease. Attention therefore focuses scientists to other research and aluminum is now possible to exclude from the list of risk factors of dementia.

Regardless of the form of dementia, personal, economic and societal consequences of this disease can be devastating. The following portion provides a comprehensive summary of the results of international studies of the risk factors of dementia using statistical methods.

22.6 Conclusions

Age was demonstrated (in accordance with literature) as the major risk factor of severe cognitive impairment. The risk of severe cognitive impairment increases with age, some studies have suggested that the highest age groups is slower increase. Pliant factors, such as. Lifestyle, can prevent and slow down the development of cognitive disorders. Lifestyle also affected by the presence of other diseases such as hypertension, diabetes, heart attack, vascular disease of the brain which are also associated with severe cognitive impairment. It can be concluded that healthy diet reduces the risk of developing severe cognitive impairment, both directly and indirectly. There is no direct correlation between the different pathologies and pursued the development of severe cognitive impairment, but generally it can be said that a combination of factors, the monitored increases the likelihood of its development. A higher level of education and healthy lifestyle appear to be the factors which delay disease incidence in the higher age group.

People with higher education had access i greater cognitive reserve and are able to work longer and with a decrease in brain function. Interestingly finding that partner coexistence indirectly protects against the development of dementia: it is well known that persons in Partnership live longer, healthier, have more social bonds more emotional stimuli aid like. Support partnerships may thus become one of the instruments preventing dementia (and other chronic diseases in the elderly).

Aging of the population with particular emphasis on more than twofold increase in the number of dementing and those with severe cognitive impairment in a population must be understood as a call for the entire company and invites public and private institutions to action. In addition to the necessary medical care must be a target for aging society, increase the capacity of long-term care. The necessity of social services depending on age and level of dependency has been discussed in the first chapter of the thesis. The company must be aware of these changes that will belong not only to increase the number of demented people and increased costs associated with the care of patients and their treatments, but also the associated problems, such as the varying structure of the population and the load, which will represent for the family caregiver or pre-set institutional care.

Acknowledgments This article was supported by the Czech Science Foundation, No. GA ČR 15-13283S under the title "Projection of the Czech Republic Population According to Educational Level and Marital Status."

References

Hallauer J. F. (2002). Epidemiologie für Deutschland mit Prognose. In J. Hallauer & A. Kurz (Eds.), *Weissbuch Demenz. Versorgungssituation relevanter Demenzerkrankungen in Deutschland, Stuttgart* (pp. 15–18). Georg Thieme Verlag.

Hebák, P. A., et al. (2015). Statistické myšlení a nástroje analýzy dat. Informatorium: 2015. Vyd. 1. 880 s. ISBN: 978-80-7333-105-4.

Jagger, C., Andersen, K., Breteler, M. M. B., Copeland, J. R. M., Helmer, C., Baldereschi, M., Fratiglioni, L., Lobo, A., Soininen, H., Hofman, A., & Launer, L. J. (2000). Prognosis with dementia in Europe: A collaborative study of population-based cohorts. *Neurology, 54*, 16.

Jorm, A. F. (1994). A short form of the Informant Questionnaire on Cognitive Decline in the Elderly (IQCODE): Development and cross-validation. *Psychological Medicine, 24*(1), 145–153.

Nikolai, T., Vyhnálek, M., Štěpánková, H., & Horáková, K. (2013). *Neuropsychologická diagnostika kognitivního deficitu u Alzheimerovy choroby.* Praha: Psychiatrické centrum Praha 2013, 64 s. ISBN: 978-80-87142-25-7.

Zweig, M. H., & Campbell, G. (1993, April). Receiver-operating characteristic (ROC) plots: A fundamental evaluation tool in clinical medicine. *Clinical Chemistry 39*, (4): 561–577.

Chapter 23
On the Measurement of Early Job Insecurity in Europe

Maria Symeonaki, Glykeria Stamatopoulou, and Maria Karamessini

23.1 Introduction

The measurement of early job insecurity and labour market exclusion is not a straightforward procedure, since 'ideal' indicators for early job insecurity don't actually exist. Different indicators though, such as the unemployment rate, the youth unemployment rate, the youth to adult unemployment ratio, or the NEET indicator can serve as useful tools, when comparing job insecurity in different countries. When one wants to compare early job insecurity (EJI) among different European countries or study the evolution of early job insecurity over time, it is difficult, if not impossible, to take into account numerous indicators simultaneously. Thus, there is a strong need to provide one single indicator of early job insecurity that takes into account all possible indices connected to EJI for which we have reliable data to depend on. In the present paper we provide a composite index of EJI based on a number of indicators that we measure using raw data drawn from the EU-LFS, in order to estimate and compare early job insecurity among European countries.

When it comes to measuring early job insecurity and patterns of school-to-work transition, several methodological approaches have been proposed. In Karamessini et al. (2015) and in Dingeldey et al. (2015) an attempt was made to provide a definition of early job insecurity and to connect early job insecurity with school-to-work transitions. Symeonaki et al. (2016a, b) studied the transition flows between

This paper has received funding from the European Union's Horizon 2020 research and innovation programme under grant agreement No 649395 (NEGOTIATE – Negotiating early job-insecurity and labour market exclusion in Europe, Horizon 2020, Societal Challenge 6, H2020-YOUNG-SOCIETY-2014, Research and Innovation Action (RIA), Duration: 01 March 2015–28 February 2018).

M. Symeonaki (✉) · G. Stamatopoulou · M. Karamessini
Department of Social Policy, School of Political Sciences, Panteion University of Social and Political Sciences, Athens, Greece
e-mail: msymeon@panteion.gr; mkarames@panteion.gr

© Springer International Publishing AG, part of Springer Nature 2018
C. H. Skiadas, C. Skiadas (eds.), *Demography and Health Issues*,
The Springer Series on Demographic Methods and Population Analysis 46,
https://doi.org/10.1007/978-3-319-76002-5_23

labour market states for young individuals based on the EU-LFS and the EU-SILC data. In Eurofound (2014) the labour market situation of young people in Europe is presented, focusing in particular on the school-to-work transition, in terms of the amount of time it takes to start the first job after education, while also monitoring the more general transition to adulthood, the age at which young people leave the parental home. In Brzinsky-Fay (2007) sequences of school-to-work transitions are studied in ten European countries using the exploratory methods of optimal matching and cluster analysis. The process of labour market entry is observed for 5 years after leaving school by examining monthly labour market statuses. Christodoulakis and Mamatzakis (2009) applied a Bayesian approach that employed a Monte Carlo integration procedure to expose the empirical posterior distribution of transition probabilities from full-time employment to part-time employment, temporary employment and unemployment and vice versa, in the EU 15. Additionally, Alvarez et al. (2008) study the labour dynamics of the population by fitting a stationary Markov chain to the Argentine official labour survey. On the other hand Betti et al. (2007) describe some aspects of school-to-work transitions by analysing the employment situation of individuals as a function of the time elapsed since the completion of education and training, with a special focus on the patterns in Southern European countries. Ward-Warmedinge et al. (2013) present information on labour market mobility in 23 European countries, using the Eurostat's Labour Force Survey data over the period 1998–2008, whereas in Flek and Mysíková (2015), the labour market flows, i.e. flows between employment, unemployment and inactivity, are analysed using Markov transition systems in order to draw conclusions on unemployment dynamics in Central Europe. Markov system analysis is also used in Symeonaki and Stamatopoulou (2015) in order to analyse labour market dynamics in Greece and in Karamessini et al. (2016) Markov systems are used to estimate the school-to-labour market entry probabilities for a number of European countries with raw data drawn from the EU-LFS datasets for 2013. Bosch and Maloney (2007) discuss a set of statistics for examining and comparing labour market dynamics based on the estimation of continuous time Markov transition processes. They then use these to establish stylised facts about dynamic patterns of movement with the aid of panel data from Argentina, Brazil and Mexico. Moreover, the socio-economic background and the degree to which it affects the transition process has also been studied in the literature, as individuals from poorer households have lower job prospects, while educational background may postpone their first entry in countries with strong family support system. Educational qualification and skills also have a strong effect on transitions from school-to-work, as low educated people hardly escape from spells of unemployment and inactivity, restricted mostly on temporary contracts (Quintini et al. 2007). Additionally, Scherer (2005) shows that compared to Germany and Great Britain, in Italy the parental educational attainments has a negative effect on young people's speed of entry, as the more educated parents support their offspring in longer searches for better jobs. Gender plays an important role in young people's integration, since young women seem to face more problems relating to their transition than their male counterparts, with higher probabilities of being inactive or in non-standard employment for longer periods of time, while caring responsibilities also delay their entrance on labour market (Sigle-Rushton and Perrons 2013; Plantenga et al. 2013). The methods most commonly used to examine school-to-work transitions as a sequence and not as a single event are the optimal matching method and the cluster analysis (McVicar and Anyadike Danes 2002; Scherer 2001; Schoon 2001). Brzinsky-Fay (2014) presents the main advantages and disadvantages of sequence analysis in comparison to event history analysis.

Here, in order to capture the whole spectrum of early job and employment insecurity we use indicators, referring to different aspects of EJI: indicators that refer to labour market outcomes and to quality of job, indicators for employment insecurity and for transition from school-to-work. These indicators, estimated for the 15–24 age group, should be considered as complementary rather than competing and are combined into a single composite indicator of EJI. The results reveal that courtiers differ when early job insecurity is considered and the values of the proposed index vary between −0.84 for Switzerland (lowest early job insecurity) to 1.01 for Greece (highest early job insecurity).

The paper is organised in the following way. Section 23.2 provides the estimations of the early job insecurity indicators for the European countries based on the EU-LFS data of 2014. Section 23.3 presents the new composite index of EJI and provides the results for these countries, sorting them from countries of low EJI to countries with high EJI. Section 23.4 provides the reader with the conclusions of the study and aspects of future work.

23.2 Indicators of Early Job Insecurity

As earlier mentioned, to capture the entire range of early job and employment insecurity we use indicators, referring to distinctive traits of EJI: indicators that refer to labour market outcomes and to quality of job, indicators for employment insecurity and for transition from school-to-work. These indicators are estimated for the 15–24 age group, from raw data drawn from the EU-LFS survey. Table 23.1 provides the indicators that are measured and their description, thus offering information of how these were actually measured.

Typical indicators used for the measurement of early job insecurity provided in the present analysis are the Youth Participation Rate (Ind1), the Youth Employment Rate (Ind2), the Youth Unemployment Rate (Ind3), the Youth Unemployment Ratio (Ind4), the incidence of long-term unemployment (Ind5) and the NEET (not in Employment, Education or Training) indicator (Ind6).

Indicators, directly linked to the quality of jobs, are the incidence of temporary and part-time employment (Ind7 and Ind8), the incidence of underemployed part-time workers (Ind9) and working intensity measured as the distribution of employees according to usual weekly hours worked (hour bands) (Ind10).

Table 23.1 Early job insecurity indicators, Ages: 15–29, EU-LFS, 2014

Indicators		Description
Ind1	Youth Participation Rate	$\frac{\text{Number of individuals in the labour force, aged 15–24}}{\text{Total number of individuals, aged 15–24}}$
Ind2	Youth Employment Rate	$\frac{\text{Number of employed individuals, aged 15–24}}{\text{Total Population, aged 15–24}}$
Ind3	Youth Unemployment Rate	$\frac{\text{Number of unemployed individuals, aged 15–24}}{\text{Number of individuals in the labour force, aged 15–24}}$
Ind4	Youth Unemployment Ratio	$\frac{\text{Number of unemployed individuals, aged 15–24}}{\text{Total population, aged 15–24}}$
Ind5	Incidence of long-term unemployment	Young unemployed (12 months or more) as % of all young unemployed
Ind6	NEET rate	The population not in employment, education or training as a percentage of total population 15–24
Ind7	Incidence of temporary employment	As % of all employees
Ind8	Incidence of part-time employment	As % of all employed
Ind9	Underemployed part-time workers	As % of total part-time workers
Ind10	Working time	Distribution of employees according to usual weekly hours worked (hour bands)
Ind11	Probability of entry to employment from education and training	Markov system
Ind12	Probability of entry to unemployment from education and training	Markov systems
Ind13	Probability of entry to inactivity from education and training	Markov systems
Ind14	Job finding rate	Percent of unemployed at time t-1, who are employed at time t
Ind15	Job separation rate	Percent of employed in time t-1, who are not employed at time t
Ind16	Youth to Total Unemployment Ratio	$\frac{\text{Youth unemployment rate (age:15–24)}}{\text{Total unemployment rate (age>15)}}$
Ind17	Relative UR low skills/high skills	$\frac{\text{UR of those ISCED<3 (HATLEV=1)}}{\text{UR of those ISCED<3 (HATLEV=2 or 3)}}$

Another important aspect is connected to the transition of young individuals from school (education or training) to work. It is well accepted that young people's pathways from school to sustained work have become more and more rough and irregular and the probability of someone who has completed full-time education to move effectively into full-time occupation decreases, whereas the probability of engaging into part-time or temporary employment increases. Therefore, it is important to highlight useful indicators that fall into the category of measuring school-to-work transitions. In this respect, we estimate the probability of an individual that has concluded education or training to enter each one of the three labour market states: employment (Ind11), unemployment (Ind12) and inactivity (Ind13). This part of analysis will be handled with the aid of Markov system theory.

Two other useful indicators for measuring employment insecurity are the job finding rate and the job separation rate. In the present paper, as is the case with

Table 23.2 Basic labour market indicators, 2014

Country	Ind1	Ind2	Ind3	Ind4	Ind5	Ind6
Austria	67.1	61.1	8.9	5.9	16.4	10.8
Belgium	49.6	41.5	16.4	8.1	40.1	14.9
Bulgaria	45.6	37.4	18.0	8.2	57.1	24.6
Croatia	51.4	34.8	32.3	16.6	51.6	22.3
Cyprus	57.5	42.5	26.2	15.1	37.2	19.7
Czech Republic	51.3	45.8	10.6	5.4	28.0	12.2
Denmark	67.4	59.7	11.4	7.7	11.8	10.3
Estonia	56.6	50.0	11.5	6.5	35.7	14.3
Finland	61.0	51.4	15.7	9.6	7.6	12.5
France	53.5	43.3	19.1	10.2	31.0	17.2
Germany	61.8	57.6	6.8	4.2	26.9	8.9
Greece	49.3	27.1	45.0	22.1	65.3	27.3
Hungary	47.3	40.8	13.9	6.6	35.9	17.2
Ireland	53.2	43.0	19.1	10.1	46.0	18.4
Italy	41.5	28.3	31.6	13.1	59.5	27.3
Latvia	58.7	50.3	14.4	8.4	27.7	15.8
Lithuania	51.8	44.2	14.7	7.6	28.2	13.2
Luxemburg	49.5	43.0	13.0	6.4	–	6.9
Netherlands	74.0	66.0	10.8	8.0	19.6	8.9
Norway	63.7	59.3	6.8	4.3	15.8	8.6
Poland	53.2	44.4	16.5	8.8	35.1	15.8
Portugal	52.3	39.0	25.4	13.3	41.8	16. 6
Romania	48.6	41.0	15.6	7.6	38.7	20.0
Slovakia	50.1	39.4	21.3	10.7	60.0	18.3
Slovenia	52.9	42.9	18.9	10.0	–	14.0
Spain	54.6	33.0	39.6	21.7	40.3	22.7
Sweden	65.9	55.0	16.7	11.0	8.4	10.4
Switzerland	75.8	70.1	7.6	5.7	21.9	8.8
UK	66.7	58.4	12.5	8.4	27.5	14.3

Notes: Not reliable results for IS. Small samples for LU, MT, SI
Sources: EU-LFS (2014)

empirical studies (Hobijn and Sahin 2007), we will use the percent of unemployed individuals at time t-1, who are employed at time t as the job finding rate (Ind14) and the percent of employed individuals in time t-1, who are not employed at time t as the separation rate (Ind15).

Moreover, two indicators regarding relative changes in unemployment rates are: the Youth to Adult Unemployment Ratio (Ind16) and the Relative Unemployment Rate of those individuals with low skills to those individuals with high skills (Ind17), as it provides evidence of how education and training influences unemployment.

Table 23.2 provides the reader with the estimations of all indicators that relate to labour market outcomes (Ind1 – Ind6), for all European countries, for 2014. In an

Table 23.3 Basic labour market indicators, 2014

Country	Ind7	Ind8	Ind9
Austria	23.7	23.8	29.6
Belgium	22.1	20.2	39.4
Bulgaria	9.3	3.4	–
Croatia	40.1	7.1	62.9
Cyprus	27.1	18.3	75.7
Czech Republic	20.3	7.2	15.5
Denmark	19.3	51.4	17.1
Estonia	7.2	13.0	11.2
Finland	34.9	29.7	28.7
France	39.6	19.0	56.3
Germany	38.4	21.8	21.6
Greece	23.3	16.6	83.4
Hungary	17.9	5.6	46.0
Ireland	21.1	30.7	34.9
Italy	40.6	25.7	23.0
Latvia	5.1	7.1	–
Lithuania	4.9	9.6	27.4
Netherlands	47.3	64.2	25.2
Norway	22.8	42.3	25.4
Poland	53.6	9.7	49.7
Portugal	49.1	14.7	65.0
Romania	3.8	10.5	57.3
Slovakia	17.6	6.3	–
Slovenia	49.7	22.7	–
Spain	54.2	28.3	67.0
Sweden	42.1	36.8	35.7
Switzerland	36.3	27.0	34.7
UK	10.6	27.5	34.5

Notes: Not reliable results for IS, LU, MT. Concerning the indicator of underemployed part-time workers, small number of part-time workers for BG, HR, EE, HU, LV, LT
Sources: EU-LFS (2014)

analogous way, Tables 23.3 and 23.4 present the values of the indicators regarding the job quality for the same year and countries (Ind7 – Ind10). The probabilities that can be used as indicators for school-to-work transition are given in Table 23.5 (Ind11 – Ind13), followed by Table 23.6, which reveals the indicators for employment (in)security (Ind14 – Ind15). Finally, Table 23.7 provides indicators concerning the relative changes in unemployment rates (Ind16 – Ind17).

Figure 23.1 displays the values of Job Finding Rates and Job Separation Rates for the European countries.

Table 23.4 Working time indicators, 2014

Country	Working time				
	1–19	20–29	30–34	35–39	40+
Austria	10.7	7.3	4.6	30.8	46.6
Belgium	7.2	10.2	6.7	49.7	26.1
Bulgaria	0.2	2.5	0.7	0.2	96.4
Croatia	0.9	3.0	1.2	0.5	94.5
Cyprus	3.6	7.5	5.1	20.1	63.6
Czech Republic	2.0	4.0	1.7	15.1	77.2
Denmark	41.4	6.9	6.1	41.5	4.0
Estonia	3.5	5.8	2.8	2.3	85.6
Finland	17.1	8.7	7.1	38.0	29.1
France	5.4	8.9	4.2	59.8	21.7
Germany	13.4	5.1	3.6	24.1	53.9
Greece	5.9	11.4	5.5	1.7	75.5
Hungary	0.7	3.4	1.7	0.5	93.8
Ireland	13.3	14.8	5.3	33.0	33.6
Italy	6.7	15.4	6.2	10.1	61.4
Latvia	0.9	4.1	2.1	0.7	92.2
Lithuania	1.3	7.7	1.4	2.2	87.5
Netherlands	41.5	12.7	10.8	13.3	21.7
Norway	28.0	8.0	6.1	51.3	6.6
Poland	2.0	4.9	2.2	1.6	89.3
Portugal	4.5	6.8	2.4	5.6	80.8
Romania	–	0.6	0.3	0.2	98.9
Slovakia	2.1	4.5	0.7	11.4	81.3
Slovenia	6.5	8.5	3.1	1.1	80.7
Spain	11.8	15.0	6.4	9.7	57.1
Sweden	16.1	9.8	10.0	12.7	51.4
Switzerland	12.1	6.3	5.3	4.1	72.2
UK	15.4	9.7	5.4	26.4	43.1

Notes: Not reliable results for IS, LU, MT. Small samples for CY, EE, LV

Sources: EU-LFS (2014)

23.3 A Composite Index of Early Job Insecurity

In the present section we define the composite index of early job insecurity and estimate its values for all European countries for which we have the necessary data (variables).

Table 23.5 Indicators for transition from school to work, 2014

Country	School-to-Work Transition Probability	School-to-Unemployment Transition Probability	School-to-Inactivity Transition Probability
AT	0.684	0.157	0.159
BE	0.566	0.257	0.177
BG	0.369	0.358	0.273
CH	0.784	0.079	0.137
CZ	0.657	0.324	0.019
DK	0.663	0.228	0.109
EE	0.600	0.185	0.215
EL	0.194	0.513	0.293
ES	0.224	0.377	0.399
FI	0.582	0.239	0.179
FR	0.583	0.310	0.107
HR	0.297	0.695	0.008
HU	0.500	0.343	0.157
IT	0.274	0.637	0.089
LT	0.643	0.217	0.140
LV	0.608	0.248	0.144
PL	0.535	0.340	0.125
PT	0.443	0.500	0.057
RO	0.358	0.528	0.114
SE	0.619	0.306	0.075

For the countries for which MAINSTAT and WSTAT1Y (or both) are EMPTY the respective transition probabilities cannot b estimated.
Sources: Own Calculations, EU-LFS (2014)

The composite index is defined as:

$$EJI = \frac{\sum_{i=1}^{d} w_{d_i} \cdot \frac{\sum_{j=1}^{d_i} w_{ij} \cdot zInd_{ij}}{\sum_{j=1}^{d_i} w_{ij}}}{\sum_{i=1}^{d} w_{d_i}}, \tag{23.1}$$

where:

d: the number of dimensions (here $d = 5$)
d_i: the number of indicators in the i-th dimension
w_{ij}: the weight of the j-th indicator in the i-th dimension
w_{d_i}: the weight of the i-th dimension
$zInd_{ij}$: the z-score of the j-th indicator in the i-th dimension.

Using Eq. (23.1) we estimate the values of EJI for the European countries. The values are presented in Table 23.8.

Table 23.6 Indicators for employment (in)security

Country	Job finding rate	Job separation rate[a]
Austria	44.45	12.5
Belgium	32.05	9.35
Bulgaria	18.20	7.75
Croatia	25.35	12.85
Cyprus	41.80	12.3
Czech Republic	59.65	4.65
Denmark	48.10	13.40
Estonia	46.70	12.15
Finland	32.00	19.50
France	33.6	15.50
Germany	–	–
Greece	14.75	13.50
Hungary	44. 10	9.05
Italy	19.60	11.85
Latvia	51.90	14.90
Lithuania	47.35	7.80
Malta	43.75	14.25
Poland	32.65	9.15
Portugal	34.85	15.60
Romania	13.80	6.05
Slovakia	32.80	9.25
Slovenia	27.85	29.00
Spain	27.05	14.10
Sweden	42.80	19.10
Switzerland	53.55	14.6

For the countries for which MAINSTAT and WSTAT1Y (or both) are EMPTY the respective rates cannot be estimated.
Sources: EU-LFS (2014)
[a]In this report, we omit inactivity-unemployment flows and focus only on employment-unemployment flows. See Shimer (2007) and Barnichon (2009) for evidence supporting this choice

23.4 Conclusions

In the present paper we provided a composite index of EJI based on a number of indicators that we measured using raw data drawn from the EU-LFS, in order to estimate and compare early job insecurity among European countries. It is obvious that early job insecurity differs among European countries. Countries with low EJI can be identified (Switzerland, Denmark, Austria for example), whereas countries of high EJI are also recognisable. Croatia, Italy, Spain and Greece are the countries

Table 23.7 Relative changes in unemployment rates

Country	Youth to total UR	Relative UR, low skills/high skills
Austria	1.58	2.12
Belgium	1.92	2.49
Bulgaria	1.58	2.46
Croatia	1.87	2.01
Cyprus	1.63	1.25
Czech Republic	1.73	3.61
Denmark	1.73	1.55
Estonia	1.57	1.87
Finland	1.82	2.34
France	1.85	2.11
Germany	1.38	2.68
Greece	1.70	1.03
Hungary	1.80	2.59
Ireland	1.69	2.41
Italy	2.49	1.29
Latvia	1.32	2.26
Lithuania	1.37	2.74
Luxemburg	2.15	–
Netherlands	1.45	2.12
Norway	1.95	2.46
Poland	1.84	1.89
Portugal	1.82	1.27
Romania	2.29	1.00
Slovakia	1.61	2.78
Slovenia	1.95	1.47
Spain	1.62	1.54
Sweden	2.09	3.06
Switzerland	1.66	1.41
UK	2.04	2.43

Notes: Not reliable results for LU and CY
Sources: EU-LFS (2014)

facing worrying EJI. Countries can be categorised into four different clusters of countries with low, moderate, considerable and high early job insecurity. Figure 23.2 provides the map of early job insecurity for 2014.

Early job insecurity can have multiple consequences: Systematic labour market young people at the very beginning of their professional careers, the growing discourses over the 'threat of a lost generation', accompanied by a multi-faceted social malaise that includes among others high risks of poverty, precarity, social exclusion, disaffection, insecurity, scarring, higher propensity towards offence and crime, as well as (mental and physical) health problems, to name but a few.

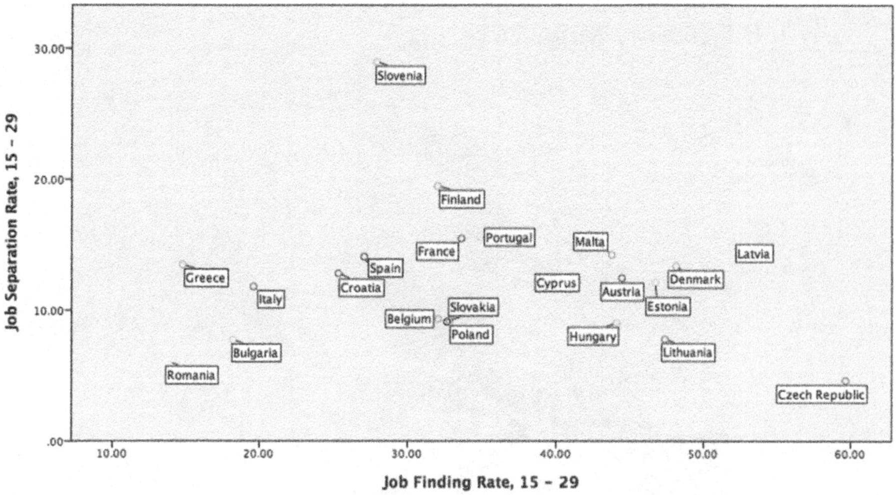

Fig. 23.1 Job finding rates and job separation rates across European countries, 15–29, EU-LFS, 2014

Table 23.8 Early job insecurity indicator, EU-LFS, 2014

	Country	Early job insecurity index
1.	Switzerland	−0.84
2.	Denmark	−0.79
3.	Austria	−0.68
4.	Estonia	−0.45
5.	Lithuania	−0.38
6.	Finland	−0.29
7.	Czech Republic	−0.41
8.	Sweden	−0.24
9.	Belgium	−0. 14
10.	France	−0.07
11.	Hungary	−0.01
12.	Poland	0.01
13.	Romania	0. 16
14.	Portugal	0.25
15.	Croatia	0.60
16.	Italy	0.61
17.	Spain	0.84
18.	Greece	1.01

Therefore, it is very important to activate effective policies that can prevent the unfavourable effects of early job insecurity and youth unemployment. In this paper we have provided evidence based on empirical data that early job insecurity exists, it can be measured and it must be tackled since it exhibits worrying trends for a lot of European countries. Further research will be perused with the EU-LFS data for 2015.

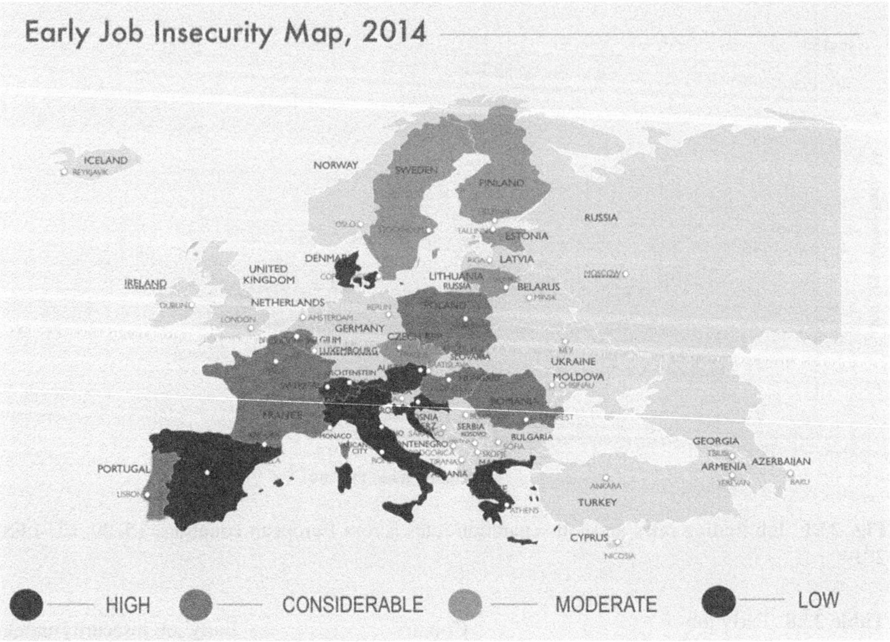

Fig. 23.2 Mapping early job insecurity

References

Alvarez, E., Ciocchini, F., & Konwar, K. (2008). A locally stationary Markov chain model for labour dynamics. *Journal of Data Science, 7*, 27–42.

Barnichon, R. (2009). *Vacancy posting, job separation and unemployment fluctuations* (Federal Reserve Board, Working Paper No 35).

Betti, G., Lemmi, A., & Verma, V. (2007). A comparative analysis of school-to-work transitions in the European Union. *Innovation: The European Journal of Social Science Research, 18*(4), 419–442.

Bosch, M., & Maloney, W. (2007). *Comparative analysis of labor market dynamics using Markov processes: An application to informality*. Discussion paper series, IZA DP, 3038.

Brzinsky-Fay, C. (2007). Lost in transition? Labour market entry sequences of school leavers in Europe. *European Sociological Review, 23*(4), 409–422.

Brzinsky-Fay, C. (2014). The measurement of school-to-work transitions as processes. About events and sequences. *European Societies, 16*(2), 213–232.

Christodoulakis, G., & Mamatzakis, C. (2009). *Labour market dynamics in EU: A Bayesian Markov chain approach*. Discussion paper series, Discussion paper no. 2009–07. Department of Economics, University of Macedonia.

Dingeldey, I., Hvinden, B., Hyggen, C., O'Reilly, J., & Schøyen, M. A. (2015), *Understanding the consequences of early job insecurity and labour market exclusion: The interaction of structural conditions, institutions, active agency and capability*. https://blogg.hioa.no/negotiate/files/2015/04/NEGOTIATE-working-paper-no-D2.1.pdf

Eurofound. (2014). *Mapping youth transitions in Europe*. Luxembourg: Publications Office of the European Union.

Flek, V., & Mysíková, M. (2015). Unemployment dynamics in Central Europe: A labour flow approach. *Prague Economic Papers, 24*(1), 73–87.

Hobijn, B., & Sahin, A. (2007). *Job-finding and separation rates in the OECD*. Federal Reserve Bank of New York, Staff Report No 298.

Karamessini, M., Papazachariou, A., Parsanoglou, D., & Stamatopoulou, G. (2015). *Indicators and data sources to measure patterns of labour market entry across countries*. https://blogg.hioa.no/negotiate/files/2015/04/NEGOTIAE-working-paper-no-D3.1.pdf

Karamessini, M., Symeonaki, M., Stamatopoulou, G., & Papazachariou, A. (2016). *The careers of young people in Europe during the economic crisis: Identifying risk factors*. https://blogg.hioa.no/negotiate/files/2015/04/NEGOTIATE-working-paper-no-D3.2-The-careers-of-young-people-in-Eurpa-during-the-economic-crisis.pdf

McVicar, D., & Anyadike Danes, M. (2002). Predicting successful and unsuccessful transitions from school to work by using sequence methods. *Journal of the Royal Statistical Society: Series A (Statistics in Society), 165*(2), 317–334.

Plantenga, J., Remery, C., & Lodovici, M. S. (2013). *Starting Fragile: Gender differences in the youth labour market*. Luxembourg: European Commission.

Quintini, G., Martin, J., & Martin, S. (2007). *The changing nature of the school-to-work transition process in OECD Countries*. IZA Discusion paper no. 2582.

Scherer, S. (2001). Early Career Patterns: A comparison of Great Britain and West Germany. *European Sociological Review, 17*(2), 119–144.

Scherer, S. (2005). Patterns of labour market entry – Long wait or career instability? An empirical comparison of Italy, Great Britain and West Germany. *European Sociological Review, 21*(5), 427–440.

Schoon, I. M. (2001). *Transitions from school to work in a changing social context*. Young-Uppsala-, 9, 4–22., 9, 4–22.

Shimer, R. (2007). *Reassessing the ins and outs of unemployment* (NBER Working Paper No. 13421).

Sigle-Rushton, W., & Perrons, D. (2013). *Employment transitions over the life cycle: A statistical analysis*. LSE Working paper series no. 46.

Symeonaki, M., & Stamatopoulou, G. (2015). *A Markov system analysis application on labour market dynamics: The case of Greece*. Athens: IWPLMS.

Symeonaki, M., Karamessini, M., & Stamatopoulou, G. (2016a, June 1–4). *Measuring school-to-work transition probabilities in Europe with evidence from the EU-SILC*. In C. Skiadas, S. Silvestrov, & T. Oliveira (Eds.), 5th Demographics workshop, Valletta, Malta. Springer.

Symeonaki, M., Karamessini, M., & Stamatopoulou, G. (2016b, June 1–4). *Gender-based differences on the impact of the economic crisis on labour market flows in Southern Europe*. SMTDA, Valletta, Malta.

Ward-Warmedinge, M., Melanie, E., & Macchiarelli, C. (2013). *Transitions in labour market status in the European Union*. LEQS paper 69.

Chapter 24
Health Estimates for Some Countries of the Rapid Developing World

Konstantinos N. Zafeiris and Christos H. Skiadas

24.1 Introduction

It was a long ago when scientists from different scientific fields tried to study the health of a population. Among the first was Chiang (1965), who introduced an *"Index of health"*, based on data from the Canadian Sickness Survey, 1950–1951. Others used life table techniques, like Sanders (1964) who tried to construct tables of *"effective life years"*, as a measure of the current health of the population based on mortality and morbidity rates. Sullivan (1966, 1971) calculated the expectation of life free of disability and the expectation of disability. Torrance (1976) developed a health status index model for the determination of the amount of health improvement created by a health care program. In these methods, the combined use of mortality and survey data in order for the health status of a population to be estimated was very common.

Today, one of the most important recent contributions to the problem of calculating the health status of a population is the one developed by the World Health Organization (WHO), which is based on the aforementioned Sullivan's (1971) approach. In this method population data on health and disability are combined in a life table (WHO 2014). For that the Global Burden of Disease Survey (GBD; Global Burden of Disease Study 2012; Murray et al. 2012a, b) is conducted aiming to quantify health loss from a high number of diseases, injuries and risk factors. However, as WHO notes, several limitations exist in this method, because of the lack

K. N. Zafeiris (✉)
Department of History and Ethnology, Laboratory of P. Anthropology, Democritus University of Thrace, P. Tsaldari 1, Komotini 69100, Greece
e-mail: kzafiris@he.duth.gr

C. H. Skiadas
ManLab, Technical University of Crete, Chania, Crete, Greece
e-mail: skiadas@cmsim.net

© Springer International Publishing AG, part of Springer Nature 2018
C. H. Skiadas, C. Skiadas (eds.), *Demography and Health Issues*,
The Springer Series on Demographic Methods and Population Analysis 46,
https://doi.org/10.1007/978-3-319-76002-5_24

of reliable data on mortality and morbidity and of the comparability of self-reported data from health interviews and the measurement of health-state preferences for such self-reporting.

In another, however very efficient, approach the stochastic theory is applied. Such a process is always described by a parent stochastic process and a boundary or barrier indicating a stopping condition for the process under consideration (see Lee and Whitmore 2006). In this case, human health is the stochastic and thus totally unpredictable process but a person dies when their health falls below a barrier. The problem then is how to model this process in order for the health status of a population to be calculated. Skiadas and Skiadas (2012), Skiadas and Skiadas (2014a, b, c) and Skiadas (2012a) have developed the relevant theory based only on life table data. In a series of publications Skiadas (2012a), Skiadas and Zafeiris (2015a) and Zafeiris and Skiadas (2015a, b) have tested this theory and showed its validity in calculating the health status of a population or in providing accurate measurements for inter-population comparisons.

Recently, another method was developed and is based on the force of mortality μ_x (see Skiadas 2012b; Skiadas and Zafeiris 2015b; Zafeiris and Skiadas 2015c).

This approach is based on a two parameters Gompertz-like model:

$$\mu_x = \left(\frac{x}{T}\right)^b$$

where (x) is the age and $\mu(x)$ the relevant mortality rate. T represents the age at which $\mu(x) = 1$ and b is a parameter expressing the curvature of $\mu(x)$. Then, the main idea is to divide the areas in the parallelogram OBAD (Fig. 24.1), into two segments - one being the mortality effect and the other the healthy part of the population, an idea which has emerged from the First Exit Time Theory approach that was described above. Thus, the area Ex under the curve OCABO in the mortality diagram of Fig. 24.1 is a measure of the mortality effect and can be estimated as follows:

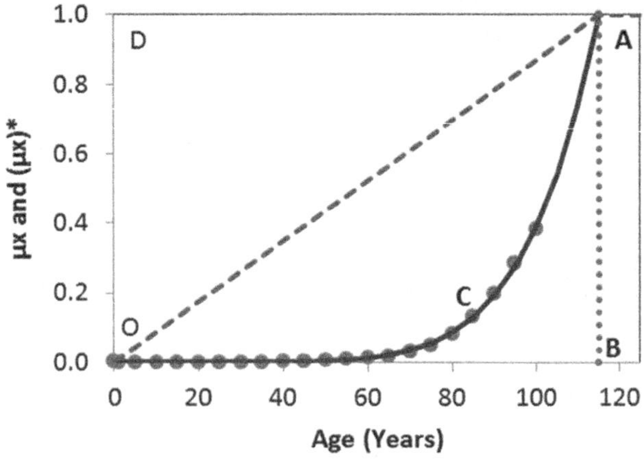

Fig. 24.1 The mortality diagram

$$E_x = \int_0^T \left(\frac{x}{T}\right)^b dx = \frac{T}{(b+1)} \left(\frac{x}{T}\right)^b$$

Based on the equation above, it is proven that the loss of healthy life years LHLY can be estimated as LHLY $= \lambda(b + 1)$, where λ is a correction multiplier which can be set to 1 in order for different countries to be compared. Accordingly, healthy life expectancy (HLE) is LEB-LHLY, where LEB is life expectancy at birth.

Then the problem of calculating healthy life expectancy with this method deals with the accuracy and precision of life table data. However, until now all the analyses done for such estimations are based on full life table data and in that way in cases in which such data are either problematic or absent, a usual phenomenon for many countries, this is not possible. The aim of this paper is to provide a method for estimating healthy life expectancy for such countries based on abridged life table data.

24.2 Methods and Data

Data come from the World's Health Organization database (WHO, http://apps.who.int/gho/data) in the form of abridged life tables. These tables contain information for the age groups <1, 1–4 and for 5-years age intervals up to the age 100 which corresponds to the open-ended one. The analysis was done for the so-called BRIICS countries: Brazil, Russia, India, Indonesia, China and South Africa. They are rapid growth economies and their population represent almost 3 billion people, nearly half the world's population (see http://www.oecd.org/tad/tradedev/globalisationandemergingeconomies.htm)/

In the analyses carried out in this paper two aspects need to be clarified further. First the method used for the estimation of healthy life expectancy and second how to expand the abridged life table into a full one.

The first aspect was confronted with the μ_x based method which was described in the introductory section of this paper. Thus, the parameter b must be estimated. It was found that an excellent estimation was made according to the following formula:

$$b = \frac{x m_x}{\sum_0^x m_x}$$

where x is the age.

The second aspect was confronted with the aid of the UNABR application of the MORTPAK (vers. 4.3) application for Windows, of the software created by the

United Nations (UN Population division) for the needs of mortality analysis. This application is based on the Heligman and Pollard (1980) formula as follows:

$$1q_x = A^{(x+B)^C} + De^{-E(lnx-lnF)^2} + \frac{GH^x}{1+GH^x} \quad (24.1)$$

where x is the age and B, C, D, E, F, G and H parameters that should be estimated. However, it must be noted that the Heligman-Pollard model has proven to be quite problematic in the fitting process of mortality data (see Kostaki 1992; Zafeiris and Kostaki 2017), but it was used here as it is a widely accepted software.

24.3 Results

The results of the analysis are seen in the diagrams 2–7. These results are also compared with several publications from the World Health Organization's point of view, namely the World's Health reports of 2000, 2001, 2002 and 2004 (World Health Organization 2000, 2001, 2004) and Salomon et al. (2012) and Murray et al. (2015) publications. The acronym used in that case is HALE, which also corresponds to healthy life expectancy as estimated by the method applied in the time of these publications.

Such comparisons bear many complications. One springs from the fact that data used in this analysis are in their current and most revised form in comparison with data used for the previous publications. Thus, deviations are expected to be found because of that and also because of the differences in the methodologies used and have been revised several times in the past. Thus, the results of the analysis should be interpreted thoroughly. Also, the use of MORTPAK was quite problematic in many cases. For example, for the year 2005 in Russian males the expansion procedure of the abridged life table gave a life expectancy at birth of 81.68 years compared with 58.6 according to the estimations of the World Health Organization. But it is worth noting that the life expectancy at birth published by WHO never coincided with the estimations of MORTPAK software.

A glimpse of such problems is given by the examination of data from Brazil, where significant deviances are found in the data used by WHO in the original publications of 2000 and 2004 and the data published currently in the web page of the organization. A general trend that describes these differences, as can be judged by life expectancy at birth, is that they become larger for the first years of the study in both genders. Thus, the estimations of WHO and related scientists are based on old data. Instead in this paper, because we have used the most recent data for the

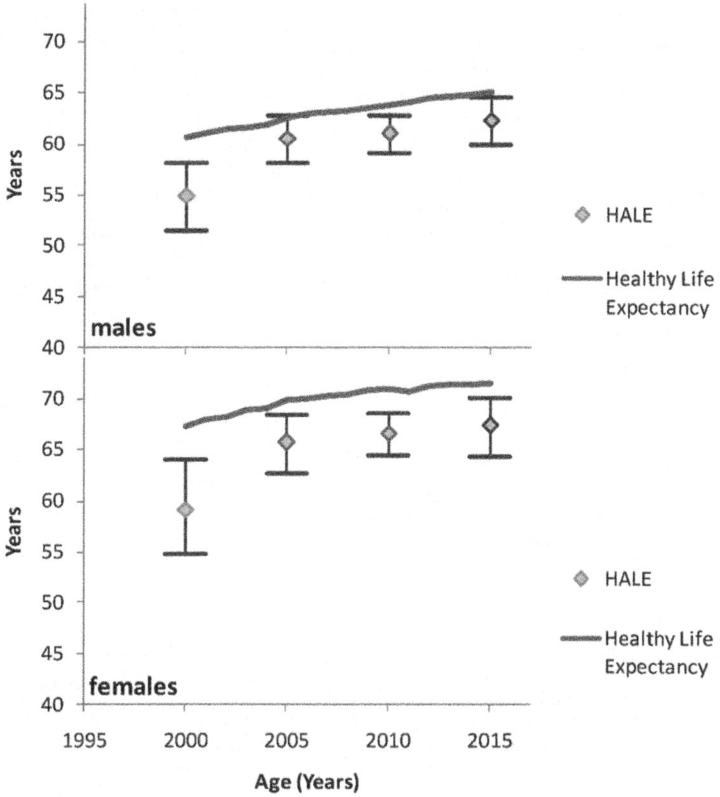

Fig. 24.2 HLE and HALE estimations, Brazil

calculations, healthy life expectancy is very close to the upper confidence interval of the published estimations (Fig. 24.2).

Population health seems to have increased almost linearly in Russia (Fig. 24.3) in both genders and the methods compared seem to be in accordance, especially in males.

In India (Fig. 24.4), the revision of data led to about +2 years increase in life expectancy for the majority of the calendar years studied, while in females it was almost +2 years for the older calendar years and less than 0.6 for the rest. The expanding procedure, concerning life expectancy at birth worked excellently, as the differences between the published by WHO results and those calculated by MORTPAK were less than 0.1 years for the majority of the calendar years studied. Healthy life expectancy, as calculated in this paper, were very close to the upper limit

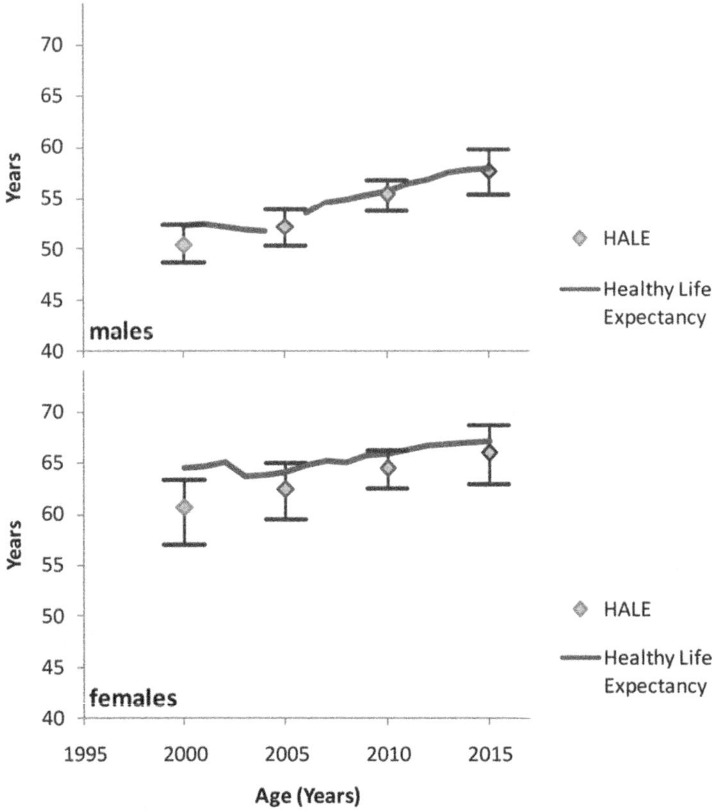

Fig. 24.3 HLE and HALE estimations, Russia

of the estimations of the World Health Organization, fact that can be attributed to the revised data used in this paper.

For Indonesia (Fig. 24.5), data were revised mostly for the most recent years (almost −2 years in life expectancy). However, the expanding process led to an underestimation of life expectancy at birth from 0.4 to 2.1 years. In that scheme, the estimation of healthy life expectancy does not differ much among the methods.

For the males from China (Fig. 24.6) the revised life table data gave a life expectancy at birth which was 0.6–1.7 years lower than that calculated from the original data. On the contrary, life expectancy at birth from the expanding process was exactly the opposite. As a result, the healthy life expectancy calculated in this paper is almost the same estimated with the other methods. The same happened with females, though, healthy life expectancy in them is somewhat lower in the most recent years studied.

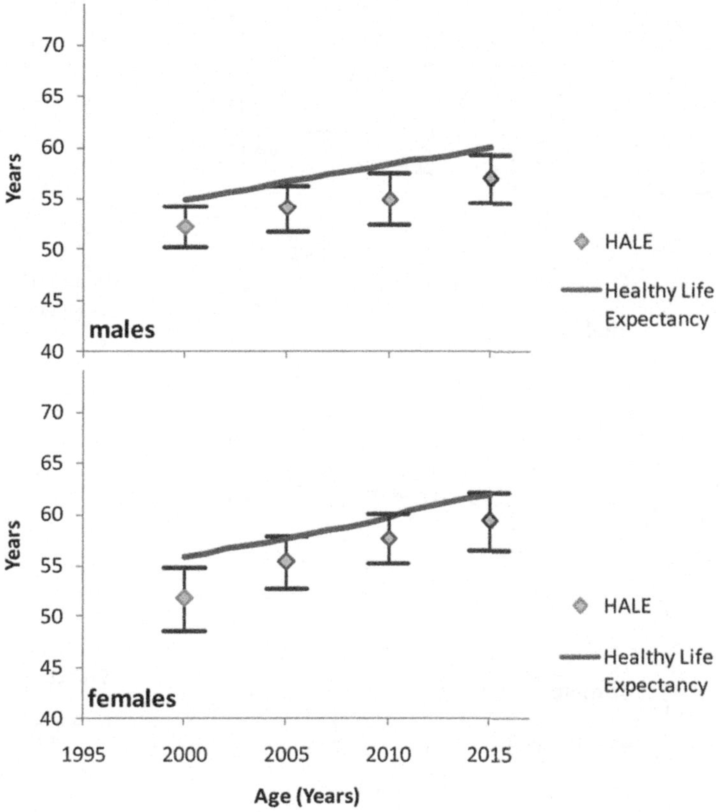

Fig. 24.4 HLE and HALE estimations, India

Finally, for South Africa (Fig. 24.7) the published results by WHO and the other connected scientists have the peculiarity that HALE is increasing constantly during the twenty-first century even though life expectancy at birth is low and remains almost unchanged in females and decreasing in males until 2005. Instead according to the methodology used in this paper, healthy life expectancy decreases up to 2005 and increases later following the temporal trends of life expectancy at birth.

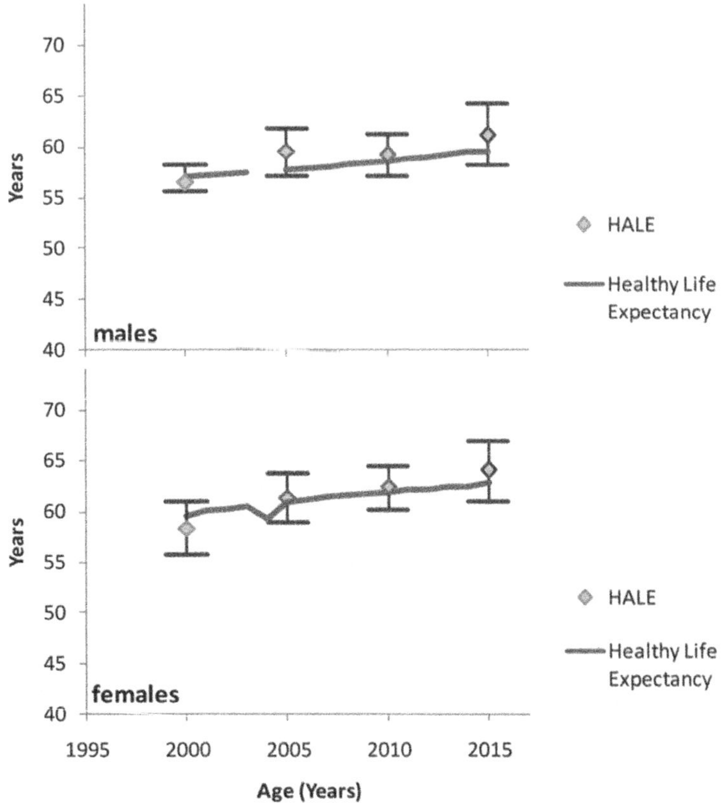

Fig. 24.5 HLE and HALE estimations, Indonesia

24.4 Conclusions

A method of calculating healthy life expectancy was applied in the BRIICS countries, based on abridged life table data from the World Health Organization. However, because the μ_x based approach described in this paper can be applied only to full life table data, the original tables were expanded to full ones with the aid of the UNABR application of the MORTPAK software, created by the Population Division of the United Nations.

The analysis revealed that the MORTPAK software is not very suitable for this purpose because significant deviations were observed in life expectancy at birth as calculated by this software in comparison with the published results of the World Health Organization. A further shortcoming was that the already published

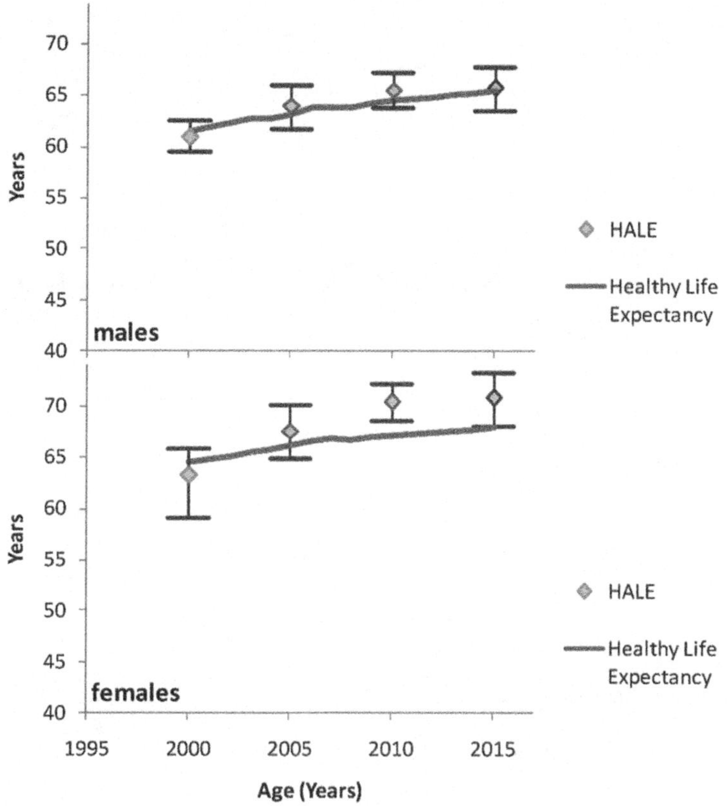

Fig. 24.6 HLE and HALE estimations, China

estimations of the World Health Organization and related agencies were made in old data, thus the ability of comparing the results of this analysis with the previous ones was problematic,

It is seen then that the μx based approach is quite efficient in estimating the healthy life expectancy and its temporal trends, as it is based solely on life table data. In that way, it is totally costless and its only limitation springs from the quality of data. In any case, it seems that a more sensitive application is needed in order for abridged life table data to be expanded and used by this method.

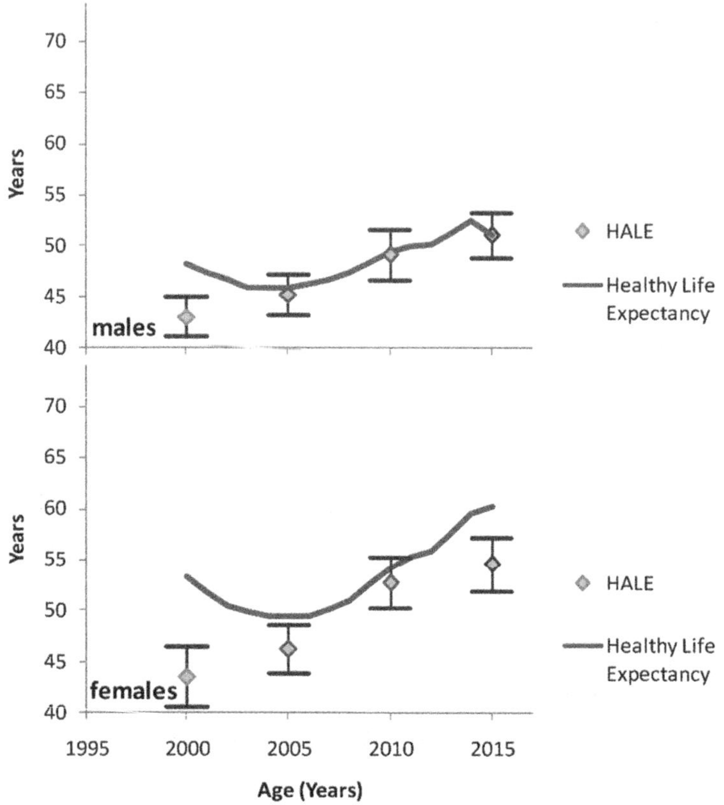

Fig. 24.7 HLE and HALE estimations, South Africa

References

Chiang, C. L. (1965). *An index of health: Mathematical models*. U.S. Department of HEW, Public Health Service, Publication No. lCXK). Series 2, No. 5.

Global Burden of Disease Study. (2012). *Global Burden of Disease Study 2010 (GBD 2010) Disability Weights*. Seattle: Institute for Health Metrics and Evaluation (IHME).

Heligman, L., & Pollard, J. H. (1980). The age pattern of mortality. *Journal of the Institute of Actuaries, 107*, 47–80.

Kostaki, A. (1992). A nine parameter version of the Heligman-Pollard formula. *Mathematical Population Studies, 3*(4), 277–288.

Lee, M.-L. T., & Whitmore, G. A. (2006). Threshold regression for survival analysis: Modeling event times by a stochastic process reaching a boundary. *Statistical Science, 21*(4), 501–513.

Murray, C. J. L., Ezzati, M., et al. (2012a). GBD 2010: A multi-investigator collaboration for global comparative descriptive epidemiology. *Lancet, 380*, 2055–2058.

Murray, C. J. L., Ezzati, M., et al. (2012b). GBD 2010: Design, definitions, and metrics. *Lancet, 380*, 2063–2066.

Murray, C. I., et al. (2015). Global, regional, and national disability-adjusted life years (DALYs) for 306 diseases and injuries and healthy life expectancy (HALE) for 188 countries, 1990–2013: Quantifying the epidemiological transition. *Lancet*. https://doi.org/10.1016/S0140-6736(15)61340-X

Salomon, J. A., et al. (2012). Healthy life expectancy for 187 countries, 1990-2010: A systematic analysis for the global burden of disease study. *Lancet, 380*, 2144–2162.

Sanders, B. S. (1964). Measuring community health levels. *American Journal of Public Health, 54*, 1063–1070.

Skiadas, C. H. (2012a). Life expectancy at birth and forecasts in the Netherlands (females). In C. H. Skiadas & C. Skiadas (Eds.), *The health state function of a population* (1st ed., pp. 47–67). Athens: National Library of Greece.

Skiadas, C. H. (2012b). The health state function, the force of mortality and other characteristics resulting from the first exit time theory applied to life table data. In C. H. Skiadas & C. Skiadas (Eds.), *The health state function of a population* (1st ed., pp. 69–92). Athens: National Library of Greece.

Skiadas, C. H., & Skiadas, C. (2012). Estimating the healthy life expectancy from the health state function of a population in connection to the life expectancy at birth. In C. H. Skiadas & C. Skiadas (Eds.), *The health state function of a population* (1st ed., pp. 97–109). Athens: National Library of Greece.

Skiadas, C. H., & Skiadas, C. (2014a). *Demographic and Health indicators for 193 countries of the World Health Organization and the United Nations.* Second supplement of the book The Health State Function of a Population, Athens.

Skiadas, C. H., & Skiadas, C. (2014b). First time exit problem. In L. Miodrag (Ed.), *International encyclopedia of statistical science* (pp. 521–523). Berlin/Heilderberg: Springer.

Skiadas, C. H., & Skiadas, C. (2014c). The first exit time theory applied to life table data: The health state function of a population and other characteristics. *Communications in Statistics-Theory and Methods, 34*, 1585–1600.

Skiadas, C. H., & Zafeiris, K. N. (2015a). Comparing WHO and first exit time theory estimations of healthy life expectancy in Europe. In A. Karagrigoriou, T. Oliveira, & C. H. Skiadas (Eds.), *Statistical, stochastic and data analysis methods and applications* (pp. 261–266). ISAST.

Skiadas, C. H., & Zafeiris, K. N. (2015b). *Population aging and healthy life lessons*. RELIK 2015 Conference proceedings. Reproduction and human capital. Available at: http://kdem.vse.cz/resources/relik15/download/pdf/45-SKIADAS-CHRISTOS-paper.pdf

Sullivan, D. F. (1966). *Conceptual problems in developing an index of health*. U.S. Department of HEW, Public Health Service Publication No. 1000, Series 2, No. 17.

Sullivan, D. F. (1971). A single index of mortality and morbidity. *HSMHA Health Reports, 86*, 347–354.

Torrance, G. W. (1976). Health status index models: A unified mathematical view. *Management Science, 22*(9), 990–1001.

WHO. (2014, March). *WHO methods for life expectancy and healthy life expectancy*. Global health estimates technical paper WHO/HIS/HSI/GHE/2014.5.

World Health Organization. (2000). *The world health report 2000 – Health systems: Improving performance*, France. Available at http://www.who.int/whr/2000/en/

World Health Organization. (2001). *The world health report 2000 – Mental Health: New understanding*, France. Available at http://www.who.int/whr/2001/en/

World Health Organization. (2004). *The world health report 2004 – Changing history*, France. Available at http://www.who.int/whr/2004/en/

Zafeiris, K. N., & Kostaki, A. (2017). Recent mortality trends in Greece. *Communications in Statistics-Theory and Methods* doi: https://doi.org/10.1080/03610926.2017.1353625.

Zafeiris, K. N., & Skiadas, C. H. (2015a). Demographic and heath indicators in the Pomaks of Rhodopi. In R. Manca, S. McClean, & C. H. Skiadas (Eds.), *New trends in stochastic modelling and data analysis* (pp. 311–324). ISAST.
Zafeiris, K. N., & Skiadas, C. H. (2015b). An application of the first exit time theory in some European populations. In A. Karagrigoriou, T. Oliveira, & C. H. Skiadas (Eds.), *Statistical, stochastic and data analysis methods and applications* (pp. 229–249). ISAST.
Zafeiris, K. N., & Skiadas, C. H. (2015c). *Some methods for the estimations of healthy life expectancy*. RELIK 2015 Conference proceedings. Reproduction and human capital. Available at: http://kdem.vse.cz/resources/relik15/download/pdf/34-Zafeiris-Konstantinos-paper.pdf

Chapter 25
Social Capital, Income Inequality and the Health of the Elderly

Maria Felice Arezzo

25.1 Introduction

Ageing is at the same time one of the greatest achievement and most difficult challenge of our times. This explains why there is an ongoing debate among researchers on this topic.

A main stream of research is around the social determinants on the healthy ageing and therefore central to the discussion surrounding the extension of active lifespan is the state of health of older adults, where "health" refers to the physical, mental and social well being.

The European Union has recently stressed the importance of maintaining autonomy and independence for older people, as a key goal in the policy frame-work for active ageing. While physical and mental health are crucial in this context, there are numerous determinants of healthy and active ageing that lie beyond the health system, having direct or indirect effects on health.

Recently, an explanation has begun to take hold: social capital (see below for the definition of the concept) can be one of the key factor to understand why some individuals are more exposed to disease and mortality than other, despite the undoubted improvement of medicine and living conditions over time. As a consequence the relationship between social capital (SC) and health is capturing the attention of an increasing number of researchers (Andrew 2005; d'Hombres et al. 2010; Folland 2007; Hawe and Shiell 2000; Islam et al. 2006; Poulsen et al. 2011; Rocco and Marc 2012; Szreter and Woolcock 2004; van Groezen et al. 2011). However, the nexus is not fully proved: some studies provide empirical evidence that these two concepts are connected (Lindstrm 2004), but there are others which

M. F. Arezzo (✉)
Università di Roma "La Sapienza", Rome, Italy
e-mail: mariafelice.arezzo@uniroma1.it

© Springer International Publishing AG, part of Springer Nature 2018
C. H. Skiadas, C. Skiadas (eds.), *Demography and Health Issues*,
The Springer Series on Demographic Methods and Population Analysis 46,
https://doi.org/10.1007/978-3-319-76002-5_25

report the absence of it (Greiner et al. 2004; Veenstra 2005; Ziersch and Baum 2004). Interestingly this association seems to hold for the population of the elderly. An explanation is that older adults are considered to have higher degree of involvement in their communities compared to other age groups (Lowe 2010). With increasing age most social contacts fade away, bonds with non-kin decrease in importance, while the bonds with children and close family members may increase; older adults could be involved in new roles within the family or in the community.

A number of studies emphasize the association between social capital and health among older people (Andrew 2005; Arezzo and Giudici 2017; Kondo et al. 2007; Veenstra 2000). Recent studies attempted to prove that this relation could be more than a simple statistical association (Arezzo and Giudici 2016; Rocco and Marc 2012) and established a causal path leading from social capital to health.

Recently, researchers pulled together the literature that explores the relation between health and social capital to the one on socioeconomic inequality and health. This is mostly done focusing on the distribution of income. The pioneer of this stream of very recent literature was (Wilkinson 1996) who demonstrated that higher income inequality is associated with lower life expectancy in wealthier countries. Wilkinson's results has awakened an enormous interest and many works have followed ever since, some supporting (Kawachi and Berkman 2000; Marmot 2002; Subramanian and Kawachi 2004; Wilkinson and Pickett 2006), some refuting (Lynch et al. 2001, 2004; Mackenbach 2002; Osler et al. 2002; Ross et al. 2000; Shibuya et al. 2002) his findings.

The contribution of this work is to try to understand if the relationship between social capital and income inequality with health exists for the population of the European elderly. The rest of the paper is organized as follows: Sect. 25.2 provides the definitions of social capital and recall some discussions around it; Sect. 25.3 illustrates the theoretical pathways from social capital to health and from income inequality to health; Sect. 25.4 covers data, variables and the models used; Sect. 25.5 provides the results. The conclusions are reported in Sect. 25.6.

25.2 Social Capital

The first glimmer of social capital as a concept dates back to the beginning of the twentieth century with the contribution of (Hanifan 1916, 1920), who emphasized the importance of social structure to people with a business. In the last 20 years a flourishing multidisciplinary literature on the topic serves to enrich and qualify the concept of social capital.

There is widespread agreement among researchers that social capital is the synthesis of three different points of view (Grootaert and van Bastelaer 2001): the first, due to Putnam, defines social capital as those characteristics of social communities, such as networks of individuals and families together with norms that create externalities for the society as a whole; the second interpretation, referred to by Coleman, defines social capital as a "variety of different entities which all consist of some aspect of social structure and which facilitate certain actions of actors -whether personal or corporate actors- within the structure"; the third is associated with Olson and North and includes the social and political environment that shapes social structure and allows for the development of norms.

Theoretical research identifies a structural and a cognitive aspect of social capital, the first being related to actions of individuals and the second to their perception. Structural aspects appear in rules and in specific behavior (such as networking or volunteering activities), whereas cognitive aspects materialize as trust, shared values, empathy and respect towards community. The former are more easily measured objectively than the latter.

Another important distinction, particularly relevant to our research, can be drawn between bonding and bridging social capital (Putnam 1995): the first refers to the relations that an individual has within his/her "inner circle" whereas the second relates to ties with people outside of the closest circle. In other words, bonding SC refers to the trusting and co-operative strong relations among individuals who recognize to be similar in terms of social identity (family ties are an important example of this category); bridging SC comprises relations among people who know they are not alike in some socio-demographic sense (Szreter and Woolcock 2004).

Another important issue discussed in theoretical literature is on the level of relevance of its tenure and measurement: the sociologist Pierre Bourdieu defines social capital as "the aggregate of the actual or potential resources which are linked to possession of a durable network of more or less institutionalized relationships" (Bourdieu 1985).

As argued by (Andrew 2005), Bourdieu's conceptualization of social capital as a durable network of relationships is consistent with the idea that social capital is a resource which can be measured at an individual level. According to Bordieu "the volume of social capital possessed by a given agent thus depends on the size of the network of connections he can effectively mobilize and the volume of the capital possessed by each of those to whom he is connected" (Bourdieu 1985).

Also according to (Lin 1999), who says that "social capital is captured from the embedded resources in social networks", social capital is more properly captured at the individual level.

In other conceptualizations, social capital is considered in purely collective terms. For example in (Kawachi and Berkman 2000) it is argued: "social capital inheres in the structure of social relationships; in other words it is an ecological characteristic" which "should be properly considered a feature of the collective (neighborhood, community, society) to which an individual belongs".

Although some authors consider social capital more relevant at an individual level (Bourdieu 1985; Dayton-Johnston 2003; Pevalin 2003; Portes 1998; Veenstra 2000) whereas others at collective level (Kawachi and Berkman 2000; Lochner et al.

1999; McKenzie et al. 2002; Szreter and Woolcock 2004) and the appropriate level at which it should be measured remains uncertain, the literature on social capital and health shows that differences in health could be better predicted by individual level social capital (De Silva et al. 2005). We follow this approach and use an individual level measurement of SC.

25.3 Theoretical Pathways from Social Capital and Income Inequality to Health

The findings of an empirical association between social capital and income inequality with health require a deeper analysis highlighting the theoretical motivations and the mechanisms underlying these nexuses.

25.3.1 Income Inequality and Health

Three mechanisms have been suggested to link income inequality and health (Kawachi et al. 1994; Lynch and Kaplan 1997): (a) the disinvestment in human capital; (b) the erosion of social capital; and (c) social comparisons.

On behalf of the first path, there is a strong evidence (Kaplan et al. 1996) that the degree of income inequality at the state level and indicators of human capital investment are negatively and significantly correlated. One reason why high income inequality may translate into lower spending in education (and other social areas) is that in countries with rising inequalities, the interests of the rich diverge profoundly from those of the typical family. Paul Krugman said that: *A family at the 95th percentile pays a lot more in taxes than a family at the 50th, but it does not receive a correspondingly higher benefit from public services, such as education. The greater the income gap, the greater the disparity in interests. This translates, because of the clout of the elite, into a constant pressure for lower taxes and reduced public services* (Krugman 1996).

Another mechanism through which income inequality may affect health is via the crumbling of social capital; in fact as the gap between rich and poor increases, the resulting social conflict leads to increasing mistrust between members of society. Kawaki et al. (1997) showed that citizens living in states characterized by high income inequalities are more mistrustful of each other.

The last pathway from income inequality to health is through social comparisons. More specifically the comparison between individuals with very different economic status and/or possibilities to have access to relevant resources, very typical in unequal societies, results in a direct negative effect on health (Dressler 1996; Dressler et al. 1998).

25.3.2 Social Capital and Health

The theoretical literature identifies two major ways in which social capital influences health (Veenstra 2005; Veenstra et al. 2005): the first, also known as "compositional" health effect of social capital, is a direct pathway to individual health whereas the second, the so called "contextual" health effect of social capital, exerts its influence only indirectly.

On behalf of the first, durable networks impact people behavior through four primary pathways: (1) social support; (2) social influence; (3) social engagement and attachment; and 4) access to resources and material goods. These behavioral processes have direct pathways to health status: (1) direct physiological stress responses, (2) psychological states and traits (for example self-esteem, self-efficacy, security), (3) health behaviors (for example they inhibit damaging habits like tobacco or alcohol consumption and foster healthy behavior such as appropriate health service utilization, medical adherence, and exercise) (Berkman et al. 2000).

Another interesting point of view that sheds lights on the compositional health effect and that is particularly suited for our purposes is given by the Social Production Function (SPF) theory applied to ageing (Ormel 2002; Ormel et al. 1999; Steverink and Lindenberg 2006). The SPF theory identifies three basic social needs: affection, behavioral confirmation, and status; the overall well being increases as these three needs are satisfied. In particular, affection is fulfilled by relationships that give the feeling of being loved, trusted and accepted; behavioral confirmation results primarily from the feeling of doing the "right" thing in the eyes of relevant others and oneself; and the need of status is fulfilled by relationships that give one the feeling to be treated with respect, taken seriously etc. In the light of the SPF theory, bonding social capital would benefit health because it fulfills affection whereas bridging SC behavioral confirmation and/or status. The variables we chose to measure SC, see Subsection 25.4.2, are consistent with this theory.

The second pathway, i.e. the "contextual" health effect of social capital, has an impact on individual health indirectly through its influence on socio-economic and environmental factors of the community as a whole. These elements are determinants of health themselves. For example social capital is known to generate overall economic prosperity and wealth (Woolcock 1998) and there is evidence for a link between community wealth and health [see for example (Kaplan et al. 1996; Lynch et al. 1998; Veenstra 2003; Wilson and Daly 1997)].

25.4 Methods

25.4.1 Data

Our study is based on the fourth wave of the survey on health and retirement in Europe (SHARE). SHARE is a multidisciplinary and cross-national panel database of micro data on health, socio-economic status and social and family networks of more than 85,000 individuals aged 50 or over. SHARE involves 18 European countries plus Israel and aims at analyzing the process of population ageing in depth.

The fourth wave (2010–11) introduces for the first time a social network module that allows for the computation of social capital and its dimensions. This is the reason why we decided to base our study on the fourth wave.

Since we are interested in the ongoing mechanisms of the older adults, we downsized the sample to the population older than 60. The countries analyzed are Austria, Germany, Sweden, Netherlands, Spain, Italy, France, Denmark, Switzerland, Belgium, Czechia, Poland, Hungary, Portugal, Slovenia, Estonia.

Our results are based on a sample is of 35,391 individuals who live (i.e. are nested) in 16 European countries and are older than 60 in 2011.

25.4.2 Variables

The dependent variable is the self-perceived health (SPH). The original five levels variable (excellent, very good, good, fair and poor) was transformed into a dichotomous one (excellent/very good/good and fair/poor). If an individual perceive to be in fair/poor health he/she is labeled with 1; otherwise it is 0. Dichotomization of self-rated health is not a seldom practice among authors and is due to the fact that the distribution of SPH is concentrated in the central values [Some examples are, (Kawachi et al. 1999; Kim et al. 2006; Nieminen et al. 2010; Pirani and Salvini 2012)]. We decided to transform SPH in a binary variable to have results comparable with other works on social capital and health.

Among the independent variables we considered age, gender, income, body mass index (BMI), years of education and social capital. Income was measured using a proxy: the ability to make ends meet. In particular, we created a binary variable which assumed value 1 if to make ends meet is easy or fairly easy and 0 otherwise.

For the measurement of social capital we proceeded in two steps. First we selected those questions from the survey relevant for our purpose; they are: frequency of family contacts, number of individuals in family network, frequency done charity or voluntary work in the last 12 months, frequency attended an educational or training course in the last 12 months, frequency gone to a club in the last 12 months. Second we performed a principal component analysis (PCA) and used the loadings of the two factors extracted as the social capital variables. The variables with the highest relative contributions to the first components are frequency of family contacts and number of individuals in family network. We therefore named the first factor as bonding social capital. The second component was named bridging social capital.

Some descriptive statistics are reported in Table 25.1.

Table 25.1 Descriptive statistics for individual and country level variables

	N	Mean Std.	Dev	Min	Max	Type[a]
Individual level variables						
SPH	35,391	0.470	0.499	0	1	B
Years of education	35,391	10.062	4.320	0	25	D
BMI	35,391	26.945	4.634	1.469	76.125	C
Age	35,391	71.475	7.733	61	102	D
Bonding SC	35,391	0.001	1.246	−2.106	5.987	C
Bridging SC	35,391	−0.059	1.125	−3.145	6.791	C
Female	35,391	0.553	0.497	0	1	B
Ends meet						
With some difficulty	35,391	0.290	0.454	0	1	B
Fairly easily	35,391	0.349	0.477	0	1	B
Easily	35,391	0.265	0.442	0	1	B
Country level variable						
Gini index[b]	35,391	28.375	3.040	23.800	33.700	C

[a] *B* Binary, *D* Discrete, *C* Continuous
[b] Obtained from the OECD Regional well-being database

25.4.3 Statistical Models

To take into account the clustered structure of the data (i.e. individuals nested into countries), we used multilevel models (Hox 2010; Rabe-Hesketh and Skrondal 2008) and to evaluate how each component influence SPH we used a sequential approach. In particular we fitted a series of four models. The first (*Null Model*) was an intercept-only model and allows to see how much of the variance in SPH is due to differences among countries. In the second model (*Compositional Model*) there are all the individual level covariates but social capital (age, gender, income, BMI, years of education). In the third (*Social Capital Model*) we added social capital and in the last (*Full Model*) it is included the Gini index for the 16 countries. In all models the intercept is random.

Formally, we write the generic model as:

$$logit(\pi_{ij}) = \beta X_{ij} + \gamma K_j + u_j + e_{ij} \tag{25.1}$$

with the distribution of the random components assumed to be normal: $e_{ij} \sim N(0, \sigma_e^2)$ and $u_j \sim N(0, \sigma_u^2)$.

Where j indicates the countries, i the individuals, π_{ij} is the probability that the ith individual who lives in jth country has a fair/poor self-perceived health, β, γ is a vector of parameters to be estimated as well as σ_e^2 and σ_u^2.

The model is a random intercept type and it assumes that each country has its own effect on self-perceived health. Note that if $\sigma_u^2 = 0$ the model reduces to the ordinary logistic regression, meaning that there is no need for setting a different intercept for each country (i.e. no country specific effect).

Table 25.2 Regression coefficients (standard errors in parentheses) of fitted multilevel models

	Null Model Coef.	Contextual Model Coef.	Soc. Cap. Model Coef.	Full Model Coef.
Costant	−0.139	−4.651	−4.495	−5.441
	(0.423)	(0.000)	(0.000)	(0.000)
Years of education		−0.061	−0.051	−0.050
		(0.000)	(0.000)	(0.000)
BMI		0.056	0.055	0.055
		(0.000)	(0.000)	(0.000)
Age		0.060	0.056	0.056
		(0.000)	(0.000)	(0.000)
Female		0.109	0.114	0.114
		(0.000)	(0.000)	(0.000)
Ends meet (ref: With great difficulty)				
With some difficulty		−0.527	−0.491	−0.491
		(0.000)	(0.000)	(0.000)
Fairly easily		−0.935	−0.878	−0.878
		(0.000)	(0.000)	(0.000)
Easily		−1.203	−1.116	−1.116
		(0.000)	(0.000)	(0.000)
Bonding SC			−0.146	−0.146
			(0.000)	(0.000)
Bridging SC			−0.208	−0.208
			(0.000)	(0.000)
Gini index				0.033
				(0.413)
Random effect estimate	0.694	0.589	0.537	0.526
Log-likelihood	−24213.164	−20922.242	−20499.139	-20498.810
Chi2		3120.65***	3380.48***	3381.76***
		(df = 7)	(df = 9)	(df = 10)

25.5 Results

The results of all models are presented in Table 25.2. We will first comment on the random component and then on the regression coefficients. The null model gives an estimated standard deviation $\left(\sigma_u^2\right)$ equal to 0.694. This indicates a substantial variation in perceived health across countries: an individual in a country which is one standard deviation above the mean have odds of perceiving a fair/poor health that is almost double than a comparable individual in an average country [exp (0.694) = 2.002]. This standard deviation indicates a correlation of 0.174 in the latent propensities to be in fair/poor self-perceived health of comparable individual in the same country. The result follows from the fact that $\rho = \frac{\sigma_u^2}{\sigma_u^2 + \pi^2/3} = \frac{0.694}{0.694 + 3.290}$ (Rabe-Hesketh and Skrondal 2008)[1].

When we insert the control variables (contextual model), the standard deviation decreases to $\hat{\sigma}_u^2 = 0.589$. Adding up the social capital variables (social capital model) lead to $\hat{\sigma}_u^2 = 0.537$. That means that bridging and bonding social capital are able to capture 8.83%[2] of the unexplained variation of the model with only the control variables. It certainly is a non-negligible percentage which testifies the importance of social capital in explaining self-perceived health.

As for the full model, the standard deviation decreases to 0.526, meaning that the introduction of the Gini index gives only a very small contribution to the reduction of the unexplained health heterogeneity.

On behalf of the regression coefficients (top part of Table 25.2), we note that all the individual level variables have a significant association with health and the sign of the coefficients is consistent with the literature: it is well known that self-perceived health worsens with age and is negatively influenced by bad physical conditions captured by the BMI. Among all the variables considered the ability to make ends meet easily appears to be the most important factor associated with self-perceived health. People with economic difficulties are more likely to report being in poor self-perceived health.

Looking at the estimates of the social capital model, we note first of all that both components of SC have a strong significant association with self-perceived health. In particular the higher the SC the lower the risk of having a poor perceived health. Secondly, the greatest effect is exerted by the bridging component. A possible explanation is that interaction with people not belonging to someone's inner circle triggers a psychological effect with positive consequences on self-perceived health. A virtuous circle can be imagined: more bridging social capital, better perceived health, more strength and willingness to interact with others, more social capital.

There is a possible existence of a reverse effect between social capital (especially the bridging component) and health: people in bad health may not feel like having contacts with others and be involved in activities. The existence of endogeneity, as well known, leads to biased estimates of the parameters which doesn't allow to properly capture the effect of the variables in the model. Therefore some caution is needed.

The regression coefficient associated with income inequality is not significant proving the lack of effect. This is also confirmed by the small variation in the estimated standard deviations passing from the social capital model to the full model.

[1]Here $\pi = 3{:}14$.

[2]It is the relative change between the two models: (0.537- 0.589)=0.589.

25.6 Conclusions

There are three main results in our analysis: the first and most important is the strong association between both bridging and bonding social capital and self-perceived health: the higher the SC the lower is the risk of having a poor perceived health; the second result is that we identify in the bridging component that with the highest effect, suggesting a sort of virtuous circle linking health and social capital; the third is that we find no significant effects of income inequality measured at country level.

Consistently with the literature on the determinants of health, we find that age, lifestyle elements, the ability to make ends meet and education are also statistically significant: overweight and difficulty to make ends meet are associated with fair/poor health ratings; a high education and the facility to make ends meet are associated with good to excellent health ratings.

Although the possibility of reverse causation in social capital claims for caution when interpreting these findings, it is not out of place to say that improvements in social capital give the potential to improve health quite considerably in Europe. In fact it might well be, and the results of other researches point in that direction (d'Hombres et al. 2010), endogeneity (Arezzo and Giudici 2016), that the nexus between social capital and health could be found stronger once the reverse causation is ruled out.

This gives room for some recommendations to policy makers. Sure enough the policies that confront the multiple impacts of population ageing should be multidimensional: they should regard labour market, social and health care, housing, education, social protection and pension schemes. The traditional political answer to the current demographic challenges mainly concerns pension and health systems, but a more comprehensive approach on health issues, which includes family, housing and other social policies is emerging. In this sense a brand new approach is the one related to the build of social capital. States cannot intervene directly: social capital is frequently a byproduct of religion, tradition, shared historical experience, and other factors that lie outside the control of any government. But, as the literature has suggested, the main objectives that policy makers should pursue in order to foster the accumulation of social capital are the reduction of inequalities (which have an impact on social capital accrual) and the accumulation of human capital. Regarding the latter, the area where governments probably have the greatest direct ability to generate social capital is education. Educational institutions do not simply transmit/increase human capital, they also pass on social capital in the form of social rules and norms.

References

Andrew, M. K. (2005). Social capital, health, and care home residence among older adults: A secondary analysis of the health survey for England 2000. *European Journal of Ageing, 2*(2), 137–148.

Arezzo, M. F., & Giudici, C. (2016). The effect of social capital on health among european older adults: An instrumental variable approach. *Social Indicators Research*, 1–14.

Arezzo, M. F., & Giudici, C. (2017). Social capital and self-perceived health among european older adults. *Social Indicators Research, 130*, 1–21.

Berkman, L. F., Glass, T., Brissette, I., & Seeman, T. E. (2000). From social integration to health: Durkheim in the new millennium. *Social Science & Medicine, 51*(6), 843–857.

Bourdieu, P. (1985). *The forms of capital*. New York: Greenwood.

Dayton-Johnston, J. (2003). *Social capital, social cohesion, community: A microeconomic analysis*. Toronto: University of Toronto Press.

De Silva, M. J., McKenzie, K., Harpham, T., & Huttly, S. R. A. (2005). Social capital and mental illness: A systematic review. *Journal of Epidemiology and Community Health, 59*(8), 619–627.

d'Hombres, B., Rocco, L., Suhrcke, M., & McKee, M. (2010). Does social capital determine health? Evidence from eight transition countries. *Health Economics, 19*(1), 56–74.

Dressler, W. W. (1996). Culture and blood pressure: Using consensus analysis to create a measurement. *Cultural Anthropology Methods, 8*, 6–8.

Dressler, W. W., Balieiro, M. C., & Santos, J. E. D. (1998). Culture, skin color, and arterial blood pressure in Brazil. *American Journal of Human Biology, 11*(1), 49–59.

Folland, S. (2007). Does community social capital contribute to population health? *Social Science & Medicine, 64*(11), 2342–2354.

Greiner, K. A., Li, C., Kawachi, I., Hunt, D. C., & Ahluwalia, J. S. (2004). The relationships of social participation and community ratings to health and health behaviors in areas with high and low population density. *Social Science & Medicine, 59*(11), 2303–2312.

Grootaert, C., & van Bastelaer, T. (2001). *Understanding and measuring social capital: A synthesis of findings and recommendations from the social capital initiative*. Working paper 24, Social Capital Initiative, World Bank.

Hanifan, L. J. (1916). The rural school community center. *Annals of the American Academy of Political and Social Science, 67*, 130–138.

Hanifan, L. J. (1920). *The community center*. New York: Silver Burdette.

Hawe, P., & Shiell, A. (2000). Social capital and health promotion: A review. *Social Science & Medicine, 51*(6), 871–885.

Hox, J. (2010). *Multilevel analysis: Techniques and applications* (2nd ed.). Hoboken: Taylor & Francis.

Islam, M. K., Merlo, J., Kawachi, I., Lingstrom, M., & Gerthan, U. G. (2006). Social capital and health: Does egalitarianism matter? A literature survey. *International Journal for Equity in Health, 5*, 128.

Kaplan, G. A., Pamuk, E. R., Lynch, J. W., Cohen, R. D., & Balfour, J. L. (1996). Inequality in income and mortality in the United States: Analysis of mortality and potential pathways. *BMJ (Clinical Research ed.), 312*(7037), 999–1003.

Kawachi, I., Kennedy, B. P., & Glass, R. (1999). Social capital and self-rated health: A contextual analysis. *American Journal of Public Health, 89*(8), 1187–1193.

Kawachi, I., Kennedy, B. P., Lochner, K., & Prothrow-Stith, D. (1997). Social capital, income inequality and mortality. *American Journal of Public Health, 87*(9), 1491–1498.

Kawachi, I., Levine, S., Miller, S. M., Lasch, K., & Amick, B. C., III. (1994). *Income in-equality and life expectancy: Theory, research, and policy, Society & health working paper series*. Boston: Joint Program in Society & Health, Health Institute, New England Medical Center and Harvard School of Public Health.

Kawachi, I., & Berkman, L. (2000). *Social epidemiology* (pp. 174–190). Oxford: Oxford University Press.

Kim, D., Subramanian, S. V., & Kawachi, I. (2006). Bonding versus bridging social capital and their associations with self-rated health: A multilevel analysis of 40 US communities. *Journal of Epidemiology and Community Health, 60*(2), 116–122.
Kondo, N., Minai, J., Imai, H., & Yamagata, Z. (2007). Engagement in a cohesive group and higher-level functional capacity in older adults in Japan: A case of the Mujin. *Social Science & Medicine, 64*(11), 2311–2323.
Krugman, P. (1996). The spiral of inequality. *Motherjones*, pp. 44–49.
Lin, N. (1999). Building a network theory of social capital. *Connections, 22*(1), 28–51.
Lindstrm, M. (2004). Social capital, the miniaturisation of community and self-reported global and psychological health. *Social Science & Medicine, 59*(3), 595–607.
Lochner, K., Kawachi, I., & Kennedy, B. P. (1999). Social capital: a guide to its measurement. *Health & Place, 5*(4), 259–270.
Lowe, P. (2010). *Ageing*. London: Newcastle University.
Lynch, J., Smith, G., Hillemeier, M., Raghunathan, T., Kaplan, G., & Shaw, M. (2001). Income inequality, the psycho-social environment and health comparisons of wealthy nations. *Lancet, 358*, 194–200.
Lynch, J., Smith, G. D., Harper, S., Hillemeier, M., Ross, N., Kaplan, G. A., & Wolfson, M. (2004). Is income inequality a determinant of population health? Part 1. A systematic review. *Milbank Quarterly, 82*(1), 5–99.
Lynch, J. W., & Kaplan, G. A. (1997). Understanding how inequality in the distribution of income a ects health. *Journal of Health Psychology, 2*(3), 297–314.
Lynch, J. W., Kaplan, G. A., Pamuk, E. R., Cohen, R. D., Heck, K. E., Balfour, J. L., & Yen, I. H. (1998). Income inequality and mortality in metropolitan areas of the United States. *American Journal of Public Health, 88*, 1074–1079.
Mackenbach, J. P. (2002). Income inequality and population health. *British Medical Journal, 324* (7328), 1–2.
Marmot, M. (2002). The influence of income on health: Views of an epidemiologist. *Health Affairs, 21*(2), 31–46.
McKenzie, K., Whitley, R., & Weich, S. (2002). Social capital and mental health. *The British Journal of Psychiatry, 181*(4), 280–283.
Nieminen, T., Martelin, T., Koskinen, S., Aro, H., Alanen, E., & Markku, T. H. (2010). Social capital as a determinant of self-rated health and psychological well-being. *International Journal of Public Health, 55*(6), 531–542.
Ormel, J. (2002). *Social production function (SPF) theory as a heuristic for under-standing developmental trajectories and outcomes* (pp. 353–379). New York: Cambridge University Press.
Ormel, J., Lindenberg, S., Steverink, N., & Verbrugge, L. (1999). Subjective well being and social production functions. *Social Indicators Research, 46*, 61–90.
Osler, M., Prescott, E., Gornbaek, M., Christensen, U., Due, P., & Engholm, G. (2002). Income inequality, individual income, and mortality in danish adults: Analysis of pooled data from two cohort studies. *British Medical Journal, 324*(7328), 13.
Pevalin, D. (2003). More to social capital than Putnam. *The British Journal of Psychiatry, 182*(2), 172–173.
Pirani, E., & Salvini, A. (2012). Place of living and health inequality: A study for elderly italians. *Statistical Methods and Applications, 21*, 211–226.
Portes, A. (1998). Social capital: Its origins and applications in modern sociology. *Annual Review of Sociology, 24*(1), 1–24.
Poulsen, T., Christensen, U., Lund, R., & Avlund, K. (2011). Measuring aspects of social capital in a gerontological perspective. *European Journal of Ageing, 8*(4), 221–232.
Putnam, R. D. (1995). Bowling alone: America's declining social capital. *Journal of Democracy, 6*, 65–78.
Rabe-Hesketh, S., & Skrondal, A. (2008). *Multilevel and longitudinal modeling using Stata* (2nd ed.). College Station: Stata Press.

Rocco, L., & Marc, S. (2012). *Is social capital good for health?* Technical report. WHO Regional Office for Europe.

Ross, N. A., Wolfson, M. C., Dunn, J. R., Berthelot, J.-M., Kaplan, G. A., & Lynch, J. W. (2000). Relation between income inequality and mortality in Canada and in the United States: Cross sectional assessment using census data and vital statistics. *British Medical Journal, 320*(7239), 898–902.

Shibuya, K., Hashimoto, H., & Yano, E. (2002). Individual income, income distribution, and self rated health in Japan: Cross sectional analysis of nationally representative sample. *British Medical Journal, 324*(7328), 16.

Steverink, N., & Lindenberg, S. (2006). Which social needs are important for subjective well-being? What happens to them with aging? *Psychology and Aging, 2*, 281–290.

Subramanian, S. V., & Kawachi, I. (2004). Income inequality and health: What have we learned so far? *Epidemiologic Reviews, 26*(1), 78.

Szreter, S., & Woolcock, M. (2004). Health by association? Social capital, social theory, and the political economy of public health. *International Journal of Epidemiology, 33*(4), 650–667.

van Groezen, B., Jadoenandansing, R., & Pasini, G. (2011). Social capital and health across European countries. *Applied Economics Letters, 18*(12), 1167–1170.

Veenstra, G. (2000). Social capital, SES and health: An individual-level analysis. *Social Science & Medicine, 50*(5), 619–629.

Veenstra, G. (2003). Economy, community and mortality in British Columbia, Canada. *Social Science & Medicine, 56*(8), 1807–1816.

Veenstra, G. (2005). Location, location, location: Contextual and compositional health effects of social capital in British Columbia, Canada. *Social Science & Medicine, 60*(9), 2059–2071.

Veenstra, G., Luginaah, I., eld, S. W., Birch, S., Eyles, J., & Elliott, S. (2005). Who you know, where you live: Social capital, neighbourhood and health. *Social Science & Medicine, 60*(12), 2799–2818.

Wilkinson, R. G. (1996). *Unhealthy societies: The affictions of inequality*. London: Routledge.

Wilkinson, R. G., & Pickett, K. E. (2006). Income inequality and population health: A review and explanation of the evidence. *Social Science & Medicine, 62*(7), 1768–1784.

Wilson, M., & Daly, M. (1997). Life expectancy, economic inequality, homicide, and reproductive timing in Chicago neighborhoods. *British Medical Journal, 314*(7089), 1271–1274.

Woolcock, M. (1998). Social capital and economic development: Toward a theoretical synthesis and policy framework. *Theory and Society, 27*(2), 151–208.

Ziersch, A. M., & Baum, F. E. (2004). Involvement in civil society groups: Is it good for your health? *Journal of Epidemiology and Community Health, 58*(6), 493–500.

Chapter 26
Life Annuity Portfolios: Risk-Adjusted Valuations and Suggestions on the Product Attractiveness

Valeria D'Amato, Emilia Di Lorenzo, Albina Orlando, and Marilena Sibillo

26.1 Introduction

The current international regulations restate the managerial perspectives in the insurance industry; as for other financial intermediaries, the managerial guide-lines are based on the choice of performance indicators suitable for determining risk capitals (cf. Dacorogna 2015).

Following the solvency approach, the identification and quantification of risk factors should be captured by appropriate indicators and subsequently translated into their implications in terms of capital. Internal models formulated for these purposes are increasingly formalized according to the logic of Enterprise Risk Management (ERM); within this context, all the risks should be recognized and treated throughout a holistic managerial context (cf. Farrell and Gallagher 2015). Solvency assessing is a compelling issue for insurance industry, also in light of the current international risk-based regulations. Internal models have to take into account risk/profit indicators in order to provide flexible tools aimed at valuing solvency.

The concept of performance measurement in the actuarial framework is becoming more and more deepened within the business valuations, due to the increasing importance of the communication of the business results at the same time synthetic

V. D'Amato (✉) · M. Sibillo
Department of Economics and Statistics, University of Salerno, Fisciano, SA, Italy
e-mail: vdamato@unisa.it; msibillo@unisa.it

E. Di Lorenzo
Department of Economic and Statistical Sciences, University of Naples Federico II, Naples, Italy
e-mail: diloremi@unina.it

A. Orlando
National Research Council, Naples, Italy

© Springer International Publishing AG, part of Springer Nature 2018

C. H. Skiadas, C. Skiadas (eds.), *Demography and Health Issues*,
The Springer Series on Demographic Methods and Population Analysis 46,
https://doi.org/10.1007/978-3-319-76002-5_26

and easy to be realized. This is the aim of the profitability ratios (cf. Easton and Harris 2007), indices that can well describe the overall efficiency of a Company as a whole or of a specific business line.

Insurance business bases on insurance and investment operations (cf. Swiss Re 2012), being the first or the second aspect predominant according to the kind of offered product. The deferred life annuity and all its variations are strongly saving products, differently from disability insurance, for example, offering a pure risk protection. As consequence, analysing the risk sources in the case of life annuities means to deepen the investment results and the premium calculation. To structure a performance metric able to provide useful information to the management about the product performance could be even more expressive if clear and easy to communicate. This aspect is going to have an increasing importance in light of the communication outside (i.e. to the stakeholders) of the company's financial results (cf. Swiss Re 2012).

Considering a variable annuity (with profit participation), we deepen this topic by means of a ratio, which properly captures both financial and demo-graphic risk drivers.

The analysis is carried out in accordance with a management perspective, apt to measure the business performance, which requires a correct risk control.

In the case of life annuity business, assessing solvency has to be framed within a wide time horizon, where specific financial and demographic risks are realized. In this order of ideas, solvency indicators have to capture the amount of capital to cope with the impact of those risk sources over the considered period.

We present a study of the dynamics of such a ratio, measuring the policy surplus in relation to its variations on fixed time intervals; these variations are restyled according to a risk-adjusted procedure.

On the other hand, we further examine the insured's point of view, measuring their perception of the contract profitability within the expected utility approach. Thanks to this analysis, it is possible to reconstruct a wider picture of the dynamics of the contract over its lifetime, taking into account both the insurers profitability, and as well as market attractiveness.

26.2 Variable Annuities with Participating Benefits

Insurance policies with profit participation are generally characterized by some contract peculiarities as the guarantee of a minimum rate of return and annual bonus based on return on investment. In the following we will consider life annuities with participation level depending on the period financial result (cf. Cocozza et al. 2011; D'Amato et al. 2011); in particular the installments are increased by a percentage ρ (participation rate) of the period financial result, when it reaches a predefined value at least. This structure involves an embedded option.

Let us consider a life annuity with deferment period T, premium payment at the beginning of each year until the time $\tau(\tau < T)$ and annual installments $\tilde{b}_s$ due at the beginning of year $s(s \geq T)$.

The structure of the contract is based on the exchange of the flow of premiums P_s, paid by the insured during the deferment period, with the flow of variable benefits $\tilde{b}_s$, paid by the insurer if the insured is alive, during the annuitization period. The benefits can be described basing on the quantity we indicate as the period financial result.

To the aim of defining the period financial result R_t obtained in the time interval $(t-1, t)$, we write the expression of the stochastic mathematical reserve at time t:

$$V_t = \sum_{i=t}^{\infty} \left(\tilde{b}_i 1_{(T \leq i \leq K(x))} - P_i 1_{(i<\tau | K(x)>i)} \right) v(t, i). \tag{26.1}$$

where $\{v(t, s)\}$ is the stochastic process describing the value at time t of one monetary unit at time s. In formula (26.1) the indicator function $1_{(T \leq i \leq K(x))}$ takes the value 1 if $T \leq i \leq K(x)$ ($K(x)$ being the random curtate lifetime of an annuitant aged x at the issue time of the contract), 0 otherwise, whilst the indicator function $1_{(i < \tau | K(x) > i)}$ takes the value 1 if $i < \tau$ if the insured is alive, 0 otherwise.

The financial result R_t of the t-th accounting period is given by:

$$R_t = \left(V_{t-1} + P_{t-1} 1_{(t-1<\tau | K(x)>t-1)} \right) v(t, t-1) - \left(\tilde{b}_t + V_t \right) 1_{(T \leq t \leq K(x))}. \tag{26.2}$$

in which the indicator function takes the value 1 if the event at subscript happens, otherwise takes the value 0.

When the period financial result R_t obtained in the time interval $[t-1, t]$, net of the administrative expenses θ is positive, $\rho(R_t - \theta)$ is added to the provision allocated in t, hence the benefits for the policyholders (cf. D'Amato et al. 2011) are increased; otherwise only the basic installments b_t are due to the insureds.

Without loss of generality, in the following we will assume that the additional benefits are added to the future installments.

Summarizing, the benefit flow $\tilde{b}_t$ payable to the insureds can be expressed. as:

$$\tilde{b}_t = \begin{cases} b_t + \rho(R_t - \theta) & if \ (R_t - \theta) > 0 \\ b_t & if \ (R_t - \theta) \leq 0 \end{cases} \tag{26.3}$$

synthetically written as:

$$\tilde{b}_t = b_t + \rho(R_t - \theta)^+$$

26.3 Internal Control Tools

Now we realize a risk adjusted performance measurement, aimed to evaluate the period financial result, so obtaining tools the insurer can use in a solvency perspective. The index we propose is referred to the end of each time interval, i.e. each year, and expresses the profit realized over the year on the overall surplus realized by the insurer at that time. It is built as a stochastic entity in which the two risk drivers are involved and gives the profit realized per unit of the total surplus of the contract at that time:

$$I(t+1) = \frac{R_{t+1} - \rho(R_{t+1} - \theta)^+}{\left[\sum_{j=0}^{\infty} P_j 1_{(j<\tau|K(x)>j)} - \tilde{b}_j 1_{(T\leq j\leq K(x))}\right] v(t+1,j)} \tag{26.4}$$

with R_{t+1} the financial result of the $(t + 1)$-th accounting period.

The denominator in formula (26.4) is the difference between the assets and the liabilities valued at time t. In this way we obtain an useful information: I(t) provides a measure apt to the purpose of evaluating the contract profitability and consequently, in a wider perspective, assessing solvency.

To the aim of providing an example of the study of the indicator we propose, we consider an immediate life annuity, issued to an insured aged 65, consisting in 10 annual anticipated unitary installments given by Eq. (26.3), where b_t is equal to 1. The single premium is paid on the basis of the technical interest rate of 2%. The survival probabilities are obtained by the Human Mortality Database web-site and are referred to the American male population. The Company invests the premium in the market and the global rate of return from investments is described by the Vasicek process:

$$dr_t = \beta(\alpha - r_t)dt + \sigma dW_t$$

with β (the long term mean), α (the reversion factor) and (the instantaneous volatility) positive constants and W_t a standard Wiener process.

We calibrated the process referring to the 3-month interest rate dataset collected by the Federal Reserve. The temporal interval ranges from 4th January 1982 to 1st December 2014, obtaining the values collected in Table 26.1.

The numerical application aims to quantify the index $I(t)$ as expressed in formula (26.4) providing its expected values. We will calculate them assuming the independence of the financial and the demographic systematic risk drivers during the annuity duration, according with the following formula:

$$E[I(t)] = \frac{E[R_t] - \rho max\{E[R_t] - \theta, 0\}]}{\left[\sum_{j=0}^{\tau-1} P_{jj}p_x - \sum_{j=T}^{\infty} \tilde{b}_{jj}p_x\right] E\left[v(t,j)\right]} \tag{26.5}$$

By way of an example, we pose the annual expenses equal to 0.02 and the participation quota ρ equal to 0.2, 0.4, 0.6. The expected values of $I(t)$ reported in

Table 26.1 The interest rate parameters

3-month time series evaluation			
Alpha	Beta	Sigma	r(0)
0.071241	0.0440	0.5781	0.021

Table 26.2 The profit index pattern over the annuity duration

	Expected values of I(t)%		
Valuation time	Rho = 0.2	Rho = 0.4	Rho = 0.6
1	−3.44789	−3.44789	−3.44789
2	−3.44615	−3.44615	−3.44615
3	2.82076	2.54378	2.07664
4	2.82001	2.52981	2.06882
5	2.67980	2.49052	2.01885
6	2.54398	2.39007	2.00981
7	2.24599	2.12432	2.00329
8	2.01754	2.00962	1.54898
9	1.11983	1.03477	0.67761
10	1.07889	0.86545	0.63456

Table 26.2, have been valued throughout the contract duration. They, as conceivable, decrease as ρ increases and in particular show a hump behavior with a maximum at time 4. In our example, the contract reveals itself to be efficient from the point of view of the insurer's solvability after the second year, following an increasing trend maximum at time 3; then the index values decrease. In this case, the weight of the future debt prevails on the fruitful power of the invested capital (single premium paid at the issue time). After the first 2 years, the premium investment and the liability lowering begin to get an ameliorative impact on the index, always positive till the end of the contract. The best snapshot of the contract solvency status corresponds to the third year: at this time, in our example, the contract displays the best solvability performance.

26.4 The Insured's Point of View

The safeguard of the consumer/policy holder covers a central role in the planning and monitoring dynamics operated by the European commission aptly set up. It is within this framework that product distribution profiles ought to be suitably examined, as well as contractual architectures, information transparency and the clients degree of financial awareness. The matter, therefore, is extremely complex and requires wider multi-disciplinary e orts. The problem is currently evident when it comes to pension products, as highlighted by the recent report by the European Insurance and Occupational Pension Authority (EIOPA) (cf. EIOPA 2016b). What EIOPA itself emphatically argued (cf. EIOPA 2016a), then, should not come as a surprise: Consumer protection is in the DNA of EIOPA. EIOPA wants to make sure that all the activities under its remit will make a tangible difference to consumers (. . .). Furthermore, EIOPA contributes to the achievement of a coordinated approach to the regulatory and supervisory treatment of new or innovative financial activities.

In a nutshell, vigilance over products and a governance system for insurance firms constitute a chief goal, as claimed by EIOPA Committee on Consumer Protection and Financial Innovation (CCPFI) (cf. EIOPA 2016c). Current literature is paying increasing attention to the problem outlined above; among others, Maurer et al. presented in 2013 German participating life annuities (PLA) with guaranteed minimum benefits and participation in insurers surpluses, paying attention to the lifetime utility of annuitants (cf. Maurer et al. 2013). Following the guidelines of Maurer et al. (2013) we will consider the utility stemming from the contract considered in Sect. 26.3, from the insureds point of view. We will adopt the CRRA utility function proposed by Maurer et al. in order to obtain an equivalent fixed life annuity.

The utility expected by the benefit stream is given by:

$$U = E\left(\sum_{i=1}^{\omega-x-1} \phi_i^i p_x \frac{\tilde{b}_i}{1-\gamma}\right) \tag{26.6}$$

with γ the relative risk aversion, ϕ the discount factor arising from the insured's subjective preferences. As suggested by Maurer et al. in (2013), we con-sider three different value of ϕ, 0.98, 0.96, 0.94, in order to represent a patient/normal/impatient individuals, conjointly with three different risk aversion levels, which represent, respectively, low, medium and high risk aversion. Moreover, we x the participation rate ρ equal to 0.40. Referring to the exemplifying contract of Sect. 26.2, in Table 26.3 we collected the utility equivalent constant annuity obtained in the case of a fixed interest rate i = 0.02, whilst in Table 26.4 the results obtained in the case of stochastic interest rates as used for the values in Table 26.2.

Table 26.3 Utility-equivalent constant flow, i = 2%

Utility-equivalent fixed annuity EA			
Subjective discount factor	Gamma = 2 low risk adverse	Gamma = 5 medium risk adverse	Gamma = 10 high risk adverse
phi = 0.98 – patient	1,192,292	1,146,691	1,092294
phi = 0.96 – normal	1,201,823	1,155,252	1,098241
phi = 0.94 – impatient	1,211,607	1,164,214	1,104,566

Table 26.4 Utility-equivalent constant flow, Vasicek process

Utility-equivalent fixed annuity EA			
Subjective discount factor	Gamma = 2 low risk adverse	Gamma = 5 medium risk adverse	Gamma = 10 high risk adverse
phi = 0.98 – patient	1,195,704	1,148,102	1,092461
phi = 0.96 – normal	1,205,041	1,156,582	1,098383
phi = 0.94 – impatient	1,214,601	1,165,446	1,104,679

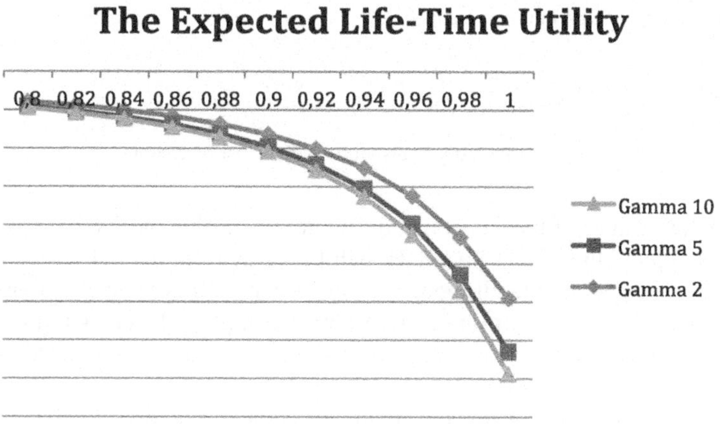

Fig. 26.1 The expected life-time utility with ϕ varying

In both cases we observe that the constant installments decrease when the risk aversion parameters increase; on the other hand, the constant installments increase when the subjective patience levels decrease. The corresponding values in Tables 26.3 and 26.4 show rather small variances, maybe due to the time horizon length.

Finally in Fig. 26.1 the behavior of the expected life-time utility is shown, for each considered value of α, when ϕ varies.

According with the application of formula (26.6), in Tables 26.3 and 26.4 the constant installment equivalent to the variable one (consisting in the unit plus the eventual result of the profit participation) has been valued, leveling the CRRA utilities coming from the two contractual forms. The first observation is that the constant installment the insured perceives as equivalent to the variable one, as proposed in the participating contract, is higher than 1, as conceivable. The utility-equivalent installment got in this way has been valued basing on detailed profiles, depicting the different levels of risk aversion and impatience of the insured.

Looking at Tables 26.3 and 26.4, fixing the impatience level, when the risk aversion increases, the constant installment considered equivalent to the participation contract decreases: the person with a high risk aversion will be satisfied with a rather low installment, provided that it is certain, so avoiding the randomness implied in the participating contract.

On the other hand, fixing the risk aversion level, it will be the less impatience person that will be satisfied with a lower installment, provided that it is fixed. The values of the fixed installment of the equivalent life annuity follow the same trends in the case of fixed interest rate and Vasicek interest rates. Basically the values in the case of a fixed interest rate are lightly lower than the corresponding ones in the Vasicek case. The differences are stronger in the case of high risk aversion.

In Fig. 26.1 the expected utility trend is reported when the subjective dis-count factor ϕ varies and for the three different levels of risk aversion, considered in the application. The expected utility takes the highest value, for any level of risk aversion, in the case of individuals characterized by a high degree of impatience,

Table 26.5 Sample of premium amounts

Annuity	Premium
Participating life annuity	9.055
Constant life annuity	7.985
Utility-equivalent annuity normal individuals with medium risk aversion	9.183

that is by low values of the subjective discount factor. This means that the more the insured is greedy, the higher his utility will be, apart from his risk aversion. When becoming more patient, the differences arising by the different level of risk aversion comes more evident. The insured preserving the highest level of utility that one having the lowest risk aversion. The expected utility trend is strictly decreasing with the subjective discount factor.

Furthermore, we observe that the annuitants choice could depend on the premium amount, if they could be able to find an utility-equivalent certain annuity, consistently with their risk aversion and impatience profile. But this may not be trivial under "normal" market conditions and surely hard enough under increasingly large market movements.

In Table 26.5 we collect, as an example, the premium amount, respectively, for the participating life annuity, the life annuity with unitary constant installments, the utility- equivalent constant annuity obtained with $\phi = 0.9$ and $\gamma = 5$.

As further research line, it is interesting to develop the insureds point of view, taking into account also behavioral considerations. This approach can be realized by means of the increasingly used laboratory experiments, which offer much unexpected food for taught concerning "emotional" aspects and "mental perspectives" (cf. Knoller 2016).

References

Cocozza, R., De Simone, A., Di Lorenzo, E., & Sibillo, M. (2011, June 7–10). *Participating policies: risk and value drivers in a financial management perspective.* In Proceedings of the 14th Applied Stochastic Models and Data Analysis Conference, Rome, pp. 41–48. ISBN: 97888467-3045-9. http://www.asmda.eu/home.html

Dacorogna, M. (2015, December). A change of paradigm for the insurance industry. *SCOR Papers.*

D'Amato, V., Di Lorenzo, E., Orlando, A., Russolillo, M., & Sibillo, M. (2011). Profit participation annuities: A business liability analysis within a demographic risk sensitive approach. *Investment Management and Financial Innovations, 10*(1), 155–165.

Easton, A.E., & Harris J.F. (2007). *Actuarial aspects of individual and annuity contracts* (2nd ed.). Winsted: Actex Publication https://eiopa.europa.eu/consumer-protection

EIOPA. (2016a) https://eiopa.europa.eu/consumer-protection

EIOPA. (2016b). EIOPACP16/001, 1 February 2016. Consultation paper on EIOPAs advice on the development of an EU Single Market for personal pension products (PPP)). http://www.slideshare.net/EthosMedia/cp-16001-eiopa-personal-pensions

EIOPA. (2016c). EIOPA-BoS-16-071, 6 April 2016. *Final Report on public consultation on preparatory guidelines on product oversight governance arrangements by insurance undertakings and insurance distributors.*

Farrell, M., & Gallagher, R. (2015). The valuation implications of enterprise risk management maturity. *The Journal of Risk and Insurance, 82*(8), 625–657.

Knoller, C. (2016). Multiple reference points and the demand for principal-protected life annuities: An experimental analysis. *The Journal of Risk and Insurance, 83*(1), 163–179.

Maurer, R., Rogalla, R., & Siegelin, I. (2013). Participating payout life annuities. Lessons from Germany. *ASTIN Bulletin, 43*(02), 159–187.

Swiss Re. (2012). *Understanding profitability in life insurance*. http://www.swissre.com/media/news releases/nr 20120207measuring life pro tability.html

Chapter 27
Flexible Retirement Scheme for the Italian Mortality Experience

Mariarosaria Coppola, Maria Russolillo, and Rosaria Simone

27.1 Introduction

For National Social Security systems, it is of growing importance to account for longevity risk in programming retirement schemes. Specifically, as the mean life expectancy is increasing, at different rates for males and females and for different cohorts, longevity risk should be dynamically managed over time.

In this framework it is clear the necessity of reforming pension systems projected in the context of lower mortality rates. The dynamics of mortality for the industrialized countries over the last 50 years show: (1) an increase in life expectancy at old ages (over 65 years); (2) an increase in the mode of the age of death distribution; (3) a decrease in mortality rates at old ages. As consequence in terms of the shape of the survival function we can observe: it tends to shift towards a rectangular shape (due to the increasing concentration of deaths around the mode (at old ages) of the curve of deaths) and it expands to the right, i.e. the mode of the curve of deaths moves towards very old ages.

From a financial point of view, rectangularization and expansion have different effects. The concentration of deaths around the mode reduces the variance of the distribution and then the related risk. The expansion phenomenon, generating the risk of systematic deviations of mortality from the assumed projected behavior, together with the accelerating trend of mortality decline at old ages, increases risk for the Social Security System (Visco 2006).

M. Coppola (✉) · R. Simone
Department of Political Sciences, University of Naples Federico II, Naples, Italy
e-mail: m.coppola@unina.it; rosaria.simone@unina.it

M. Russolillo
Department of Statistics and Economics, University of Salerno, Salerno, Italy
e-mail: mrussolillo@unisa.it

© Springer International Publishing AG, part of Springer Nature 2018

C. H. Skiadas, C. Skiadas (eds.), *Demography and Health Issues*,
The Springer Series on Demographic Methods and Population Analysis 46,
https://doi.org/10.1007/978-3-319-76002-5_27

From these considerations emerges the need of accurate mortality projections based on stochastic analysis in order to provide reliable measures of mortality and of its uncertainty which are essential for proper pension reforms.

In this vein, we propose a flexible retirement scheme based on the indexation of the retirement age to reach a prescribed Expected Pension Period Duration (EPPD) (Bisetti and Favero 2014). In particular, we test such approach considering two stochastic projection mortality models: the classical Lee Carter Model (no cohort effect) and the Renshaw–Haberman model specifying the cohort effect. We refer to Italian male and female population. The aim is measuring the impact of the mortality model selection on the retirement age settings by gender. The paper is organized as follows: in Sect. 27.2 we introduce the stochastic mortality models that will be used for our analysis. Section 27.3 describes the Italian pension system and discusses the proposal of an indexed retirement mechanism. Section 27.4 is devoted to apply our proposal to the Italian mortality experience. Concluding remarks on forthcoming developments end the paper.

27.2 Stochastic Mortality Models

The aim of this contribution is to compare the impact that mortality projection for males and females has on a flexible retirement scheme when different stochastic mortality models are considered. In particular, we refer to the Lee-Carter model and the Renshaw–Haberman model (RH), because the LC model has become a milestone and it is largely used in the actuarial literature, whilst the RH model allows us to take into account the cohort effect.

They both are two of the stochastic mortality models belonging to the GAPC (Villegas et al. 2016) class. The unifying design for these models prescribes a predictor $\eta_{x,t}$ which is related to mortality rates according to a log or logit link, generally. In this framework, the predictor structure proposed by Lee and Carter (1992) is given by:

$$\eta_{x,t} = \alpha_x + \beta_x k_t$$

where α_x denotes age effects, k_t the period effects, $\beta_x$the age-period modulating terms.

The LC model is widely used because of its simplicity and robustness despite its inability to model specific cohort effects. In 2006, Renshaw and Haberman proposed an extended version of the LC model by introducing one of the first stochastic models for population mortality with a cohort effect to obtain the predictor:

$$\eta_{x,t} = \alpha_x + \beta_x k_t + \gamma_{t-x}$$

where γ_{t-x} denotes the cohort effects.

In order to project mortality, the time index k_t and the extra parameter γ_{t-x} are modelled and forecasted using ARIMA processes.

27.3 A Flexible Retirement Scheme

Societies across the world are ageing, with challenges for sustainable adequate pension systems. Governments and pension funds have largely responded by postponing pension ages and by discouraging early retirement. In many countries, for example, pension legislations have been reformed during the last decade, moving from Defined Benefits (DB) to Notional Defined Contributions (NDC) system, the latter highly relying on the rules to take into account life expectancies and their changes in the pension formulae (Belloni and Maccheroni 2006). The Italian pension system is composed by three pillars: (1) Public, compulsory and unfunded pay-as-you-go system (PAYG); (2) The private, voluntary and collective funded system; and (3) Private, voluntary and individual savings related to social security schemes. The first pillar, the dominant one in Italy, passed through two main reforms during the nineties. The first reform, introduced by Law 335/95, determined a shift from DB to NDC scheme, in which notional accumulated contributions on individual accounts were converted into an annuity at retirement. Unlike the previous method, the latter takes into account the amount of contribution paid throughout the whole working life accumulated at the expected GDP (Gross Domestic Product) growth rate, the life expectancy of the pensioner at retirement age and the number of years that a survivor's benefit will be withdrawn by any widow or widower, according to actuarial equivalence principle. The second reform, introduced by Fornero with Law 214/2011, had two directives: the rise of the pensionable age and the calculation of the requirements for retirement on the basis of the number of years of social security contributions made and no longer on the average salary earned in the last years before retirement. In particular, among the others, the reform will see the retirement age increased to 66 years and 7 months for both men and women in the public and private sector by 2018; future retirement ages increasing in line with life expectancy from next year. For all workers, in accordance with Law Number 122/2010, age and service requirements will be periodically reviewed based on the actual increases in life expectancy published by ISTAT, the Italian National Institute for Statistics. Moreover, pensions calculated under the NDC system will be affected by the application of periodically reviewed annuity conversion factors. In this framework, we propose an indexing mechanism for retirement age based on the period life expectancy $e^{(M)}_{x_0,C}$ at age $x_0 = 65$, for selected cohorts and the chosen stochastic mortality model M. We consider cohorts of males/females born from 1952 to 2012, setting the cohort 1952 as benchmark. Those individuals will be aged 65 in 2017, which was the retirement age prescribed by law until the Fornero Reform.

We follow an age-period approach in the sense that life expectancy is considered as a function of the age x and the calendar year t. Specifically, let us consider an individual belonging to the cohort C, aged x_0 on the first of January of year t_0, when the expected lifetime provided by a given stochastic mortality model M is equal to $e_{x_0,C}^{(M)}$. Let us suppose that the pension system we refer to foresees that $x_0$is the fixed retirement age for all subsequent cohorts. The individual aged $x_0$receives a constant monthly payment B as long as he/she survives. We can say that $e_{x_0,C}^{(M)}$ represents the Expected Pension Period Duration according to model M (EPPD$^{(M)}$), that is the expected number of years during which pension payments are due.

Then, for a fixed mortality model M and for each of the selected cohorts C, we determine the age at which life expectancy equals the EPPD$^{(M)}$. Specifically, we evaluate $e_{x_0+j,C}^{(M)}$ for increasing age span j = 1,2. . . ., and we index the retirement age x_0 by shifting it by the minimal amount $s_C^{(M)}$ to reach the EPPD$^{(M)}$, that is:

$$s_C^{(M)} = \min\left\{j : e_{x_0+j,C}^{(M)} \leq EPPD^{(M)}\right\}. \tag{27.1}$$

In this way, the Social Security System will be obliged for an expected number of years that does not exceed the fixed EPPD$^{(M)}$ and will keep pension costs to budgeted level.

27.4 Application: Italian Dataset

As aforementioned, we consider cohorts of individuals born from 1952 to 2012 for ages from 55 up to 89 years. The data are downloaded from the Human Mortality Database (2014) by single calendar year and by single year of age. We focus on ages 55–89 since we are interested in mortality dynamics at old ages. The numerical application is performed considering the LC and RH mortality models according to the following steps: we fit the selected models, assess goodness of fit, forecast mortality and calculate the indexed retirement age both for males and females.

The goodness-of-fit of mortality models is typically analyzed by inspecting the residuals of the fitted model.

In Figs. 27.1 and 27.2 scatter plots of residuals for the LC and RH models are reported, respectively, by age, period and cohort for both males and females. As well known, regular patterns in the residuals indicate the inability of the model to describe all the features of the data appropriately. In our case the scatter plots of deviance residuals show the inability of LC model to capture a not negligible cohort effect. On the contrary the residuals of RH model look more reasonably random.

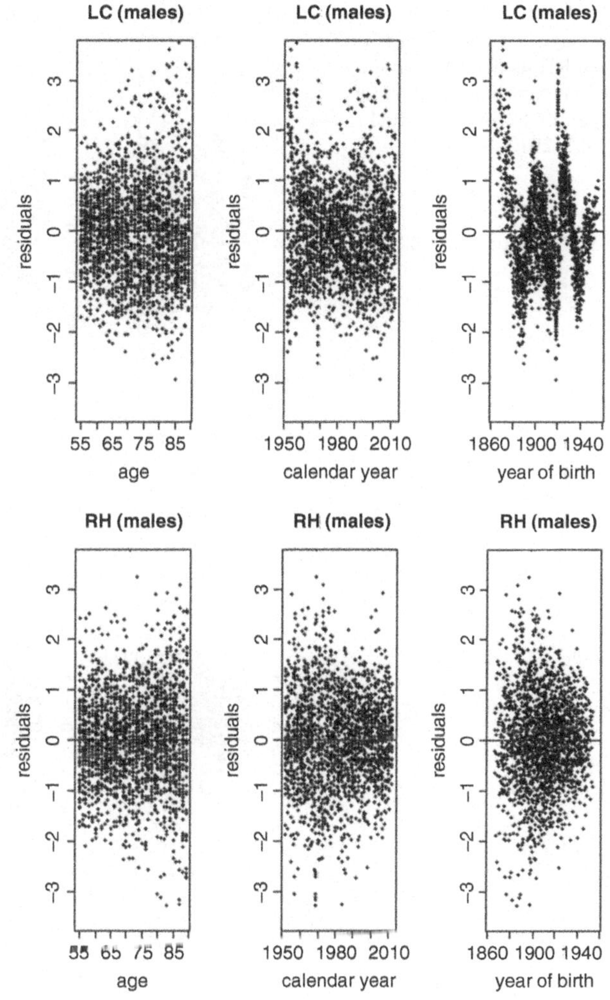

Fig. 27.1 Scatter plots of deviance residuals for LC and RH models fitted to the Italian male population for ages 55–89 and the period 1952–2012

The better performances of the RH model are supported also by pursuing model selection on the basis of the BIC index, reported in Table 27.1 both for females and males.

For mortality projections, we consider a forward time span of h = 30 years. As customarily, we assume that the period index $k_t$follow a random walk with drift and the cohort index γ_{t-x} follows a univariate ARIMA process, independent of the period indexes. Then, for each mortality model, the forecasting procedure is based on the best ARIMA process fitting the observed data, as obtained from the auto. arima() function of the R Package "forecast" (Hyndman et al. 2008). Table 27.2 reports the ARIMA(p,d,q) process that are assumed for the cohort effects both for females and males.

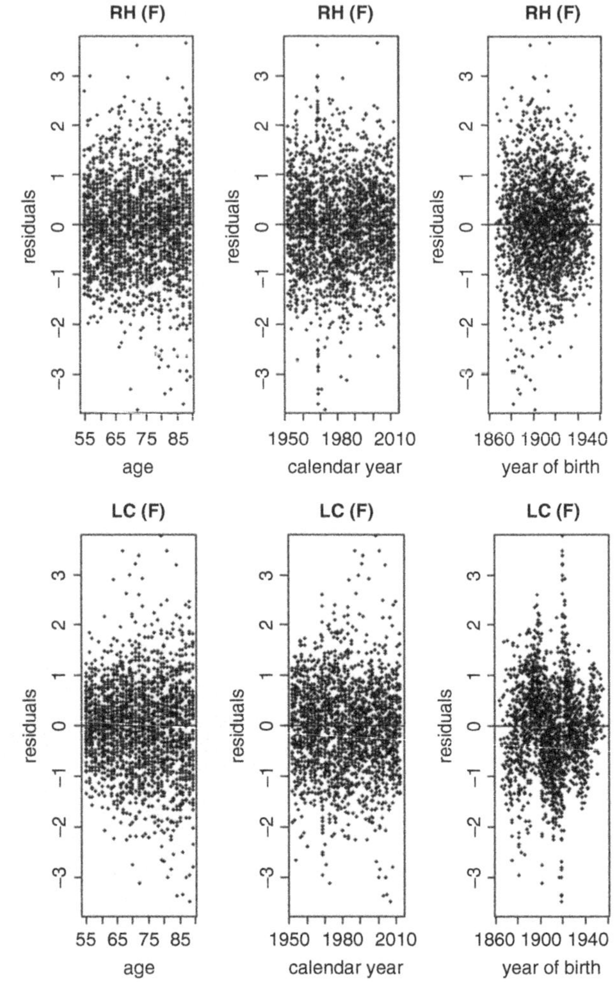

Fig. 27.2 Scatter plots of deviance residuals for LC and RH models fitted to the Italian female population for ages 55–89 and the period 1952–2012

Table 27.1 BIC index for selected mortality models

	Males	Females
RH	27839.01	27584.65
LC	43772.54	29778.88

Table 27.2 Selected ARIMA process for forecasting cohort effect

Males		Females	
RH	ARIMA (1,2,2)		ARIMA(1,2,2)

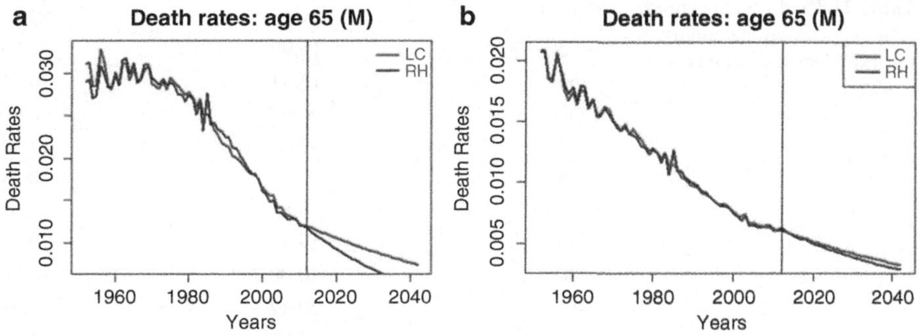

Fig. 27.3 (**a**) Fitted and forecasted death rates for males aged 65. (**b**) Fitted and forecasted death rates for females aged 65

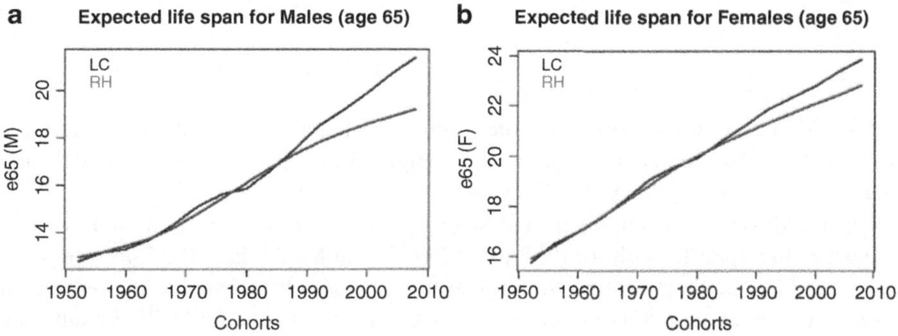

Fig. 27.4 (**a**) Life expectancy for males aged 65. (**b**) Life expectancy for females aged 65

Table 27.3a Life expectancy at age 65 for male cohorts for the selected mortality models

Cohort	LC	RH
1952	12.97	12.80
1956	13.16	13.16
1960	13.42	13.31
1964	13.74	13.70
1968	14.22	14.37
1972	14.81	15.12
1976	15.47	15.63
1980	16.11	15.86
1984	16.73	16.61
1988	17.30	17.52
1992	17.82	18.55
1996	18.24	19.20
2000	18.59	19.89
2004	18.91	20.71
2008	19.23	21.40

Table 27.3b Life expectancy at age 65 for female cohorts for the selected mortality models

Cohort	LC	RH
1952	15.90	15.76
1956	16.41	16.51
1960	16.97	16.98
1964	17.57	17.54
1968	18.22	18.28
1972	18.85	19.05
1976	19.47	19.56
1980	20.00	19.95
1984	20.47	20.58
1988	20.91	21.18
1992	21.32	21.88
1996	21.71	22.35
2000	22.08	22.80
2004	22.46	23.40
2008	22.84	23.86

According to these forecasts, the central projections of death rates and the expected residual life span at age 65 are computed for the two selected models and gender (see Figs. 27.3a and b, 27.4a and b; Tables 27.3a and 27.3b).

The indexation mechanism will assume, for each mortality model M, the expected life span for cohort 1952 as $EPPD^{(M)}$. Tables 27.4a and 27.4b report the computed lag as the minimum forward shift that should be applied to the retirement age (say, set at age 65), in order to reach the threshold $EPPD^{(M)}$. Results are represented in Fig. 27.5a and b. Different patterns are observed for different genders. Specifically, for females residual life expectancy is globally higher than for males, although the specification of the cohort effects (which is supported by the data) yields a steeper increase in expected lives for males than for females. This circumstance yields that in the case of RH model the lags requested for females are lower than for males for younger generations. Finally, we note that the cohort effect is stronger for the male population (lags are higher in case of RH model respect the LC model for males), and also the RH more sharply improves the fitting performances for males than for females.

27.5 Conclusions

The paper suggests a flexible pension scheme based on the expected residual life to adjust the retirement age for keeping a constant Expected Pension Period Duration (EPPD) and containing the pension costs to a fixed level. In this context the choice of the stochastic mortality model is crucial. So, we applied the indexing mechanism to the Italian male and female populations in case of the LC and RH models. In this way

Table 27.4a Required lags by the indexation mechanism for Males

Lag	1956	1960	1964	1968	1972	1976	1980	1984	1988	1992	1996	2000	2004	2008
LC	1	1	2	3	4	5	5	6	7	7	8	8	8	9
RH	1	1	2	3	4	5	5	6	8	9	10	10	11	12

Table 27.4b Required lags by the indexation mechanism for Females

Lag														
	1956	1960	1964	1968	1972	1976	1980	1984	1988	1992	1996	2000	2004	2008
LC	1	2	3	4	4	5	6	6	7	7	7	8	8	9
RH	2	2	3	4	5	5	6	7	7	8	8	9	10	10

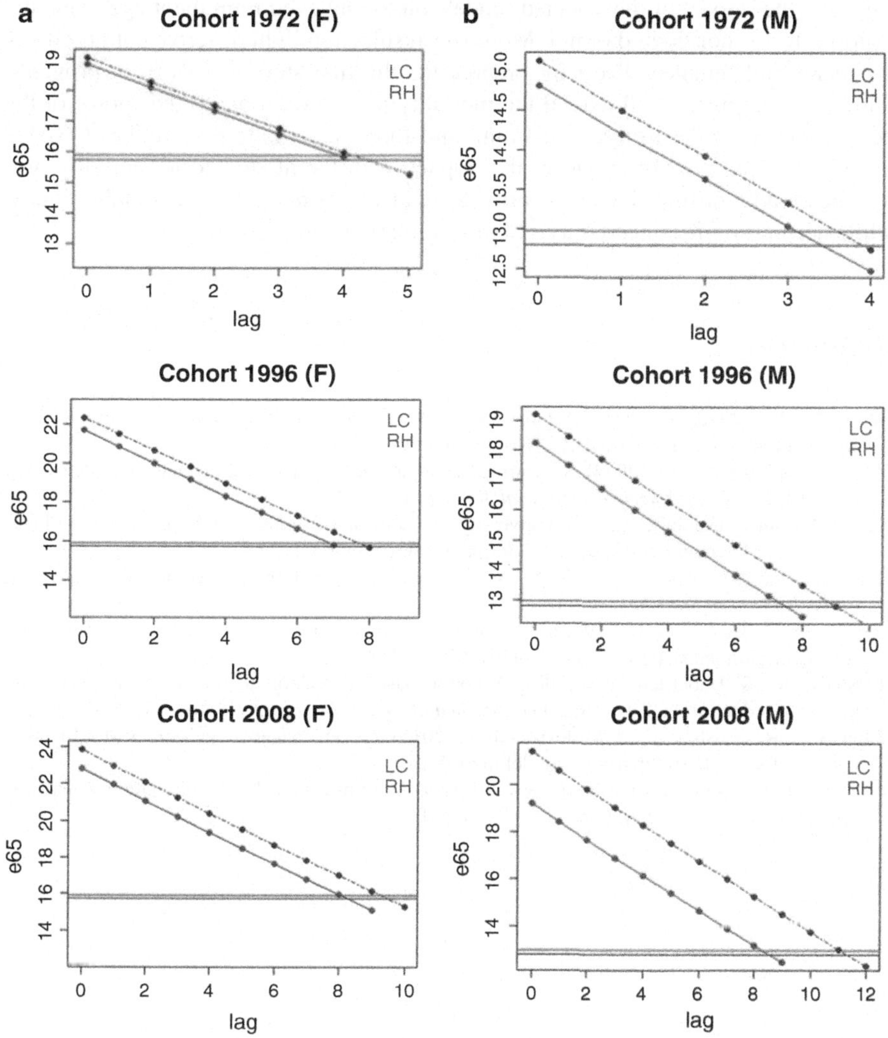

Fig. 27.5 (**a**) Lag to reach EPPD for LC (red) and RH (blue) females. (**b**) Lag to reach EPPD for LC (red) and RH (blue) males

we show the impact of the selected models on the indexed retirement age when the cohort effect is considered or not. Moreover results highlight different cohort effects for males and females. The paper represents the first step of a work in progress. Future developments will extend the mortality projection topic to the choice of the best mortality model in terms of fitting and forecasts among the family of GAPC models. Finally, we will measure the impact of different stochastic mortality projection models on the Social Security System costs introducing a suitable index, while accounting for uncertainty of both estimation and prediction.

References

Belloni M., Maccheroni C. (2006). *Actuarial neutrality when longevity increases: An application to the Italian Pension System* (CERP, Working Paper 47/06).

Bisetti, E., & Favero, C. A. (2014). Measuring the impact of longevity risk on pension systems: The case of Italy. *North American Actuarial Journal, 18*, 1.

Human Mortality Database. (2014). University of California, Berkeley (USA), and Max Planck Institute for Demographic Research (Germany). www.mortality.org

Hyndman, R. J., & Khandakar, Y. (2008). Automatic Time Series Forecasting: the forecast Package for R. *Journal of Statistical Software, 27*(3).

Lee, R. D., & Carter, L. R. (1992). Modeling and forecasting U.S. mortality. *Journal of the American Statistical Association, 87*(419), 659–671.

Renshaw, A., & Haberman, S. (2006). A cohort-based extension to the lee-carter model for mortality reduction factors. *Insurance: Mathematics and Economics, 38*(3), 556–570.

Villegas, A. R., Kaishev, V., & Millossovich, P. (2016). *Under review or revision*. StMoMo: An R Package for stochastic mortality modelling (38 p).

Visco I. (2006). *Longevity risk and financial markets*. https://www.bancaditalia.it/pubblicazioni/interventi-vari/int-var-2006/visco_12_10_06.pdf

Chapter 28
Sibling Death Clustering Among the Tribes of Central and Eastern India: An Application of Random Effects Dynamic Probit Model

Laxmi Kant Dwivedi and Mukesh Ranjan

28.1 Introduction

The Infant mortality rate (IMR) has been considered as a highly sensitive measure of population health. This reflects the apparent association between the causes of infant mortality and other factors that are likely to influence the health status of populations such as their economic development, general living conditions, social wellbeing, rates of illness, and the quality of the environment (Whitehouse 1982). There were around 4.6 million deaths (74% of all under-five deaths) occurred within the first year of life (WHO 2011). Globally, IMR has decreased from an estimated rate of 63 deaths per 1000 live births in 1990 to 34 deaths per 1000 live births in 2013 (UNICEF 2014).

One of the targets under United Nations Millennium Development Goals (UNMDGs) is to reduce IMR by two-thirds between 1990 and 2015. For India, it translates into a goal of reducing IMR from 88 infant deaths per thousand live births in 1990 to the level of 29 infant deaths per thousand live births by 2015. The recent figure of IMR for India, is 37 infant deaths per 1000 live births (Sample Registration System (SRS) 2015). Hence, it clearly reflects that India lagged far behind in achieving mortality related UNMDGs goal. In India, the issue of high IMR exists with a lot of regional variations across the states. For example, among the bigger states and UTs, IMR varies from 12 in Kerala to 50 in Madhya Pradesh (SRS 2015). In view of these statistics, child survival in India needs sharper focus. This includes better managing neonatal and childhood illnesses, improving child survival, particularly among vulnerable communities and we need a different approach to tackle the IMR & under 5 mortality rate (U5MR). Survival risk remains a key challenge for the disadvantaged who have little access to reproductive and child health services.

L. K. Dwivedi · M. Ranjan (✉)
International Institute for Population Sciences (IIPS), Mumbai, Maharashtra, India

© Springer International Publishing AG, part of Springer Nature 2018

C. H. Skiadas, C. Skiadas (eds.), *Demography and Health Issues*,
The Springer Series on Demographic Methods and Population Analysis 46,
https://doi.org/10.1007/978-3-319-76002-5_28

Major states in the heartland of India fell significantly short of UNMDGs targets related to infant mortality, by more than 20 points.

In the backdrop of high mortality situation prevailing in the developing nations across the world including India, the situation of high mortality is not only an issue of concern itself but it also have a strong linkages with the intra-family clustering of deaths in a particular region. In other words, there may be a situation when there is a high mortality in the region but deaths are not randomly distributed in the entire exposed families of the area rather there are certain high- risk families which only experiences deaths frequently and other families in the nearby in spite of sharing the similar socio-cultural environment do not experience frequent child loss. This situation is known widely among researcher as death clustering. This phenomena was first highlighted by Das Gupta (1990) in her paper while studying child mortality in rural Punjab. Since then it is on the research agenda while studying infant mortality and also a new dimension of familial component got added and entire research community has seen this phenomena as another important approach for studying infant and child mortality.

Among various social groups, it has been found that on average, an Indian child has 25 percent lower likelihood of dying under age five as compared to an Adivasi or Tribal child (Das et al. 2010). According to the third round of the National Family Health Survey (IIPS 2007), in rural areas where a majority of *adivasi* children live, contributed about 11 percent of all births and almost one-fourth of all deaths under the age of 5 years. Children born to women from scheduled castes (SCs) and scheduled tribes (STs) have higher mortality rates than children born to women from other backward classes and other than these classes (i.e., general/advanced classes). A nationally representative study of India based on the 1981 census also indicated that under-five mortality among STs and SCs was significantly higher than non-tribal population (Das et al. 2014). The gap in infant mortality between tribal and non-tribal populations was substantial in the early months after birth, narrowed between the fourth and eighth months, and enlarged mildly afterwards (Ranjan et al. 2016). In a study on clustering of infant deaths in families in central and eastern region of India, it was found that among SCs & STs, infant death clustering is mainly affected by the scarring factor that is effect of previous infant deaths in families on the survival status of index child in Jharkhand and Madhya Pradesh,while mother-level unobserved factors were important in Odisha and both scarring and mother-level unobserved factors were key factors in Chhattisgarh (Ranjan et al. 2018).

Tribes are varied in terms of their socio-economic and political development. The term "Scheduled Tribes" refers to specific indigenous peoples whose status is acknowledged by the Constitution of India. The tribal population in India, according to the 2011 census, was 87 million and it constitutes around 8.2 percent of the total Indian population. Around 80 percent of them found in central India and a large part of the rest in the north-eastern states. The maximum share of tribal population is contributed by Madhya Pradesh (14.7%), followed by Odisha (9.2%), Jharkhand (8.3%) and Chhattisgarh (7.5%) to the India's population. A majority of tribal population living in these states are the Particularly Vulnerable Tribal Groups (PVTGs) (Ministry of Tribal Affairs 2015). They are socially as well as economically backward in the sense that they have little access to the resources for their development, low rate of literacy, relatively small population size, dwindling in numbers and some of the groups are at the verge of extinction. They are distributed in various ecological zones beyond the state boundaries with immense variation in subsistence pattern, technological development, ways of living and contact with outside world as well as with different worldviews in respect with neighborhoods called mainstream population. Accordingly, the present research was undertaken to investigate the extent of clustering of infant deaths among tribal families by rural-urban in the central and eastern states of India. This paper also explores whether infant deaths are uniformly distributed among tribal mothers across different states of this region after adjusting the confounding variables using random effects dynamic probit model. Lastly, the reduction in infant deaths will be worked out by changing the level of scarring factor and literacy status of women.

28.2 Materials and Methods

In order to examine the family level infant death clustering bivariate analysis was carried out and for capturing the linkages between survival prospects of siblings and mother specific unobserved heterogeneity, the random effects dynamic probit model was applied. The random effects dynamic probit panel data model has the advantage of simultaneously capturing unobserved heterogeneity and the causal positive or negative scarring mechanisms at the same time in the model. The model also accounted for the endogeneity factor which arose due to the inclusion of previous sibling-survival status in the model, thus avoiding the potential bias in previous studies.

The potential problem which has been found in the empirical specification of the earlier models include the problem of left truncation & endogeneity, measurement error and time inconsistency (Bolstad and Manda 2001; Curtis et al. 1993; Guo 1993; Sastry 1997). It would be very important to understand these unaddressed problems of the earlier models. First, left truncation is the problem associated with retrospective data. It means an age cut-off is used to select the respondents. The interviewees may be a representative sample at survey date, but they will not be so for earlier years (Rindfuss et al. 1982).This non-representativeness of the sample over the years along with the recall bias, a common practice in previous research has been to discard information on children who were born before an arbitrarily selected date, such as 10 or 15 years before the date of the survey (Bhargava 2003; Bolstad and Manda 2001; Curtis et al. 1993; Guo 1993; Madise and Diamond 1995; Sastry 1997). This left truncation of the data by calendar time occurs at the different points in the birth history, creating additional complications. Many studies have even discarded the first-born child in every family. This will result in a severe loss of information. Moreover, left truncation of the data, whether by calendar time or by birth order of child, will lead to the problem that the start of the sample does not coincide with the start of the stochastic process under study. The next issue is of measurement error as it can be seen that the risk of mortality among index child is a function of the preceding child's survival status. Positively correlated measurement in these variables will tend to create an upward bias in the scarring coefficient that is coefficient of previous child survival. This potential problem is addressed in the present model. The other problem related with variables inconsistent with time has been sorted out in the present model. It is usually seen that data in retrospective surveys with regard to child, year of birth and death is available for the larger number of years. In our case, information was available for more than 35 years before the survey date. These surveys typically gather information on variables such as household assets, toilet facilities, electricity or access to piped water at the date of the survey. The time inconsistency problem is that, in such cases, data that pertain to the survey date are less informative. It means the information of certain predictors which are though important one are not available for all the children under study. In the present analysis, where the entire birth history of each tribal mother was used, the problem was even more severe. We, therefore, did not include any currently dated variables as explanatory variables in the model.

By ignoring these potential problems, bias will be created because previous child's survival status and its correlation with survival status of index child will confound the causal interpretation of previous death in the family. In order to avoid these biases, modelling of the initial condition (mortality risk for first-born children) jointly with the dynamic mortality process for the second and higher-order births need to be applied (Arulampalam and Bhalotra 2006, 2008; Heckman 1987; Manski and McFadden 1981; Oettinger 2000; Wooldridge 2010). The present study used the dynamic panel data model along with the initial condition to assess the death clustering among tribes of central and eastern India. Model with such initial condition will estimate the scarring effect that is effect of previous death in families on the survival status of the index child without bias and establish the true impact in studying the death-survival relationship among siblings. The relative contribution of social factors, that is, literacy status vis-à-vis biological factors, that is, survival status of sibling is examined in explaining the infant deaths.

28.2.1 Data Source

The data used in the study is taken from National Family health Survey-3 which was conducted in 2005–06. It interviewed 124,385 ever married women aged 15–49 at the time of the survey. It has a complete retrospective history of births together with a record of child deaths for each mother, for a period spanning more than 35 years (1970–2006). Thus, it would give sufficient number of cases for analysis as well as we would be able to construct (unbalanced) panel data for mothers. Further full retrospective birth history has been used for all the statistical analysis in the study.

28.2.2 The Empirical Model

The dependent variable that is infant death of index child and the main covariates survival status of the preceding child (i.e. lagged variable) were both coded as binary variables -one if a child died before the age of 12 months and zero otherwise. By taking child specific and mother specific covariates along with preceding child (lagged variable), the random effect dynamic probit model was applied. Children who were younger than 12 months at the time of the survey were dropped from the sample because they had not 12 months of exposure to mortality risk. When the index child was not singleton but instead twins they were also dropped from the model so that siblings should be identified properly.

28.2.3 Choice of Independent Variables

The predictors like, sex and birth order of the child, mother's education, religion, caste and place of residence, exposure to mass media, availability of toilet facility, type of fuel used for cooking and standard of living, mother receiving tetanus immunization during pregnancy and preceding birth interval were considered as the main determinants of infant and child mortality for most of the Indian states (Pandey and Tiwary 1993). Apart from the above factors, the tribal children, in fact, face certain adverse realities like insufficient food intake, frequent infections, and lack of access to health services. They also have the lack of awareness about environmental sanitation and personal hygienic practices, proper child rearing, breastfeeding and weaning practices (Pandey and Tiwary 1993; Reddy 2008). Women's autonomy, social class, mother's education and quality care received by the children has been cited as some of the reasons for clustering (Madise and Diamond 1995). Causal factors that determine equality levels in the distribution of mortality risks for children between families or between mothers may conveniently be divided into two factors: Bio-demographic differentials and differentials in other socioeconomic characteristics of the families (and/or the mother) (Zaba and David 1996). Bio-demographic factors include mother's age, fertility levels, and birth-spacing patterns, as well as inherited genetic disorders and the mother's medical condition and disease profile. Socioeconomic differentials includes characteristics of the families like income, occupation, and social class, and level of education, as well as factors relating to the wider environment of the child, such as the community, the neighbourhood, and the family's ecological and disease environment. The socio-economic category also contains the much-discussed "maternal competence" factor (breastfeeding behaviour and behaviours or attitudes that affect the child health). Other authors have likewise stressed the connections among clustered mortality, family size, and fertility patterns (Ronsmans 1995). Taking the idea that the death of one child 'scars' the family, making the next child in that family more vulnerable

(Arulampalam and Bhalotra 2006). Studies often attribute death clustering to socio-demographic covariates: either a causal scarring effect (the previous sibling's survival status being included as a covariate) or unobserved heterogeneity (with family or community-specific effects) (Reddy 2008). Some studies included both, but without accounting for the bias induced by potential correlation between the unobserved heterogeneity and previous child's survival-status (Bolstad and Manda 2001; Curtis et al. 1993; Ronsmans 1995; Sastry 1997). The present study is using econometric dynamic panel data model which at the same time capture both the unobserved heterogeneity and the causal positive or negative scarring mechanisms. This model has also been used in few of the earlier studies referred to as 'state dependence' if panel data are used (Arulampalam and Bhalotra 2006, 2008; Heckman 1987; Manski and McFadden 1981; Wooldridge 2010). This model accounts for the endogeneity of previous sibling-survival status, thus avoiding the potential bias in previous studies.

The child-specific covariates considered in the model are Sex of the index child, Survival status of the previous sibling;

mother specific covariates in the model include Educational attainment, religion of the mother, mother's age at the birth of index child and wealth status of the household; *and community level variables* are state of residence and place of residence.

The educational attainment of respondent's partner has been categorized into two categories viz. literate and illiterate. Wealth status of the household has been divided into three categories poor, middle &rich. Mother's age at child birth was taken as continuous variable as it will take into account both mother's age and child's birth interval. Religion was taken in two categories hindus and others.

28.2.4 Statistical Model

The dynamic panel data model was:

$$Y_{ij}^{*} = X_{ij}^{*}\beta + \gamma Y_{ij-1} + \alpha_i + u_{ij} \tag{28.1}$$

Let there be n_i children of mother *i*. For child *j* $(j = 1,2\ldots,n_i)$ of mother *i* $(i = 1,2,\ldots,N)$, the unobservable propensity to experience an infant death, Y_{ij} * is specified in Eq. (28.1). Where *X* is a vector of strictly exogenous observable child-specific and mother-specific characteristics and β is the vector of coefficients associated with *X*. The dynamic panel data model of Eq. (28.1) has the panel consisting of a naturally time ordered sequence of siblings within mothers. A child is observed to die when his or her propensity for death crosses a threshold; in this case $Y_{ij}^{*} > 0$. The model has a random intercept α_i, to account for time-invariant mother specific unobserved characteristics. This picks up any correlation of death risks among siblings arising, for example, from shared genetic characteristics or from innate ability of their mother.

The model also includes the observed survival status of the previous siblings, Y_{ij-1}, the coefficient which picks up scarring. The estimated parameter γ should be interpreted as the 'average' effect of scarring over the time period considered. In models of this sort, the previous sibling's survival status, Y_{ij-1} is necessarily correlated with unobserved heterogeneity, α_i. In order to identify a causal effect, we need to take account of this correlation in the estimation. This is referred to as the 'initial conditions' problem (Heckman 1987; Wooldridge 2010). We are thus able to model the initial condition of the process as a natural extension of the model given in Eq. (28.1). We specify the equation for the first-born child of each mother as

$$Y*_{i1} = Z_i' \lambda + \theta\, \alpha_i + u_{i1} \tag{28.2}$$

$i = 1 \ldots N$ and $j = 1$.

Where, Z_i is a vector of strictly exogenous covariates. In general, Eq. (28.2) allows the vector of covariates Z to differ from X in Eq. (28.1). However, we set the two vectors of covariates to be the same given that we observe the process from the start. Eqs. (28.1) and (28.2) together specify a complete model for the infant survival process. In this way, the endogeneity of the 'lagged dependent variable', that is, the previous child's survival status is taken into account. The effect of unobservable mother's characteristics in Eqs. (28.1) and (28.2) to be correlated by specifying this unobservable as $\theta\alpha_i$. We assume that u_{ij} is independently distributed as a logistic distribution, and that the mother specific unobservable, α_i, are independent and identically distributed as normal. Marginalizing the likelihood function with respect to α_i, gives for mother i. Previous analyses of dynamic models with unobserved heterogeneity have shown the potential sensitivity of the estimates to the assumption made about the distributional form for unobserved heterogeneity, α_i (Heckman and Singer 1984). A weakness of the normality assumption is that it may not be flexible enough to account for the fact that some families never experience any child deaths and that, in some families, all children die (the mover-stayer problem). Our sample does not contain any families in which all children die in infancy. However, there are many families that experience no infant deaths, and this is accommodated by allowing for a single (empirically determined) mass at minus infinity: a very large negative value for α_i gives a very small value for Y_{ij}^*, and hence a very small probability of observing death of the index child (Narendranathan and Elias 1993). A test of H_0: $\sigma_\alpha^2 = 0$ is a test that there is no unobservable characteristics of the mother in the model.

This can be tested by using a likelihood ratio test (or a standard normal test) but the test statistic will not have a standard chi-square (or a standard normal) distribution since the parameter under the null hypothesis is on the boundary of the parameter space. The standard likelihood ratio (normal) test statistic is 0.5 χ^2 (1) (0.5 $N(0, 1)$) for positive values.

In addition to mother-specific unobserved heterogeneity, community level random effects were included in the model to account for the sampling design, which involved clustering at the community level. Failure to allow for community level unobserved heterogeneity in the likelihood maximization would provide consistent parameter estimators but inconsistent standard errors (Deaton 1997). Although the model is multilevel, we have chosen to treat the community level effect as a nuisance parameter. This is because we cannot interpret a time invariant community level effect in any meaningful manner. To the extent that families migrate or the infrastructure of different communities develops at different rates, the assumption of a time invariant community effect is restrictive: we expect that children of the same mother, who are born at different dates, may experience different community level effects. In any case, in this paper, the focus is not on estimation of the variance that is associated with mothers versus communities but, rather, on robust estimation of the scarring effect, which is captured in the parameter γ.

28.3 Results

28.3.1 Sample Characteristics of Tribal Mothers and their Children

Table 28.1 shows the characteristics of 2494 sampled tribal mothers (or families) and their 9069 children in the central and eastern region of India. From the table it is observed that 70 percent families never experienced any infant deaths while rest 30 percent families experienced all infant deaths. Among 30 percent families, nearly 10 percent families experienced clustered of infant deaths (families with at least two deaths) and rest 20 percent had only one infant death. Nearly 90 percent families belong to Hindus. Of total families, most of them were illiterate (89%). Almost substantial proportion (94%) of tribe mothers resides in rural areas. Nearly, 89 percent families were poor while less than 5 percent families falls in rich wealth group. A majority of tribe mothers (96%) did not have improved sanitation facilities and defecated in open or have unhealthy disposal of stool. Nearly 60 percent families receive safe drinking water. The child characteristics shows that there were 9069 total children born during 1970–2006, nearly 12 percent died as infant. There were 10 percent such children whose sibling also died as infant. Of total births of central and eastern regions, nearly 43 percent and 20 percent births took place in Madhya Pradesh & Odisha, respectively. More than half of the children were male. Births with first order contributed 27 percent of the total sampled children. Nearly 17 percent births born as second or higher order and the gap between two successive births were less than 24 months while 56 percent births were of second or higher order and had birth interval more than 24 months.

Table 28.1 Sample characteristics of Tribal mothers & their children, central & eastern India, 2005–06

Mother/Family Characteristics #	Percent	Number
State		
Jharkhand	19.2	**464**
Odisha	23.7	**617**
Chhattisgarh	18.8	**696**
Madhya Pradesh	38.3	**717**
Families with		
No infant death	70.3	**1782**
One infant death	20.5	**494**
At least two infant death	9.2	**218**
Religion		
Hindu	89.5	**2226**
Others	10.5	**268**
Mother's education		
Illiterate	80.8	**1970**
Literate	19.2	**524**
Place of residence		
Urban	6.2	**278**
Rural	93.8	**2216**
Wealth index		
Poor	88.6	**2129**
Middle	6.8	**189**
Rich	4.7	**176**
Sanitation Facility		
Improved	3.6	**151**
Not improved	96.4	**2343**
Drinking water		
Safe	59.9	**1514**
Unsafe	40.1	**980**
Total	**100.0**	**2494**
Child characteristics $	**Percent**	**N**
Infant death		
No	88.5	8045
Yes	11.5	1024
Previous infant death		
No	10.0	896
Yes	90.0	8173
State		
Jharkhand	18.5	1655
Odisha	21.1	2028
Chhattisgarh	17.9	2456

(continued)

Table 28.1 (continued)

Mother/Family Characteristics #	Percent	Number
Madhya Pradesh	42.5	2930
Sex of the child		
Male	50.6	4616
Female	49.4	4453
Birth interval		
Birth order 1	26.9	2494
BO> = 2 & BI<24 months	17.0	1497
BO> = 2 & BI> = 24 months	56.1	5078
Total	**100.0**	**9069**

Note: # is based on sample of mother and $ is based on sample of children who born between 1970 and 2006

28.3.2 Distribution of Infant Deaths among Tribes by Background Characteristics in Central and Eastern India

Table 28.2 shows the distribution of 1024 infant deaths and 8045 births who survived at least age 12 months among tribal families by selected background characteristics in the central and eastern India. Of total infant deaths, Madhya Pradesh experienced 45%, Odisha observed 20%, Chhattisgarh and Jharkhand each contributed nearly 17% infant deaths. A majority of infant deaths took place among Hindus. 87% tribal children who died during infancy had mothers as illiterate. Most of the deaths took place in rural areas. Nearly 91% infant death occurred in poor families. Among total infant deaths, 20% infant deaths also had a prior sibling who died as infant.

28.3.3 Clustering of Infant Deaths among Families in the Central and Eastern India

Tables 28.3a and 28.3b shows the clustering of infant deaths among tribal families by region of residence in the central and eastern India. In urban areas it is noticed that among 278 families who had one or more live births, nearly 78% families never experienced any infant deaths while remaining 22% families experienced all infant deaths. Of 22% families who have experienced any infant deaths, nearly 7% families have contributed 52% clustered infant deaths (2 or more infant deaths). In the Rural areas, of total 2216 families, nearly 85% families have given two or more births which accounted for 96% of total 8179 children. Further, of total 938 infant deaths in rural areas, there were 71% families who never experienced any infant deaths, 20% families experienced exactly one infant deaths and had 48% of total infant deaths

Table 28.2 Distribution of births that not died as infant & Infant deaths among tribal families by background characteristics, Central & eastern India, 2005–06

Variables	Percent	Number	Percent	Number
State				
Jharkhand	17.0	173	18.7	1482
Odisha	20.4	221	21.2	1807
Chhattisgarh	17.7	277	17.9	2179
Madhya Pradesh	44.9	353	42.2	2577
Religion				
Hindu	90.1	923	89.7	7188
Others	9.9	101	10.3	857
Mothers education				
Illiterate	87.1	891	85.5	6773
Literate	12.9	133	14.5	1272
Place of residence				
Urban	5.3	86	5.7	804
Rural	94.7	938	94.3	7241
Wealth index				
Poor	91.2	908	89.3	6957
Middle	6.8	77	6.7	599
Rich	2.1	39	4.0	489
Previous infant death				
Yes	80.0	817	91.3	7356
No	20.0	207	8.8	689
Sex of the child				
Male	54.3	570	50.1	4046
Female	45.8	454	49.9	3999
Birth interval				
Birth order 1	34.2	359	25.9	2135
BO> = 2 & BI<24 months	29.4	294	15.4	1203
BO> = 2 & BI> = 24 months	36.5	371	58.7	4707
Total	**100**	**1024**	**100.0**	**8045**

while remaining 9% families experienced two or more infant deaths and the extent of clustered infant deaths in such families was 52%.

28.3.4 Result of Random Effects Dynamic Probit Model & Unobserved Heterogeneity

Table 28.4 shows the results of random effects dynamic probit model of infant deaths among tribes in the central and eastern India. After adjusting for mother, child and community level characteristics in the model, it is observed that infant deaths is more

Table 28.3a Clustering of infant deaths among tribal families in urban areas of central& eastern India, 2005–06

Total Children ever born	Infant deaths per family					Total Families	Children	% Children
	0	1	2	3	5			
1	45	2	0	0	0	47	47	5.3
2	58	7	0	0	0	65	130	14.6
3	55	5	2	0	0	62	186	20.9
4	34	12	4	1	0	51	204	22.9
5	13	7	4	1	0	25	125	14.0
6	7	3	2	0	0	12	72	8.1
7	3	1	1	0	1	6	42	4.7
8	1	4	2	0	0	7	56	6.3
9	0	1	0	1	0	2	18	2.0
10	1	0	0	0	0	1	10	1.1
Families	217	42	15	3	1	**278**	**890**	
% families	78.1	15.1	5.4	1.1	0.4	**6.8**		
Infant deaths	0	42	30	9	5	**86**		
% infant deaths	0.0	48.8	34.9	10.5	5.8	**51.2**		

likely to occur in families who experienced prior infant deaths in comparison to those families who never experienced any prior infant loss and result was statistically significant ($p < 0.01$). Infant deaths was more likely to occur in the states of Madhya Pradesh in comparison to Jharkhand ($p < 0.05$). Mothers age at birth of index child was found to be negatively associated with infant deaths and as mother's age at child's birth increases, infant deaths is less likely and it is statistically significant ($p < 0.01$). Further, infant deaths among female child was less likely to be seen in comparison with male child. Religion, mother's education, place of residence and household wealth was found to be statistically not significant factors affecting infant deaths in this region. The value of intra class correlation which represent intra mother correlation coefficient by value of theta was found to be statistically not significant which represent that mother level unobservable characteristics do not affect the child mortality outcome and the initial condition problem was empirically unimportant in the region. This was further supported by the fact that intra class correlation was not significant which also make the estimated mother specific unobservable to be not significant as was depicted in the model. Further, mother level unobserved factors was also found to be not significant in all four states of the central and eastern India. The insignificant value of theta and mother specific unobserved heterogeneity and similar significant value of coefficient of previous death in both random effect dynamic probit model and the probit model suggest that probit model was equally better model to capture infant deaths. So, we have used the probit model based simulation to examine the effect of scarring and literacy on infant deaths in the region and in its four states.

Table 28.3b Clustering of infant deaths among tribal families in rural areas of central& eastern India, 2005–06

Total children ever born	Infant deaths per family									
	0	1	2	3	4	5	6	Family	Children	% Children
1	290	28	0	0	0	0	0	318	318	3.9
2	345	51	7	0	0	0	0	403	806	9.9
3	362	67	10	2	0	0	0	441	1323	16.2
4	251	83	20	4	0	0	0	358	1432	17.5
5	163	87	27	6	3	0	0	286	1430	17.5
6	90	65	31	8	0	0	0	194	1164	14.2
7	44	35	15	6	6	1	0	107	749	9.2
8	10	16	12	6	4	0	0	48	384	4.7
9	7	15	9	6	4	0	0	41	369	4.5
10	3	4	4	3	0	2	1	17	170	2.1
11	0	1	1	0	0	0	0	2	22	0.3
12	0	0	1	0	0	0	0	1	12	0.1
Family	1565	452	137	41	17	3	1	**2216**	**8179**	
% family	70.6	20.4	6.2	1.9	0.8	0.1	0.0	**9.0**		
Infant deaths	0	452	274	123	68	15	6	**938**		
% infant deaths	0.0	48.2	29.2	13.1	7.2	1.6	0.6	**51.8**		

Table 28.4 Result of random effects dynamic probit model of infant death by selected background characteristics among tribes, central & eastern India, 2005–06

Covariates	Coefficient	95% Confidence interval	
Previous death			
No ®			
Yes	0.516***	0.376	0.656
States			
Jharkhand®			
Odisha	0.112	−0.057	0.280
Chhattisgarh	0.113	−0.055	0.280
Madhya Pradesh	0.212**	0.048	0.375
Mothers age at child birth	−0.020***	−0.029	−0.010
Sex			
Male ®			
Female	−0.097**	−0.183	−0.010
Religion			
Hindu®			
Others	0.156	−0.030	0.342
Education			
Literate®			
Illiterate	0.092	−0.049	0.234
Place of residence			
Urban®			
Rural	0.054	−0.128	0.235
Wealth			
Poor®			
Middle	0.070	−0.105	0.244
Rich	−0.124	−0.373	0.126
Constant	**−1.165*** **	**−1.504**	**−0.827**
Rho	**0.0447**	**0.0105**	**0.1716**
Theta	**2.384**	**0.5199**	**10.9325**
Estimated variance of mother specific unobservable	**0.154**		
N	**9069**		

Note*p < 0.01; **p < 0.05;*p < 0.1;** ® refers to reference category; The model also included interactions of all regressors with a dummy for first-born child (not shown)

28.3.5 Probit Model based Simulation Results of Effects of Scarring and Literacy on Infant Deaths in Central & Eastern India

Table 28.5 shows the probit based simulation results of predicted probability of infant deaths among tribes in the central and eastern India and its four selected states.

Table 28.5 Simulation results based on probit model of reduction in infant deaths among tribes of infant deaths, Central and eastern India, 2005–06

States	Overall Predicted Probability (a)	Predicted Probability when no scarring (b)	Percent reduction (b-a/a) *100	Predicted Probability when all mothers were literate (c)	Percent Reduction (c-a/a) *100
Central & eastern India	0.113***	0.100***	11.5	0.098*	0.13
Jharkhand	0.105***	0.097***	6.9	0.117	12.24
Odisha	0.109***	0.101***	7.5	0.071**	34.68
Chhattisgarh	0.113***	0.094***	16.3	0.085*	24.84
Madhya Pradesh	0.120***	0.106***	11.7	0.115	4.95

Note***$p < 0.01$; **$p < 0.05$;*$p < 0.1$

It can be concluded that overall predicted probability of infant death was 0.113 for central and eastern region but when we removed the clustering of deaths in families the predicted probability reduced to 0.100 leading to a decline of 11%. It shows that scarring contributed 11% decline in the family level clustering of infant deaths in the central & eastern India. Similarly for states within this region scarring factor was statistically significant for all states and the family level clustering of deaths attributed due to scarring factor was maximum in Chhattisgarh (16%) and Madhya Pradesh (12%) respectively. In Jharkhand and Odisha, 7% and 8% clustering could be reduced by eliminating the effect of scarring factor at family levels respectively. As literacy was found to be a significant factor affecting infant deaths so we have also predicted the situations where it is assumed illiterate women as literate and examined the reduction in predicted probability of infant deaths. For central & eastern Indian region, literacy led to a reduction of 13 infant death though it was moderately significant ($p < 0.1$).On the other hand the states like Odisha and Chhattisgarh experienced a 34% and 25% reduction in infant deaths only if we would provide education to illiterate women.

28.4 Discussion & Policy Implications

In the present paper, an attempt has been made to examine the clustering of infant deaths at family level for aboriginal's (tribal population) living in the forested hill tracts of peninsular India in four states of the central and eastern India. Most of these tribes are the Particularly Vulnerable Tribal Groups. The challenge of inaccessibility to health services and their health care seeking behaviour seem to dominate the discourse in tribal health (Balgir 2006).

In the present research article, the discussion is primarily based on the findings related to clustering of infant deaths from the study. We started examining the level of infant death clustering where we have estimated the extent of death clustering among scheduled tribes by region of residence. It has been found that among various caste groups, the scheduled tribes have the highest number of families with at least two infant deaths (9%) where nearly more than half of the total infant deaths are concentrated. State wise clustering of infant deaths in families suggest that Madhya Pradesh has the highest level of clustered deaths as nearly 11% families experienced 57% of two or more infant deaths (table not shown) suggesting clearly the existence of clustering in the central and eastern Indian region. Since most of the tribal families are located in rural areas, so we have also examined the extent of clustering by region of residence which suggest that for rural areas the clustering is more pronounced than urban areas as the number of vulnerable families (those experienced two or more infant deaths) were higher in rural areas.

The scarring effect (both positive as well as negative) has played an important role in intra-family death clustering in all states. In the first model, random effects dynamic probit model, obtained from the estimate for scarring by taking endogeneity and mother specific unobserved heterogeneity into account which indicated the positive influence of previous infant death in families on infant death of the index child. In this model, mother specific unobserved heterogeneity did not influence the child survival and the coefficient for previous death was almost same in both random effect dynamic probit model and probit model. Insignificant mother level unobserved factor suggests that the biological and other implicit characteristics of women in the central and eastern India are homogeneous leading to no variation between mother in terms of these characteristics. It clearly indicate that tribal women constitute a homogenous group across different regions of India and follow the similar socio-cultural practices. The simulation analysis suggests that for central and eastern region, scarring factor alone can reduce the infant mortality by 12%. However, for the state like Odisha illiteracy plays a greater role than scarring. The infant deaths in the state like Chhattisgarh is much influenced by scarring mechanism as it has contributed maximum in reducing the infant deaths once the effect of scarring has been eliminated. Eliminating illiteracy among tribal women in Chhattisgarh also resulted into reduction in infant death but the effect is lesser than scarring.

The findings suggest that, in the states like Odisha and Chhattisgarh the infant deaths among tribal families could be reduced to a significant level if we address both education and previous deaths in families.

It's a consequential findings from the study because, if we control the risk of death for the children of first and second order, the experience gained by mother in rearing of these two children would automatically help in reducing the risk of infant death of the next child and this would reduce infant deaths significantly. The findings of scarring effects suggest a higher pay-off to interventions designed to reduce mortality than previously recognized. It is known as the activation of a social multiplier (Manski 1999). So it indicates that reducing the risk of death of a child automatically implies in reducing the risk of death of his or her succeeding siblings. It is seen that once scarring effect is eliminated from the model, it would also underestimate the mortality levels up to certain extent.

A study conducted by Monica Das Gupta on twentieth-century in rural Punjab, demonstrated that families who had already experienced the loss of other children stood an increased chance of losing further children (Das Gupta 1990). This relationship applied to a child's survival chances at all stages of childhood following the neonatal period. It is understandable that, siblings share a large number of highly relevant demographic characteristics of the mother, such as the mother's age; her breastfeeding patterns; and her level of fecundity, which strongly correlates with length of birth interval. These factors are already well documented in previous studies on infant and child mortality (Hobcraft et al. 1983). Arulampalam and Bhalotra (2006) have argued that deaths may cluster in families not only because of unobserved heterogeneity—because of siblings share certain traits—but also as a result of a causal process driven by the scarring effects on mothers and families from an earlier child death, making the next child in the family more vulnerable. One of the ways in which interfamilial scarring occurs is when a mother quickly conceives again after the death of an infant through either resumed fecundity or the wish to replace the child that was lost. In addition, scarring may occur when an infant death causes the mother to become depressed, which may also have serious deleterious health effects on the next infant, either after its birth or in the womb. The mother level, insignificant unexplained variation in all four states in the region can be attributed due to homogeneity in culture, poverty and hazardous environmental factors in all states. Income, occupation, "Maternal competence" factor which concerns the mother's breastfeeding behaviour or other attitudes and behaviours that affect her children's health, inherited genetic disorders and the mother's medical condition and disease profile may be other factors which explain the significant but no inter-family unobserved heterogeneity. Some of the previous studies too shown that the unexplained variation between families or mothers cannot always be found, or, in some cases, it appears to be very modest (Das Gupta 1990; Guo 1993). Guo (1993) also came out with the similar findings by conducting the study in a Latin American developing country, Guatemala. that the variation between mothers was only slight once family income level and mother's educational attainment were controlled for. Sastry (1997) too found that inter-family heterogeneity to be small and unimportant in his study on Brazilian population, but only after controlling for heterogeneity at the community level. Sastry, therefore, argued, much in line with Guo that shared environmental conditions were more important determinants of shared frailty than either parental competence or genetic and biological factors.

Scarring involves responsive behaviour which may be amenable as it is shown that there is some causal process whereby frequent infant death in the family is affected by the previous sibling's death. If the causal process works through the fecundity mechanism, policies that improve the uptake of contraception are likely to reduce death clustering among the tribes. More specific policy insight depends on identifying the mechanism underlying scarring. While unobserved heterogeneity involves largely untreatable factors like genes or fixed behaviour and unalterable family specific traits is central to the nature-nurture debate (Pinker 2003). There is a need for systematic and comparative research in the different tribal communities at different time periods to understand the role of scarring mechanisms and to examine the conditions of appearance or disappearance of this hazards. In India, as in many other developing countries, health services are made available largely in response to demand. If child deaths are heavily concentrated in some families, this would suggest that substantial improvements in child mortality could be achieved by adopting the more cost-effective techniques of focusing healthcare resources specifically on the sub-group of families with a high risk of child death.

It can also be useful in targeting interventions at the most vulnerable households. The government should not only try to reduce scarring mechanism among tribes, but it should also promote education, awareness among tribes about modern health facilities and infrastructure development in the tribal areas. The policy initiatives should be pro tribe culture and it should be encouraging. Mass media based information about government policies should be promoted.

References

Arulampalam, W., & Bhalotra, S. (2006). Sibling death clustering in India: State dependence versus unobserved heterogeneity. *Journal of the Royal Statistical Society: Series A (Statistics in Society), 169*(4), 829–848.

Arulampalam, W., & Bhalotra, S. (2008). The linked survival prospects of siblings: Evidence for the Indian states. *Population Studies, 62*(2), 171–190.

Balgir, R. (2006). *Tribal health problems, disease burden and ameliorative challenges in tribal communities with special emphasis on tribes of Orissa.* Paper presented at the Proceedings of National Symposium on "Tribal Health" 19th–20th October.

Bhargava, A. (2003). Family planning, gender differences and infant mortality: Evidence from Uttar Pradesh, India. *Journal of Econometrics, 112*(1), 225–240.

Bolstad, W. M., & Manda, S. O. (2001). Investigating child mortality in Malawi using family and community random effects: A Bayesian analysis. *Journal of the American Statistical Association, 96*(453), 12–19.

Curtis, S. L., Diamond, I., & McDonald, J. W. (1993). Birth interval and family effects on postneonatal mortality in Brazil. *Demography, 30*(1), 33–43.

Das Gupta, M. (1990). Death clustering, mothers' education and the determinants of child mortality in rural Punjab, India. *Population Studies, 44*(3), 489–505.

Das, M. B., Kapoor, S., & Nikitin, D. (2010). *A closer look at child mortality among Adivasis in India.* World Bank Policy research working paper series.

Das, M. B., Hall, G. H., Kapoor, S., et al. (2014). Chapter 6—India: The scheduled tribes. In G. H. Hall & H. A. Patrinos (Eds.), *Indigenous peoples, poverty and development* (pp. 205–248). New York: Cambridge University Press.

Deaton, A. (1997). *The analysis of household surveys.* Washington, DC: Johns Hopkins University Press.

Guo, G. (1993). Use of sibling data to estimate family mortality effects in Guatemala. *Demography, 30*, 15–32.

Heckman, J. J. (1987). *The incidental parameters problem and the problem of initial conditions in estimating a discrete time-discrete data stochastic process and some Monte Carlo evidence.* University of Chicago Center for Mathematical studies in Business and Economics.

Heckman, J., & Singer, B. (1984). A method for minimizing the impact of distributional assumptions in econometric models for duration data. *Econometrica: Journal of the Econometric Society, 52*, 271–320.

Hobcraft, J., McDonald, J. W., & Rutstein, S. (1983). Child-spacing effects on infant and early child mortality. *Population Index*, 585–618.

International Institute for Population Sciences (IIPS) and Macro International. (2007). *National Family Health Survey (NFHS), 2005–06: India: Volume 1*. Mumbai: International Institute for Population Sciences and Macro International.

Madise, N. J., & Diamond, I. (1995). Determinants of infant mortality in Malawi: An analysis to control for death clustering within families. *Journal of Biosocial Science, 27*(1), 95–106.

Manski, C. F. (1999). *Identification problems in the social sciences*. Cambridge, MA: Harvard University Press.

Manski, C. F., & McFadden, D. (1981). *Structural analysis of discrete data with econometric applications*. Cambridge, MA: MIT Press.

Ministry of Tribal affairs. (2015). Retrieved from http://tribal.nic.in/

Narendranathan, W., & Elias, P. (1993). Influences of past history on the incidence of youth unemployment: Empirical findings for the UK†. *Oxford Bulletin of Economics and Statistics, 55*(2), 161–185.

Oettinger, G. S. (2000). Sibling similarity in high school graduation outcomes: Causal interdependency or unobserved heterogeneity? *Southern Economic Journal*, 631–648.

Pandey, G., & Tiwary, R. (1993). Demographic characteristics in a tribal block of Madhya Pradesh. *Social Change, 23*(2/3), 124–131.

Pinker, S. (2003). *The blank slate: The modern denial of human nature*. New York: Penguin.

Ranjan, M., Dwivedi, L. K., Mishra, R., et al. (2016). Infant mortality differentials among the tribal and non-tribal populations of central and eastern India. *International Journal of Population Studies, 2*(2), 26–43. https://doi.org/10.18063/IJPS.2016.02.004.

Ranjan, M., Dwivedi, L. K., & Mishra, R. (2018). Caste differentials in death clustering in central and eastern indian states. *Journal of Biosocial Science, 50*(2), 254–274. https://doi.org/10.1017/S0021932017000219.

Reddy, S. (2008). Health of tribal women and children: An interdisciplinary approach. Indian. *Anthropologist, 38*, 61–74.

Registrar General of India. (2015). *Sample Registration System (SRS) Statistical Report 2015*. New Delhi: Registrar General of India. Retrieved from http://www.censusindia.gov.in/vital_statistics/SRS_Reports_2015.html

Rindfuss, R. R., Palmore, J. A., & Bumpass, L. L. (1982). *Selectivity and the analysis of birth intervals from survey data*. Paper presented at the Asian and Pacific Census Forum.

Ronsmans, C. (1995). Patterns of clustering of child mortality in a rural area of Senegal. *Population Studies, 49*(3), 443–461.

Sastry, N. (1997). Family-level clustering of childhood mortality risk in Northeast Brazil. *Population Studies, 51*(3), 245–261.

UNICEF. (2014). *Levels & trends in child mortality*. Report. Retrieved from http://www.unicef.org/media/files/Levels_and_Trends_in_Child_Mortality_2014.pdf

Whitehouse, C. (1982). The health of children. A review of research on the place of health in cycles of disadvantage. *British Journal of General Practice*.

Wooldridge, J. M. (2010). *Econometric analysis of cross section and panel data*. Cambridge, MA: MIT Press.

World Health Organization. (2011). *Global health observatory data repository*. See http://apps.who.int/ghodata

Zaba, B., & David, P. H. (1996). Fertility and the distribution of child mortality risk among women: An illustrative analysis. *Population Studies, 50*(2), 263–278.

The manufacturer's authorised representative in the EU is Springer Nature Customer Service Centre GmbH, Europaplatz 3, 69115 Heidelberg, Germany. If you have any concerns regarding our products, please contact ProductSafety@springernature.com

Printed and bound by CPI Group (UK) Ltd, Croydon, CR0 4YY
30/09/2026
02225494-0017